THE AUTOIMMUNE CONNECTION

ESSENTIAL INFORMATION FOR WOMEN ON DIAGNOSIS, TREATMENT, AND GETTING ON WITH YOUR LIFE

Revised and Updated Edition

RITA BARON-FAUST, MPH

WITH

JILL P. BUYON, MD

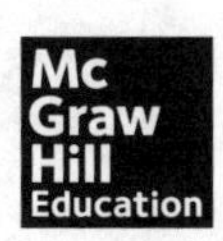

New York Chicago San Francisco Athens London Madrid Mexico City
Milan New Delhi Singapore Sydney Toronto

1 2 3 4 5 6 7 8 9 0 QFR/QFR 1 2 1 0 9 8 7 6

ISBN 978-0-07-184122-1
MHID 0-07-184122-9

e-ISBN 978-0-07-183587-9
e-MHID 0-07-183587-3

Illustrations by Marina Terletsky

For my Mother, who always believed in me. I miss you every day.
—RBF

Contents

Foreword

by Virginia T. Ladd

We at the American Autoimmune Related Diseases Association are delighted to present this updated and revised edition of *The Autoimmune Connection.* Rita Baron-Faust and Dr. Jill Buyon have distilled more than a decade's worth of new research into autoimmunity to expand and enhance their groundbreaking overview of a disease category that affects more than 50 million Americans.

In the 25 years AARDA has been advocating for people with autoimmune diseases, there have been great strides in understanding and treating these diseases, in which the body attacks the very organs it is supposed to protect.

As the nation's only nonprofit organization dedicated to bringing a national focus to autoimmunity as a category of disease and as a major women's health issue, we have been pleased to offer *The Autoimmune Connection* at our patient forums, scientific meetings, and advocacy summits across the country. It has contributed greatly to our ongoing mission to educate patients, elected officials, and the medical and scientific communities about the more than 100 different autoimmune diseases and the toll they take on lives each day.

Among those afflicted with autoimmune diseases, 75 percent are women. In fact, these diseases represent the third largest cause of chronic illness among women in the United States. Even more alarming, autoimmune diseases are among the top 10 leading causes of all deaths among U.S. women ages 65 and younger. It's no wonder that autoimmune diseases have been named a major women's health issue and a research priority by the National Institutes of Health's Office of Research on Women's Health.

Even now, too few women know about autoimmune diseases or the threat they pose until they are faced with a diagnosis. The public, patients, and even the medical community suffer from a lack of information and a plethora of misinformation and myths about these disorders, making early recognition difficult. Tragically, many women are not diagnosed until illness has progressed, and some become very ill before their symptoms are taken seriously.

Even as new research and groundbreaking biological treatments have changed outcomes for autoimmune patients, too many physicians are still quick to dismiss women's symptoms. A 2015 survey conducted by AARDA and the National Coalition of Autoimmune Patient Groups (NCAPG) found that many women were still being labeled as chronic complainers in the earliest stages of their illnesses. The time wasted costs hundreds of lives, untold suffering, and billions of dollars in healthcare costs.

The updated edition of this book will make great strides toward educating women about an important area affecting their health, well-being, and families. It will encourage women to be their own advocates and to learn more about their own family history of autoimmune disease, especially when family members can be affected by seemingly different diseases (which may not even be recognized as autoimmune).

Giving women the facts and new insights into autoimmunity will provide reassurance that their symptoms are not an "all in your head" problem to be pushed aside but rather a problem that needs to be taken seriously—and that can be helped. In this book, women will learn how biological therapies for conditions like rheumatoid arthritis are now able to change the course of illnesses like RA that once meant certain disability and disfigurement.

The next stage of AARDA's mission is the creation of the Autoimmune Disease Patient Registry Research Network—ARNet—a comprehensive central database of anonymous patient information, including diagnoses, clinical data, and perhaps even tissue and blood samples along with key demographics. ARNet's database currently encompasses eight patient groups and provides information on almost 70,000 patients with 2.34 million data points.

It is our hope that this book will encourage patients and clinicians to contribute to this "big data" effort to fully understand and ultimately eradicate autoimmune diseases.

Progress is being made every day. This book will enable more women with autoimmune diseases to find help—and hope.

Virginia T. Ladd
President, American Autoimmune Related Diseases Association

Acknowledgments

This was a book literally "years in the making"—and years in the *re*making.

It has been a challenge to keep up with autoimmune disease research since the first edition of this book was published in 2002. Over the past decade I have attended countless medical meetings, talked to dozens of clinicians and researchers, and spoken with scores of autoimmune patients at educational forums. While research has advanced, new medications have been approved, and treatment strategies have improved, I find that one thing has *not* changed: the needs of women with autoimmune diseases for information, prompt diagnosis, and effective treatments that take their real lives into account. And, most important, to be listened to and *heard* by their physicians.

At the same time, a major change has taken place in the way we talk about these diseases. At scientific and medical meetings the terms *autoimmune* and *disease clusters* are now commonplace. When I was first diagnosed with hypothyroidism in 1971, no one ever said the word *autoimmune*.

It wasn't until 1992 that I learned about autoimmune diseases when I covered the First Annual Congress on Women's Health in Washington, D.C., as a medical journalist.

It was there I first met Virginia Ladd, founder and president of the then-fledgling American Autoimmune Related Diseases Association (AARDA). She has been a mentor and friend since then, and I cannot sufficiently express my deep gratitude to her for supporting this book. I'm privileged to speak alongside her as a national educator for AARDA.

A special shout-out to Sharon Harris and Pat Barber of AARDA and Cindy Carway and Stephanie Hornback of Carway Communications for their tireless work on behalf of AARDA.

It was also through AARDA that I met Dr. Noel Rose, whom I'd like to especially thank for his continuing help and support. He's a gentleman and a scholar but, most important, a wise and compassionate physician.

Heartfelt thanks go to all the women who shared with me their personal experiences over the years: Kathleen Turner, who graciously took the time during her Broadway run in *The Graduate* in 2002 to talk with me; Hannah Wallace for sharing her story and the names of other women; Mary Kay Blakely, author of *Wake Me When It's Over*, now a professor emeritus at the University of Missouri; Lori Silverman; Annemarie Johnson, who sadly passed away in 2014; Joy Simon-Palmer; and my old friend Ann Gold, as well as the scores of other women I have met at AARDA patient forums and advocacy conferences since the first edition of this book came out. I'm in your debt and in awe of your courage.

One note about these personal stories. They are included in this book not to criticize doctors but to demonstrate the very real problems many women still experience in trying to get an accurate diagnosis. I am also deeply grateful to the Logan Science Journalism Program at the Marine Biological Laboratory at Woods Hole, Massachusetts, for affording me the opportunity to attend a postdoctoral course on neuroimmunological diseases as a Fellow in 1997, which proved invaluable in researching this book.

There are so many people who provided resources and assistance during the years of research and writing that went into this book that it is impossible to thank them all. Special mention to: Bonny Senkbeil, Jocelyn Givens, and Erin Latimer at the American College of Rheumatology; Christine Chapman, and Francesca Russo in the press office of the European League Against Rheumatism; Aaron Lohr and Jenni Glenn Gingery at the Endocrine Society; Joan Young, founder of the Platelet Disorder Support Association; Mary Lou Ballweg, the indefatigable president and executive director of the Endometriosis Association; Phyllis Greenberger, president of the Society for Women's Health Research; and to those at the National Multiple Sclerosis Society; the Myasthenia Gravis Foundation; the Arthritis Foundation; and the American Diabetes Association who have kept me up to date. Thanks also to my colleague Trudy Lieberman of the Association of Health Care Journalists, who graciously reviewed the health policy information in this book.

I am especially grateful to James Darrow, administrative director of the Division of Rheumatology at NYU Langone Medical Center, who facilitates my continued attendance at the annual NYU Seminar in Advanced Rheumatology and keeps me connected to the NYU online Health Sciences Library.

I also want to acknowledge St. Francis College in Brooklyn Heights and Dr. Kathy Nolan, who chairs the department of biology and health promotion, who gave me the opportunity to be an adjunct. Teaching introductory biology and having to explain the immune system to my students gave me a wonderful refresher.

My agent, Vicky Bijur, always understood the concept of this book and recognized its potential from the outset. Vicky, thanks for never giving up on making an updated edition of this book happen.

Christopher Brown of McGraw-Hill and my former editor at Contemporary Books, Judith McCarthy, both understand the importance of educating women about autoimmune diseases and appreciate how these diseases can impact women during various life stages. Thanks to both of you!

What can I say about my coauthor, Dr. Jill Buyon? She's a dedicated clinician and passionate researcher. When I first approached her with the idea of a book on women and autoimmune diseases years ago, she was immediately enthusiastic. When I became overwhelmed with other work, she spurred me on, despite the fact that she herself was knee-deep in writing research grants. Even as she assumed the chair of rheumatology at NYU Langone, Jill has made time for this book. She strives always for excellence and holds me to her own high standards. Ours was the first book on autoimmune diseases written expressly for patients, and I am proud that our efforts have paved the way for others that followed.

Of course, I could never have done any of this without the love and support of my husband Allen and my son Alex. They have cheered me—and cheered me on—through six books, studying for a master's degree, and countless late nights working at my computer. I love you guys; you make it all worthwhile.

I only wish my mother were here to see this new edition on bookstore shelves. This is for you, Mom.

RBF

Above all, I wish to thank each and every one of my patients with SLE, who have taught me more about lupus than any textbook and to be humble, caring, and involved. These individuals manage to cope with the ever-present uncertainty of a chronic disease that can lie dormant for months to years only to explode at the most inopportune times.

Working on this book has certainly been a major departure from the basic and clinical research activities that I hold so dear. Despite hours of my obsessive editing and struggling with the right words to communicate to the lay public extraordinarily complex medial issues, some of which are rapidly evolving, Rita Baron-Faust continued to put up with me. I believe she has managed to capture the depth of autoimmune diseases in an extraordinarily reader-friendly way. I salute her incredible tenacity in putting this omnibus book together once again and updating all the exciting recent discoveries that offer new hopes for our patients. I am confident that this final product will provide an invaluable reference to patients and their families.

On a personal note, I would like to thank my husband, Dr. Robert Clancy, who has put his heart and soul into pursuing the basic science that drives lupus. He has commented so many times that "putting out the fires in this disease can be hard." Throughout the editing of this book, he reminded me that Excedrin works quite well just being in your pocket. I thank my son Shane for keeping me company in the wee hours of the night and trying to distract me by engaging our mutual interest in real estate, and my daughter, Chelsea, for her own extraordinary passion for science and healing, relentlessly inquisitive mind, and often uncanny insights. Finally I thank my best friend in the world, Joan Emerald Merrill, for always being "on call" for me and giving every success and failure the right perspective.

My contributions to this book are dedicated to the loving memory of my mother, Harriet Buyon, who took great pride in bragging to her friends whenever she found my name in print.

JPB

Contributors

The authors wish to express gratitude to the following people who have provided insight, information, and peer review on the ever-evolving subject of women and autoimmunity during the research, writing, and updating of this book.

William P. Arend, MD
Distinguished Professor Emeritus
Division of Rheumatology
Anschutz Medical Campus
University of Colorado School of Medicine
Aurora, CO

Henry C. Bodenheimer, Jr., MD
Professor of Medicine
Hofstra North Shore-LIJ School of Medicine
Medical Director Medicine Serviceline
North Shore Health System
Manhasset, New York

Laurence A. Bradley, PhD
Professor of Medicine
Division of Clinical Immunology and Rheumatology
University of Alabama at Birmingham

D. Ware Branch, MD
Professor and Chair, Department of Obstetrics and Gynecology
University of Utah School of Medicine
Salt Lake City, UT

James Bussel, MD
Professor of Pediatrics
Weill Medical College of Cornell University
New York, NY

Vivian P. Bykerk, BSC, MD
Director of the Inflammatory Arthritis Center of Excellence
Hospital for Special Surgery
Associate Professor of Medicine
Weill Cornell Medical College
New York, NY

Daniel J. Clauw, MD
Professor of Anesthesiology, Medicine (Rheumatology), and Psychiatry
Director, Chronic Pain and Fatigue Research Center
University of Michigan
Ann Arbor, MI

Janine Austin Clayton, MD
Director, Office of Research on Women's Health (2012)
Associate Director for Research on Women's Health
Former Deputy Clinical Director, National Eye Institute (NEI)
National Institutes of Health (NIH)
Bethesda, MD

Terry F. Davies, MB, BS, MD
Florence and Theodore Baumritter Professor of Medicine
Icahn School of Medicine at Mount Sinai
Attending Physician
The Mount Sinai Hospital
New York, NY
Director, Division of Endocrinology and Metabolism
James J. Peters VA Medical Center
New York, NY

Madeline Duvic, MD
Professor of Medicine, Interim Chair, Department of Dermatology
Director, National Alopecia Areata Registry
MD Anderson Cancer Center
University of Texas
Houston, TX

Denise L. Faustman, MD, PhD
Director of Immunobiology
Massachusetts General Hospital
Boston, MA
Associate Professor of Medicine
Harvard Medical School
Cambridge, MA

Christine L. Frissora, MD, FACOG
Assistant Professor of Medicine
Weill Medical College of Cornell University
New York, NY

Allan Gibofsky, MD, JD
Professor of Medicine and Public Health
Weill Cornell Medical College
Attending Rheumatologist
Co-Director, Center for Inflammatory Arthritis and Biologic Therapy
Hospital for Special Surgery
New York, New York

Barbara S. Giesser, MD
Associate Clinical Professor of Neurology
University of California, Los Angeles

Peter H. R. Green, MD
Clinical Professor
Columbia University College of Physicians and Surgeons
Director, Celiac Disease Research Center
New York, NY

Bevra H. Hahn, MD
Chief, Rheumatology and Arthritis
Vice Chair, Department of Medicine
University of California, Los Angeles

Eon Nigel Harris, MPhil, MD, DM
University of the West Indies (Retired)
Kingston, Jamaica

Sunanda V. Kane, MD, MSPH
Professor of Medicine, Gastroenterology and Hepatology
Mayo Clinic
Rochester, MN

John H. Klippel, MD
Former President and Medical Director
Arthritis Foundation
Atlanta, GA
Chief Medical Officer
Focus Diagnostic Medicine
Boston, MA

Paul W. Ladenson, MD
John Eager Howard Professor of Endocrinology
Professor of Medicine, Pathology, and Oncology
Director, Division of Endocrinology and Metabolism
The Johns Hopkins Medical Institutions
Baltimore, MD

Mark Lebwohl, MD
Professor and Chairman of Dermatology
Mount Sinai School of Medicine
New York, NY
President, American Academy of Dermatology

Arnold I. Levinson, MD
Emeritus Professor of Medicine and Neurology
Perelman School of Medicine
University of Pennsylvania
Philadelphia, PA

Carol J. Levy, MD
Associate Professor of Medicine, Endocrinology, Diabetes and Bone Disease
Director of the Diabetes Center,
Associate Professor of Obstetrics, Gynecology, and Reproductive Science
Director, Type 1 diabetes/diabetes in Pregnancy Program
Mount Sinai Hospital, New York, NY

Michael D. Lockshin, MD, MACR
Director, Barbara Volcker Center for Women and Rheumatic Diseases
Hospital for Special Surgery
Weill Cornell Medical Center
Professor of Medicine and Obstetrics-Gynecology
Joan and Sanford Weill College of Medicine of Cornell University
New York, NY

Mary Loeken, PhD
Assistant Professor of Medicine
Harvard Medical School
Cambridge, MA
Investigator, Research Division
Joslin Diabetes Center
Boston, MA

Judith Luborsky, PhD
Research Scientist
Department of Biology
Woods Hole Oceanographic Institute
Woods Hole, MA

Susan Manzi, MD, MPH
Co-Director, Lupus Center of Excellence
Chair, Department of Medicine
West Penn Allegheny Health System
Pittsburgh, PA
Vice Chair and Professor, Temple University

Janice M. Massey, MD
Professor of Neurology
Chief of the Division of Neuromuscular Diseases
Duke University Medical Center
Durham, NC

Lloyd Mayer, MD (1952–2013)
Dorothy and David Merksamer Professor of Medicine
Director, Center for Immunobiology
Mount Sinai School of Medicine
New York, NY

Maureen D. Mayes, MD
Professor of Internal Medicine
Division of Rheumatology
University of Texas Health Science Center
Houston, TX

Philip J. Mease, MD
Director of Rheumatology Research
Swedish Medical Center
Clinical Professor of Medicine
University of Washington
Seattle, WA

Joan T. Merrill, MD
Professor
Head, Clinical Pharmacology Research Program
Oklahoma Medical Research Foundation
Oklahoma City, OK

Hal J. Mitnick, MD
Clinical Professor of Medicine
New York University Medical Center
New York, NY

Lila E. Nachtigall, MD
Professor of Obstetrics and Gynecology
New York University School of Medicine
NYU Langone Medical Center
New York, NY

J. Lee Nelson, MD
Professor and Director, Immunogenetics Program
Fred Hutchinson Cancer Research Center
University of Washington
Seattle, WA

David L. Olive, MD
Director, Wisconsin Fertility Institute
Middleton, WI

Melissa Palmer, MD
Clinical Professor of Medicine
New York University School of Medicine
New York, New York
Global Head, Clinical Development in Hepatology
Shire Pharmaceuticals
New York, New York

Ann L. Parke, MD
St. Francis Hospital and Medical Center
Hartford, CT

Michelle Petri, MD
Director, Lupus Clinic
Associate Professor of Medicine
Johns Hopkins Medical Institutions
Baltimore, MD

David Pisetsky, MD, PhD
Professor of Medicine
Duke University Medical Center
Co-director, Duke University Arthritis Center
Durham, NC
President, United States Bone and Joint Initiative

Anthony T. Reder, MD
Associate Professor, Department of Neurology
University of Chicago
Chicago, IL

Robert A. S. Roubey, MD
Associate Professor of Medicine
Division of Rheumatology and Immunology
University of North Carolina, Chapel Hill

Jane E. Salmon, MD
Professor of Medicine and Obstetrics and Gynecology
Weill Cornell Medical College
Collette Kean Research Professor
Hospital for Special Surgery

S. Gerald Sandler, MD
Professor of Medicine and Pathology
Georgetown University Medical Center
Washington, DC

Jasvinder A. Singh, MD, MPH
Professor of Medicine
University of Alabama, Birmingham

Daniel W. Skupski, MD
Associate Professor of Obstetrics and Gynecology
Weill Medical College of Cornell University
New York, NY

Virginia D. Steen, MD
Professor of Medicine
Division of Rheumatology, Allergy and Immunology
Georgetown University
Washington, DC

David A. Sullivan, PhD
Senior Scientist, Schepens Eye Research Institute
Associate Professor, Department of Ophthalmology
Harvard Medical School
Cambridge, MA

Rhonda Voskuhl, MD
Professor, UCLA Department of Neurology
Jack H. Skirball Chair for Multiple Sclerosis
Director, UCLA Multiple Sclerosis Program
University of California, Los Angeles

Yusuf Yazici, MD
Assistant Professor of Medicine
New York University School of Medicine
NYU Hospital for Joint Diseases
New York, NY

Introduction

A New View of Autoimmunity

It is a great pleasure for me to welcome the revised and updated edition of the very first book on autoimmune diseases written for a general audience. Since the first edition was published, patients and their families have eagerly awaited news of the latest advances in the field. Many physicians are now using this book for reference in their practices.

Considered separately, most of the autoimmune diseases are relatively uncommon. But collectively, this group of related disorders actually represents the third most common category of disease in the United States. Many of these diseases start at a relatively young age and have a disproportionate effect on well-being. Patients usually require a lifetime of care because autoimmune diseases are currently incurable. Moreover, the diseases often have great impact on families, particularly if the patient is a young wife and mother. There are, therefore, many societal reasons for considering the autoimmune diseases a major public health problem. One of the unique features of this book is to discuss the impact of these diseases on the various stages of a woman's life.

It is only relatively recently that we have begun to think of autoimmune diseases as a single category, much as we think of cancer or cardiovascular diseases—different manifestations of an underlying problem. Because they are regarded separately, autoimmune diseases are typically seen and treated by different medical specialists, and it has not been the mindset of either doctors or their patients to begin to think of these diseases together. Yet there are important reasons to do so.

One of the common features of autoimmune diseases is a bias toward women. This observation emphasizes the important interrelationship between the hormonal system and immune responses. The fact that there are a few autoimmune diseases that are not more common among women may provide valuable clues that the problem actually began before puberty. This book outlines some of the latest theories as to why there is a female preponderance in autoimmunity.

Clinically, these diseases also travel together. A single patient may have more than one autoimmune disorder. This is quite common and important for patients and their physicians to know. Autoimmune diseases also cluster in families. And while that is an indication that genetics are involved, environment must also play a role.

When we study genetics, we compare twins who are genetically identical with those who are nonidentical. If a disease is caused by an environmental factor, there should be no difference between identical twins and nonidentical twins since, theoretically, both would be exposed to the same factor or factors. If there *is* such a difference, it suggests that genetics plays a role. In studies of the autoimmune diseases, we have found that for identical twins the chances of the second twin developing an autoimmune disease are about 30 percent, as opposed to 4 or 5 percent among nonidentical twins. This also tells us that even in identical twins, where genes are the same, the immune system does not react in identical ways.

Overall, genetics may account for about half the risks for autoimmune disease. However, what is inherited is not a specific gene that causes a defect that leads to disease, but several genes that collectively increase vulnerability or susceptibility.

While it is clear that there are environmental triggers for autoimmune disease, we still don't know much about them or how they might cause disease. Probably the best documented triggers are drugs, such as those that cause lupus, and there is strong (but not conclusive) evidence that viruses and bacteria can also serve as triggers. Foods, such as gluten, can also serve as a trigger, as can hormones.

Even if one is genetically predisposed, the possibility exists that autoimmune disease can be avoided if the environmental trigger is eliminated. Indeed, as we continue to learn more about them, the victory over the autoimmune diseases may come from strategies to prevent rather than treat disease.

One of the common threads uniting all of the autoimmune diseases is the presence of *autoantibodies*. Finding autoantibodies in blood serum is a key first step in the diagnosis of autoimmune disease. We now know that some of those antibodies may have been present years before symptoms arise. So there may be a period when we can intervene early enough to avoid or lessen chances of full-blown disease.

At the same time, the presence of autoantibodies is not a sufficient criterion for a diagnosis. It is a combination of clinical findings with laboratory data that helps a physician make a final diagnosis. In fact, many normal individuals have autoantibodies in their serum without any clinical evidence of disease.

Scientifically, we now know that many of the mechanisms involved in the production of one autoimmune disease also pertain to others. Therefore, studying the common factors in these diseases may help us understand the underlying causes of autoimmune disorders as a whole—and begin to treat the underlying causes of these diseases, not just the symptoms.

The common threads that connect the autoimmune diseases are woven throughout this important book, enabling readers to obtain a greater understanding of these illnesses individually and collectively.

Together with new information contained in this volume about diagnostic and treatment advances, patients and their families will get help to be better able to cope with these diseases and, as the title states, get on with their lives.

Noel R. Rose, MD, PhD
Department of Pathology,
Brigham and Women's Hospital
Harvard Medical School,
Boston, MA
Director, PAHO/WHO Collaborating Center for Autoimmune Disorders

1

Autoimmune Disease—Facing Our Intimate Enemy

I had never heard the word autoimmune *before I was told that I had antiphospholipid syndrome. And that diagnosis was scary enough. Imagine having normal checkups all of your life, then having a stroke from an illness you never even heard of. You have to learn a whole lot in a very short time to understand what's happening to you and feel in control and not frightened.*

ELAINE, 58

You probably bought this book because you've been diagnosed with an autoimmune disease or you suspect you may have one. Perhaps someone in your family has an autoimmune disease, such as rheumatoid arthritis or lupus, and you're worried about your own risk.

Maybe you're even wondering how it is that the body can declare war on itself. Simply put, somewhere along the line, your immune cells got the wrong message. Your body dispatched the battalions of cells that normally recognize and eliminate foreign invaders such as bacteria to instead destroy healthy tissue. The attack can target any area, including the joints (causing rheumatoid arthritis), the thyroid gland (causing it to become overactive or underactive), or nerve cells (leading to multiple sclerosis).

Often it's not a single assault; immune attacks may have several targets. If you have one autoimmune disease, you're at risk for a second or even a third disease. The specialist treating your particular problem may not be looking for these additional diseases, so it's important to be aware that they can occur.

Immune attacks may also come in waves, often referred to as *flares*, with lulls in between; you can have symptoms for weeks and then feel perfectly fine.

This book is designed to give you the inside story of the battle within your body. We're focusing on what makes you special as a woman and why simply being female may put you at risk of autoimmune disease. We'll examine those diseases that are more common in women and explore how they're interrelated. We'll look at treatments—some of them brand-new and generating excitement and optimism—and discuss the impact of autoimmune diseases during different stages of your life.

Most important, you'll learn some of the key signs and symptoms of autoimmune diseases, which may help you get the right diagnosis more quickly. The absence of knowledge can lead to tragedy, such as the one endured by AARDA spokeswoman and actress Kellie Martin and her family in 1998. Martin recounts the story of her 19-year-old sister Heather, whose flulike symptoms initially led doctors to think she had a severe virus. But Heather had lupus, and by the time she was diagnosed, her kidneys had been irreparably damaged by the disease. Kellie recalls:

> *A few days after finishing her sophomore year at college, my sister Heather couldn't get out of bed. She experienced severe abdominal pain and leg cramping, had numerous sores in her mouth that prevented her from eating, and had a temperature of 102. The doctor said it was the flu, or just stress from her recent final exams. So we were told to wait it out; a flu or virus just needs to run its course. "There's nothing we can do, except give her some painkillers," they said. Three emergency room visits and three days later, the doctor finally admitted Heather to the hospital for observation and testing. In the hospital she was examined by an internist, an infectious disease doctor, and a hematologist. After running several tests and concluding that she did indeed have an unusual virus, the doctor discharged Heather.*
>
> *They discharged Heather even though she still couldn't walk, eat, or sleep. After she was home for a few days, my mom and I took Heather to another doctor's office, where her condition was suspected two minutes after our arrival. The doctor looked disturbed at Heather's charts and medical history. After a brief physical exam, the doctor simply sat down and talked to Heather. He listened thoughtfully as she described exactly how she was feeling. The doctor suspected that she had an autoimmune disease called lupus.*

The following day she was again admitted to the hospital because of dehydration and kidney failure, both caused by lupus.

We were given the list of treatments Heather would be receiving: steroids, vitamins, and fluids. During her first week at the hospital, the blood vessels in her lungs began to burst, and her breathing became increasingly labored. The doctors, who now included a pulmonary specialist, three rheumatologists, and an oncologist (and those are just the doctors I can remember at this point), found that the lupus had affected Heather's liver and bone marrow. Therefore, the list of treatments increased to antibiotics and chemotherapy. My family believed that once Heathers condition had a name, she would receive the treatment necessary to make her better. Unfortunately, that diagnosis came too late. She died not long afterward in 1998, at age nineteen.

Unfortunately, it's common to encounter difficulty in getting a diagnosis of an autoimmune disease. A survey conducted by the Lupus Foundation of America found that more than half of people with lupus had symptoms for at least four years and saw three or more doctors before they were correctly diagnosed. Misdiagnosis or late diagnosis, due to being unaware and not knowing what diseases the symptoms might be a sign of, is a leading cause of death in autoimmunity. So it's imperative that you, the patient, be informed and alert.

At the same time, physicians are becoming more and more knowledgeable about diseases such as lupus with major campaigns across the country and educational efforts directed at medical students. It's not that a particular disease may be hard to diagnose, but rather that it requires knowledge of different signs and symptoms that don't appear at the same time but rather occur over time.

To truly understand your disease and the others for which you may be at risk, you need to become familiar with the fundamentals of autoimmunity. So that's where we'll begin. Think of this chapter as Autoimmunity 101.

Our Immune System—and How It Goes Awry

Our immune system has several layers. The first line of defense from outside invaders is a physical barrier—the skin and mucous membranes. Harmful organisms such as bacteria can breach this perimeter when, for example, we get a cut.

Once inside, these bacteria must face a second line of defense called the *innate immune system*, white blood cells produced by the bone marrow. If you remember the old video game Pac-Man (or in this case, Ms. Pac-Man), you'll recall those little smiley circles that gobbled up everything in their path. The Ms. Pac-Men of the innate immune system are *neutrophils* and *macrophages* (in Latin, *macro* means "big," *phage* means "to eat"; this cell is literally a "big eater"). Billions of neutrophils patrol the bloodstream at any given time. When neutrophils see an invader (like bacteria from that cut), they grab it, suck it in, and chew it up into little pieces that are destroyed by enzymes within the cell. They are messy eaters, though. They burp back fragments of their meal, and those "crumbs" can signal other immune cells to join the fray. Not only that, but as they chomp away, neutrophils produce chemicals that also cause inflammation that helps to heal but, if allowed to go on too long, can also hurt.

Now we come to the third (and most complicated) layer of the immune system, the one that's mainly involved in autoimmunity. It's called the adaptive immune system—cells in this system must be told how to do their job. All of these cells are intended to recognize what is self and what is nonself or foreign.

When a nonself entity like a bacteria or virus enters the bloodstream, the neutrophils and macrophages sound the alarm and battalions of other white blood cells (*lymphocytes*) are mobilized to search out the invader, referred to as an *antigen*.

There are several types of lymphocytes in the adaptive immune system, and each has a specific job to do: T cells help identify and eliminate antigens, and B cells produce antibodies that attach to one special antigen and help destroy it.

B cells, which develop in the bone marrow, must be activated in order to produce antibodies. First, B cells encounter antigens in the circulation. Then, after a special signal from "helper" T cells, B cells multiply and intensify their antibody response, making it more specific and lethal. In autoimmune diseases, susceptible women produce autoantibodies, antibodies that attack self. We make many different autoantibodies that can interfere with the normal function of tissues and destroy them. Some antibodies specifically react with material inside the nucleus of a cell (think of the nucleus as the yolk of an egg). These are classified as *antinuclear antibodies*, or *ANAs*. These antibodies are associated with autoimmune diseases such as *systemic lupus erythematosus (SLE)*.[1] While ANAs can be an indication you may have an autoimmune disease, they're not diagnostic in and of themselves and can be found in up to about 15 percent of healthy people who do not have any autoimmune diseases. Some antibodies attack the fluid of the cell surrounding the nucleus, called the *cytoplasm* (the white of the egg); these antibodies are also seen in SLE, and in *Sjögren's syndrome.*

Many other antibodies attack the surface or membrane of a cell—such as a red blood cell or platelet, or in a specific tissue such as the thyroid—causing the cell (or the target tissue) to malfunction. For example, an autoimmune assault on the thyroid gland can cause it to become overactive and produce too much thyroid hormone (*Graves' disease*), or to become underactive and secrete too little thyroid hormone (*Hashimoto's thyroiditis*). In *multiple sclerosis (MS),* the target is the protective coating called *myelin* that's wrapped around nerve cells in the brain and spine, disrupting communication between nerves and causing disability. In myasthenia gravis, the immune system targets the nerves that control muscles, causing progressive damage and weakness.

It is important to keep in mind that not all autoantibodies are bad. In fact, researchers have found that there are natural or protective antibodies. These antibodies are often of a type called IgM[2] whereas IgG is the type that is most associated with autoimmune diseases.

There are three main types of T cells:

- Helper T cells (e.g., Th1 and Th2). Th1 cells are associated with cellular immunity and maximize the killing efficiency of macrophages. Th2 cells signal B-cells to produce stronger antibodies
- Natural killer (NK or cytotoxic) T cells produce molecules that destroy cells carrying antigens
- Tregs, regulatory T cells (formerly called suppressor T cells) downregulate other immune responses
- Th17 are developmentally distinct from Th1 and Th2 cells. These cells create inflammation and can cause tissue injury in autoimmune diseases, an example being multiple sclerosis.

T cells are activated when they encounter an antigen, "recognizing" it through a kind of antenna on their surface, called a *receptor*, which receives signals from molecules sitting on the surface of the antigen. Cells that signal the T cells in this process are called antigen-presenting cells (APCs).

A normal helper T cell might signal a B cell that it has found a rhinovirus (which causes the common cold); the B cell would then produce the appropriate antibody to get rid of that virus. A *self-reactive* (also called *autoreactive*) T cell would tell the B cell to produce an antibody against the body's own healthy tissue. An NK T cell might mistake the body's cells for a bacterium or a virus and target it for destruction. A Treg might hamper protective immune responses. Many autoimmune diseases are *cell mediated*, meaning the T cells cause damage, not antibodies.

We encounter millions of antigens during our lifetime, and we have a vast array of T cells capable of recognizing, responding to, and remembering these antigens.[3] T cells mature in the thymus gland, where their receptors are programmed to react against foreign antigens and tolerate *self-antigens* (also called *autoantigens*); T cells with receptors that react to self-antigens are usually eliminated in the thymus. But sometimes self-reactive T cells aren't eliminated, or, as some researchers speculate, the thymus may not properly eliminate enough self-reactive T cells. Whatever the cause, rogue T cells are able to roam at will around the body, attacking healthy tissue or sending the wrong signals to B cells. New subsets of T cells are still being discovered.

T cells send signals through messenger molecules called *cytokines* and chemokines, which can also be key players in autoimmune disease. Cytokines are proteins that can activate immune cells (including other T cells) and affect nonimmune processes, directly causing inflammation and damage. A common inflammatory cytokine in autoimmune disease is *tumor necrosis factor alpha (TNFα)*. Drugs that can slow or halt the progress of rheumatoid arthritis, Crohn's disease, and other autoimmune diseases block the destructive effects of TNFα (see page 10). *Chemokines*, substances manufactured by cells and tissues, act like a magnet for other immune cells. Overproduction of chemokines attracts neutrophils and macrophages (both of whom never refuse a meal), and when these cells invade tissues, inflammation and destruction can ensue.

As we mentioned, macrophages and neutrophils (also called *phagocytes*) normally patrol the body, killing foreign cells by engulfing them and destroying them with toxic molecules. After digesting antigens, neutrophils spit out tiny bits of the antigen on their surface to alert T cells to the presence of an enemy. Neutrophils also fight off infectious agents by releasing granules of potent chemicals that destroy the invaders. In autoimmune diseases, these cells become overactive and release too many of these toxic molecules, which damage surrounding tissue and contribute to inflammation. This happens in rheumatoid arthritis, lupus, multiple sclerosis, and other autoimmune diseases.

Another cause of inflammation in autoimmune disease is the formation of *immune complexes*, latticelike structures created when antibodies bind to antigens. These immune complexes cause activation of what's called the *complement cascade*.

If you think of antibodies as the "guns" of the immune arsenal, complement proteins function as the "bullets." The complement cascade can be thought of as nine different bullets that can make antibodies more effective in destroying foreign invaders. When complement is activated, there is a domino effect in which one complement protein makes another one active, and this cascade winds up calling in neutrophils and macrophages, which block blood flow in small blood vessels, destroying instead of nourishing tissues and organs.

As you can see, a lot is going on in autoimmunity, which is why treatment for autoimmune disease is not as simple as a single antibiotic pill that kills bacteria. These diseases may require multidrug therapies to affect the different processes that are causing symptoms and organ damage.

What Causes Immune Mistakes?

Because the immune system is so complicated, it's hard to pinpoint a single cause for any autoimmune disease. You may need to be susceptible (usually a matter of genes), you may need to encounter some kind of environmental trigger (maybe sunlight or even an infection), but for sure your immune cells have to misfire.

We normally have small numbers of autoreactive B cells and T cells floating around the immune system, but self-tolerance is usually maintained. However, in susceptible people, that tolerance can be disrupted. Some people may be genetically programmed to produce large numbers of overreactive immune cells or too many damaging cytokines. Some genes may also result in problems with T cell education in the thymus. Some T cells may turn traitor after exposure to viruses or other environmental factors.[4] Infections, environmental toxins (such as mercury), medications, and even sun exposure may also activate B cells. For example, excess iodine can be toxic to thyroid tissue, causing autoantibody production and thyroid disease. Some studies have tied exposure to *Epstein-Barr virus (EBV)*, which causes infectious mononucleosis, to lupus, MS, and other autoimmune diseases.

Recent research suggests that bacteria and other organisms normally found in our body, called the *microbiome*, may play a role in autoimmunity.

Our gastrointestinal system (the GI tract or "gut" for short) is around 30 feet long, stretching from the mouth to the anus. The gut is home to more than 500 species of bacteria, as well as yeast and other organisms. Some bacteria are harmless and some are even "friendly" helping us to digest food and maintain the health of the GI tract, such as *Lactobacillus* (also found in live yogurt cultures). But some bacteria are not so friendly. Certain types of the coliform bacteria *Escherichia coli (E. coli)* can cause serious infections when ingested in contaminated food.

The delicate balance of good and bad organisms in the microbiome can be upset by toxins, infections, and antibiotics that kill off beneficial bacteria and allow potentially harmful types to increase. Even stress can disrupt the balance. The resulting *dysbiosis* activates T cells and triggers overproduction of inflammatory cytokines that can leak into the bloodstream.[5]

The single layer of *epithelial* cells lining the intestines is usually tightly joined together, forming a barrier against outside toxins. These cellular junctions open and close when signaled by antigens, allowing properly digested fats, proteins, and carbohydrates to pass into the bloodstream. When dysbiosis occurs, the "tight junctions" between the epithelial cells may loosen and become "leaky," allowing inflammatory cytokines and harmful bacteria to slip through.

Gut dysbiosis, or "leaky gut," is thought to underlie inflammatory bowel disease (see page 243).[4] Recent research also suggests that an immune reaction to certain GI bacteria may trigger type 1 diabetes,[6] and a reaction to the oral bacteria that cause gum disease could be linked to rheumatoid arthritis (RA).[7]

The shape of some cells in the body actually resembles viruses or bacteria, so T cells may mistake one for the other and attack both. Such *molecular mimicry* happens in rheumatic fever; proteins on the surface of strep bacteria have a similar structure to proteins in cardiac muscle. Molecular mimicry is thought to be involved in a number of autoimmune diseases.

Genes also play a role, and more than one gene may be to blame for a single disease. Think of genes as minicomputers, packed with complex codes that deliver instructions to cells, telling them which proteins to produce to grow and which proteins to produce to perform different functions.

The genetic code is made up of sequences of building blocks, or bases, often referred to by the first letters of their names: A (adenine), T (thymine), C (cytosine), and G (guanine). These are the basic components that make up DNA. Sometimes there's a "typo," a missing or transposed letter or letters in a particular DNA sequence that results in a genetic mutation. Genes that predispose people to autoimmune diseases are often those called human leukocyte antigens (HLAs), which contain the codes for proteins that label a cell self or nonself. In some autoimmune diseases, these HLA genes mistakenly identify cells as nonself, setting off an attack. Several autoimmune diseases may have genes in the same HLA group in common; for example, genes in the DR4 group are linked to both rheumatoid arthritis and type 1 diabetes, among other diseases. Other genes regulate cytokines, causing too many or too few to be produced.

Autoimmune diseases and their related genes can run in families, but the same faulty genes don't always produce the same problem. One family member may have immune cells that react against the thyroid, while another may suffer an autoimmune attack on the joints. Even if you're an identical twin, your chances of developing the same autoimmune disease can vary.

All told, autoimmune reactions either cause or are involved in more than 100 chronic illnesses. The most common of these are thyroid disorders, including Hashimoto's thyroiditis and Graves' disease, which affect at least 3 percent of all adult women.

Autoimmunity: Some Common Threads

Many of these illnesses share the same autoantibodies, feature tissue or organ destruction caused by the same hordes of immune cells and inflammatory molecules, or have common genes. And the same medication can be used to treat different diseases.

For example, long before the concept of autoimmune disease (or the common factor of inflammation) was recognized, the corticosteroid drug *prednisone* was used to treat a variety of these disorders. The fact that the same drug might be used to treat diseases that vary in what organs they attack does not necessarily mean autoimmunity represents a single disorder. However, these diseases do have some key elements in common.

Medications developed to target a specific mechanism in one disease have been found to effectively combat that same factor in others. For example, patients with some autoimmune diseases have high levels of *tumor necrosis factor-alpha (TNFα)*, an inflammatory molecule that contributes to organ and tissue damage. One anti-TNF drug, *etanercept (Enbrel)*, soaks TNF up like a sponge, inactivating it; another drug, *infliximab (Remicade)*, uses a "smart bomb" molecule called a monoclonal antibody to disable TNFα. Etanercept is not only approved as a treatment for rheumatoid arthritis but is also used to treat people with Crohn's disease, autoimmune inflammatory bowel disease, and vasculitis. Remicade was initially approved for patients with Crohn's disease but is now being used to treat rheumatoid and psoriatic arthritis.

Newer medications that target the cytokine *interleukin-6 (IL-6)*, such as *tocilizumab (Actemra)*, and the *Janus kinase (JAK)* inhibitor *tofacitinib (Xeljanz)* are approved for RA and are also being tested against other autoimmune diseases. Additional target-specific drugs are currently under development.

While autoimmune diseases may target different areas of the body, the genes that affect immune responses may be the same. For example, genes that govern cytokines may have a mutation that causes too many inflammatory molecules to be released. Defective genes common to autoimmune diseases may also affect the way T cells are programmed to recognize antigens, the number of receptors they carry, the number of T cells with a faulty memory, or how many defective T cells are eliminated. Gene therapy to correct these mistakes may one day be possible.

Many autoimmune diseases have the same inflammatory molecules and immune cells that cause damage. For example, one small study found the same autoreactive T cells in people with type 1 diabetes and multiple sclerosis, targeting similar antigens in the pancreas and in the central nervous system (CNS).

Canadian researchers studied T cell autoreactivity in 38 people with MS, 54 children newly diagnosed with type 1 diabetes, and 105 of their close family members, comparing them to a group of healthy controls. To their surprise, they found T cells from the MS patients also targeted self-antigens on insulin-producing islet cells in the pancreas, and T cells from two-thirds of the children with diabetes and their parents or siblings also showed responses to at least one autoantigen seen in MS—including myelin basic protein, one of the building blocks of the "insulation" around nerve cell fibers.[8] The research suggests not only that type 1 diabetes and MS may be more closely linked than anyone thought but also that there may be a lengthy "clinically silent" phase in both diseases that could be a potential target for future preventive therapy. In fact, emerging knowledge about autoimmunity as a cause of disease may lead to treatments that could halt such reactions before they have a chance to cause serious damage.

Why Are Women More Vulnerable?

As you can see from the following table, women are prime targets for many autoimmune diseases (although disease severity doesn't always differ between the sexes). While the ratios can vary according to geography[9] and differing research,[10] one reason for the high incidence of some diseases may be that women may be exposed more often to possible triggers, like viruses,

Autoimmune Disease: Female-to-Male Ratios

Hashimoto's thyroiditis	10:1
Systemic lupus erythematosus	9:1
Sjögren's syndrome	9:1
Primary biliary cirrhosis	9:1
Graves' disease	9:1
Chronic active hepatitis	8:1
Mixed connective tissue disease	8:1
Antiphospholipid syndrome	3:1
Scleroderma	3:1
Rheumatoid arthritis	2.5:1
Myasthenia gravis	2:1
Multiple sclerosis	2:1
Immune thrombocytopenia	2:1
Autoimmune hemolytic anemia	2:1

Sources: *Frontiers in Neuroendocrinology*, 2014; *Arthritis Research & Therapy*, 2009; Institute of Medicine, 2001; American Autoimmune Related Diseases Association

medications, or even cosmetics.[11] Some explanations are likely found in sex-related biological differences in certain immune functions.

But it may all begin with the very thing that makes us female in the first place: having two X chromosomes.

Humans inherit two sets of 23 chromosomes—one set of 22 *autosomes (non-sex chromosomes)*, plus an X or Y, the *sex chromosomes*—from each parent. In a developing embryo, having two X chromosomes promotes expression of female hormones and female sex characteristics. Embryos that have one X and one Y chromosome develop as males. Being a double X may also affect autoimmune responses.

Studies of the X and Y chromosomes in mice at the University of California Los Angeles found that female mice have higher levels of autoantibodies than males. When male mice were genetically altered to have two X chromosomes, it resulted in greater disease severity and organ damage in lupus and other experimental models of autoimmunity than having the XY combination.[12]

Autoimmune disease–specific genes may also be associated with the X chromosome. Scientists at the Arthritis Research UK epidemiology unit at the University of Manchester examined DNA samples from more than 27,000 patients with and without RA, most of whom were women, and found 14 genes associated with RA.[13] This discovery may help explain why women are three times more likely than men to develop RA, the researchers say.

Of course, one biological difference is our ability to bear children. During pregnancy we're able to carry a baby in the womb without the immune system attacking a technically half-"foreign" body (a fetus has genes and immune components from both parents).[14] Recent research suggests that fetal cells from past pregnancies can survive in some women's bloodstreams for more than 20 years and may trigger an immune response akin to the rejection of a transplanted organ—perhaps causing diseases like scleroderma or rheumatoid arthritis.

Key elements in this reaction are the *human leukocyte antigens (HLAs)*, which, as you'll recall, are governed by genes. In a bone marrow transplant, the donor and recipient must have compatible HLAs (also called *histocompatibility antigens*), otherwise the transplanted cells will see the recipient's body tissues as "foreign" and attack. This is called graft-versus-host disease, which can often resemble autoimmune disease. In fact, the HLA genes involved in graft-versus-host disease are also involved in autoimmune diseases.

While our own HLAs are self-antigens, the combination of self and nonself HLAs in fetal cells means they are part foreign. The fact that fetal cells remain in a woman's circulation results in a condition called *chimerism*, a word that derives from the mythical creature called a chimera that has the head of one animal and the tail of another. The existence of these fetal cells is called *microchimerism*, and it may contribute to an autoimmune reaction by confusing the immune system.[15]

The greatest risk for some autoimmune diseases seems to occur when there's a close but not identical match between HLA molecules. This confusion between the two sets of HLA molecules may disrupt normal communication within the immune system and provoke a wrongful attack on self. "You can directly inherit genes from your mother or father that put you at risk for disease. But these are genes that come from your prior pregnancy that are in your bloodstream," explains J. Lee Nelson, MD, of the Immunogenetics Program at the Fred Hutchinson Cancer Research Center and a professor at the University of Washington in Seattle.

Those same HLA genes (some of which may be linked to susceptibility to autoimmune disease) may also determine whether fetal cells that survive in the mother's blood have a detrimental effect on the mother. For example, if a child has the same HLA gene as the mother, it seems to be a strong risk factor for some diseases in the woman. In her research, Dr. Nelson found 20 times more persistent fetal cells in women with scleroderma, compared to women who'd also had children but didn't have the disease. Similar evidence of persistent fetal cells has been found in women with other diseases such as lupus, multiple sclerosis, and autoimmune thyroid disease. It may be that in some women these cells gravitate to certain sites in the body, the thyroid for example, and contribute to an autoimmune reaction.

However, the effects of persistent fetal cells are not all adverse. "Interestingly, for rheumatoid arthritis, which usually gets better during pregnancy, women carrying a child that is not HLA-compatible have a better chance of a remission," says Dr. Nelson.[16] Recent research by Dr. Nelson and her colleagues find that while having had a baby provides a modest protective effect against RA,[17] a complicated pregnancy (such as having a premature or very low-birthweight baby) may mean a higher risk of RA.[18]

The same foreign cell "transfer" might occur from maternal cells that get into fetal circulation while the immune system is developing, Dr. Nelson adds. Maternal cells may also transfer to male offspring, increasing their risk of some autoimmune diseases, or sometimes decreasing risk, depending on the specific HLAs.

But microchimerism is only a small piece of the puzzle. Our immune systems are unique in other ways. Women produce more antibodies and autoantibodies than men, which may be related to those X chromosomes.[13] Men and women also have differing responses to organ transplantation. Organs donated by women are more likely to be rejected, and women receiving transplants have a lower survival rate compared to men.[19] This could be partly due to genes, partly due to hormonal influences, or perhaps caused by differences in cellular immune responses.

Estrogen can stimulate certain immune responses. For example, it can stimulate the production of helper T cell cytokines and enhance the production of others, remarks Michael Lockshin, MD, director of the Barbara Volcker Center for Women and Rheumatic Diseases at the Hospital for Special Surgery in New York City. Estrogen can also increase agents that protect cells against programmed cell death and foster a break in B cell tolerance.

Estrogens also increase antibody production, promoting B cell mediated autoimmune diseases like RA. In contrast, androgens act as natural immunosuppressants.[9] However, emphasizes Dr. Lockshin, estrogen alone cannot explain sex differences in autoimmune diseases.

Some autoimmune diseases may worsen in pregnancy, while rheumatoid arthritis and multiple sclerosis get better. High estrogen levels during pregnancy may improve disease through decreased T cell mediated immune responses. On the other hand, pregnancy can trigger other autoimmune diseases, such as thyroid disease and myasthenia gravis.

In some instances, the elevations in estrogen during the first part of your menstrual cycle (the *follicular* phase) may coincide with disease flares. In multiple sclerosis or myasthenia gravis, symptoms may worsen premenstrually (when progesterone is elevated). However, early data suggest that women do not have an increased risk of flares when undergoing ovulation induction (where potent hormones are given to stimulate the ovary to produce several eggs for assisted reproduction). Also, in pregnancy, very few lupus patients have a serious flare, even with estrogen levels 100 times as high as during the peak menstrual cycle. Some diseases, like Sjögren's, occur more often after menopause, when estrogen levels are decreased.

"The effects of pregnancy on the different diseases, and of the menstrual cycle, menopause, or hormone therapy, are different in different diseases, and that isn't consistent with a single cause, like hormones," stresses Dr. Lockshin. "What's more likely is that hormones may act as an on-off switch in some autoimmune diseases."

That on-off switch may be estrogen or other hormones influenced by estrogen. For instance, research at the National Institutes of Health (NIH) suggests that inflammatory autoimmune diseases are influenced by corticotropin releasing hormone (CRH), produced by the hypothalamus in the brain and by the placenta and immune tissues. CRH triggers release of stress hormones like *cortisol* (a natural steroid) when we're under stress and during pregnancy. Cortisol modulates certain aspects of immune activity in the body, including an increase in inflammatory cytokines. Research suggests that CRH may also stimulate production of a protein that helps shield the fetus from an immune attack.[20]

On the other hand, male hormones (androgens) like testosterone appear to be protective, acting as natural immunosuppressants in some autoimmune diseases.[9]

For example, women with Sjögren's syndrome are known to have lower levels of testosterone, and correcting the imbalance may help symptoms. There are now eyedrops containing androgen for women with Sjögren's.

What makes things more difficult for women is that many of the symptoms of autoimmune disease are nonspecific.

You just know that you're bone tired, and you can't seem to get yourself out of bed. And everything seems worse because of it. You get your period, and the cramps seem much worse—every little muscle ache and pain seems intensified. Your joints hurt . . . but is it water retention or is the RA worse? You often don't know what's arthritis, what's PMS, what's fibromyalgia . . . and what's simply being tired. Any new symptom that crops up, you often just don't know what to make of it. Most of the time your doctor just says, "Oh, it's your RA." And unless you make it your business to learn everything you can, you probably would think that, too.

Cate, 30

Recognizing the Enemy Within

While immune attacks may produce similar symptoms early on, they don't always point to a particular disease. Early symptoms can be vague and transitory; illnesses often overlap and mimic each other. For instance, fatigue and joint pain can be symptoms of rheumatoid arthritis, lupus, and thyroid disease.

When doctors talk about diagnosis, they use the terms *signs* and *symptoms*. What's the difference? Signs are things that can be *seen* during a physical exam, in blood tests, and on x-rays. Symptoms are what you *experience*, which can be very individual.

Sometimes there's a gap in time between your symptoms and the clinical signs of disease that doctors look for to help make a specific diagnosis. The day you see your doctor your joints may not look swollen and red if you have early rheumatoid arthritis. This may account for a time lag between the actual onset of a disease and a formal diagnosis. And that time lag can be considerable. The signs of autoimmune disease may be misdiagnosed and treated as another condition, such as depression and fatigue in MS or lupus. Or, in women like Cate, fatigue and pain may be mistaken for worsening symptoms of rheumatoid arthritis when they're actually due to fibromyalgia, a nonautoimmune disorder that often occurs with autoimmune diseases.

Virtually every woman with an autoimmune disease experiences fatigue that can be so debilitating it affects every aspect of life, according to a 2015 online survey by AARDA and the National Coalition of Autoimmune Patient Groups.

Many women suffer infertility, miscarriages, and pregnancy complications because of autoimmune-related problems, even if they don't have a diagnosable disease. For example, autoantibodies that lead to blood clots in the placenta may cause second-trimester pregnancy loss. These same autoantibodies, called *antiphospholipid antibodies*, are found in women who have lupus or antiphospholipid syndrome, as well as other autoimmune diseases.

Tests for autoantibodies such as *rheumatoid factor (RF)* or *anti-cyclic citrullinated peptides (anti-CCPs)* can help your doctor in making a diagnosis. For instance, a positive test for rheumatoid factor can be one indication of rheumatoid arthritis (and also of Sjögren's syndrome). It usually takes a combination of blood test results, an assessment of clinical signs and symptoms, and sometimes diagnostic imaging to make a definite diagnosis.

These autoantibodies and inflammatory cytokines may be present long before you start having symptoms and may signal a *preclinical* stage of a disease. An exciting area of research involves ways to figure out which marker (or group of markers) may help predict which women will eventually develop disease and tell them apart from women whose level of biomarkers is benign. The hope is to one day be able to prevent autoimmune disease even before it begins.

How This Book Can Help You

As you read each chapter of this book, you'll learn more about the kinds of tests you need to obtain a correct diagnosis and what the results mean. We'll also detail the diagnostic criteria doctors use.

If you're suffering from seemingly vague and unrelated symptoms, we'll help you sort them out and tell you where to go for help. A survey by the Sjögren's Syndrome Foundation (SSF) found that as many as three out of four women under age 35 may suffer at least two potential symptoms of Sjögren's, including dry eyes or dry mouth, yet never tell their doctor, or simply hope the problems will go away. The more quickly you act, the better your chances for a successful treatment.

This book is designed to give you the tools you need to manage your own diagnosis. But, again, be aware that having one autoimmune disease puts you at risk for others that cluster with it. So you need to be alert for other symptoms that can crop up.

We'll also tell you how autoimmune diseases—and their treatments—can affect you during different stages of your life. Some autoimmune diseases, like antiphospholipid syndrome, can make it hard to sustain a pregnancy. A frequent treatment for autoimmune disease, corticosteroid drugs, may put you at risk for osteoporosis or high cholesterol, especially if you're older. Corticosteroid drugs can also produce psychological symptoms such as depression and explosions of anger that can be extremely upsetting if you're not aware that they can occur. They also increase appetite, which can contribute to excessive weight gain.

Throughout this book, you'll learn about the latest scientific and medical research, including research into genetics, environmental and viral triggers, possible ways of altering immune responses, and potential new therapies such as stem cell transplants and gene therapy. We've called on the expertise of immunologists, rheumatologists, endocrinologists, neurologists, hematologists, and gastroenterologists from institutions leading the way in investigating these diseases. Autoimmunity continues to be a rapidly evolving field, but we've tried to include the latest information available. Each chapter will feature sections on early signs and symptoms, provide answers to commonly asked questions about fertility and pregnancy management, and detail special considerations for midlife, menopause, and later life.

Drug Information for Pregnancy, Lactation, and Fertility

In 2014, the U.S. Food and Drug Administration (FDA) made changes in the way it labels drugs for use during pregnancy and lactation. The new system will eventually replace the categories A, B, C, D, and X with three new sections, so the information sheets that you receive with your medications may look different. The risks that are detailed remain basically the same—it's the way they are presented that will change. Here's what to expect in package inserts and online information:

- *The section called "Pregnancy" will cover prenatal considerations, potential fetal risks, and subsections dealing with drug effects during labor and delivery.*
- *The section on "Lactation" (formerly a section within the letter-based system called "Nursing Mothers") discusses the amounts of drugs that may reach breast milk and potential effects on a child.*
- *A third section, called "Females and Males of Reproductive Potential," will deal with pregnancy testing, contraception, and infertility as they relate to the medication.*

These changes will affect all new prescription drug submitted for FDA approval and are being phased in gradually for those drugs already approved for autoimmune diseases. In this book, we'll use the general risk definitions used for the letter-based system.

In this book, you'll find advice on getting the latest treatments and finding an appropriate specialist in the landscape of the U.S. healthcare system laid out by the Affordable Care Act (ACA) of 2010. In the back of this book you'll find an extensive list of resources, support groups, and information on the Internet. We've also included selected current references for each chapter.

This continues to be an exciting era for autoimmune research. New treatments are emerging that may make these diseases easier to manage and maybe even stop them in their tracks. Basic science is informing clinical decision making every day. Armed with knowledge, you can take charge of your healthcare as understanding of autoimmune diseases continues to evolve.

Notes

1. Tan EM. Antinuclear antibodies defining autoimmune pathways. *Arthritis Res Ther.* 2014;16(1):104–108. doi:10.1186/ar4482.
2. Grönwall C, Vas J, Silverman GJ. Protective roles of natural IgM antibodies. *Front Immunol.* 2012;2:3–66. Published online Apr 4, 2012. doi:10.3389/fimmu.2012.00066.
3. Kuchroo VK, Ohashi PS, Sartor RB, and CG Vinuesa. Dysregulation of immune homeostasis in autoimmune diseases. *Nat Med.* 2012;18:42–47.
4. Tiniakou E, Costenbader KH, Kriegel MA. Sex-specific environmental influences on the development of autoimmune diseases. *Clin Immunol.* 2013;149:182–191.
5. Campbell AW. Autoimmunity and the gut. *Autoimmune Dis.* 2014. Article ID 152428. doi:10.1155/2014/152428.
6. Yeung W-CG, Rawlinson WD, Craig ME. Enterovirus infection and type 1 diabetes mellitus: systematic review and meta-analysis of observational molecular studies. *BMJ.* 2011;342:d35.
7. Scher JU, Abramson SJ. Periodontal disease, *Porphyromonas gingivalis*, and rheumatoid arthritis: what triggers autoimmunity and clinical disease? *Arthritis Res Ther.* 2013;15:122.
8. Winer S, Astsaturov I, Cheung RK, et al. Type I diabetes and multiple sclerosis patients target islet plus central nervous system autoantigens; nonimmunized nonobese diabetic mice can develop autoimmune encephalitis. *J Immunol.* 2001;166(4):2831–2841. doi:10.4049/jimmunol.166.4.2831.
9. Ngo ST, Steyn FJ, McCombe PA. Gender differences in autoimmune disease. *Front Neuroendocrinol.* 2014;35:347–369.
10. Oliver JE, Silman AJ. Why are women predisposed to autoimmune diseases? *Arthritis Res Ther.* 2009;11(5):252–261. doi:10.1186/ar2825.
11. Sverdrup BM, Källberg H, Klareskog L, Alfredsson L, and the Epidemiological Investigation of Rheumatoid Arthritis Study Group et al. Usage of skin care products and risk of rheumatoid arthritis: results from the Swedish EIRA study. *Arthritis Res Ther.* 2012;14:R41. doi:10.1186/ar3749.
12. Smith-Bouvier DL, Divekar AA, Sasidhar M, et al. A role for sex chromosome complement in the female bias in autoimmune disease. *J Exp Med.* 2008;205:1099–1108. doi:10.1084/jem.20070850.

13. Eyre S, Bowes J, Diogo D, et al. High-density genetic mapping identifies new susceptibility loci for rheumatoid arthritis. *Nat Genet.* 2012;44:1336–1340. doi:10.1038/ng.2462.
14. Mor G, Cardenas I. The immune system in pregnancy: a unique complexity. *Am J Reprod Immunol.* 2010;63(6):425–433. doi:10.1111/j.1600-0897.2010.00836.x.
15. Nelson JL. The otherness of self: microchimerism in health and disease. *Trends Immunol.* 2012;33(8):421–427.
16. Nelson JL, Hughes KA, Smith AG, Nisperos BB, Branchaud AB, Hansen JA. Maternal-fetal disparity in HLA class II alloantigens and the pregnancy-induced amelioration of rheumatoid arthritis. *N Engl J Med.* 1993;329:466–471.
17. Guthrie KA, Gammill HS, Madeleine MM, Dugowson CE, Nelson JL. Parity and HLA alleles in risk of rheumatoid arthritis. *Chimerism.* 2011;2(1):11–15.
18. Ma KK, Nelson JL, Dugowson CE, Gammill HS. Adverse pregnancy outcomes and risk of subsequent rheumatoid arthritis. *Arthritis Rheum.* Accepted article, Dec 23, 2013. doi:10.1002/art.38247.
19. Zeier M, Bernd Döhler B, Opelz G, Ritz E. The effect of donor gender on graft survival. *J Am Soc Nephrol.* 2002;13:2570–2576. doi:10.1097/01.ASN.0000030078.74889.69.
20. Makrigiannakis, A, Zoumakis, E, Kalantaridou, et al. Corticotropin-releasing hormone (CRH) promotes blastocyst implantation and early maternal tolerance. *Nat Immunol.* 2001;2:1018–1024.

2

Those Aching Joints—Rheumatoid Arthritis

I was doing a film, Serial Mom *(in 1997), and my feet started to swell terribly; all of the shoes that we had bought for the character suddenly seemed painfully small. I thought I must be retaining water or something, even though retaining water didn't explain the pain. And it hurt terribly. It hurt to put my feet in the shoes, it hurt to put anything on my feet. I would rip the bottoms of the covers off the bed because I couldn't stand to have the weight of the blanket on my feet. When I finished the film and came home, I found that I couldn't get into my own shoes. Even sneakers; I had to take the laces out. So I went to the head of podiatry at one of the major New York hospitals and he took x-rays, felt my feet, and told me I needed bigger shoes. He wasn't very helpful.*

Then it went to my neck; I couldn't turn my head. So I went and had an x-ray of my neck, and the doctors told me that I had lost the curvature of the first four vertebrae, and they had no idea why and there was nothing they could do. Then I couldn't open my left arm; it was locked in position. So I went to a hotshot doctor, a sports medicine specialist who treats some New York teams, supposed to be the best in the city. He took an MRI as well as an x-ray and couldn't see anything. He said perhaps we should do exploratory surgery. It was at this point that I got really freaked out. And by then I was feeling so ill, so tired, and so sick—like having the flu all the time. This was over the space of eight or nine months. Back then I wasn't that aggressive about my own health; I had never had anything seriously wrong with me. But I was frightened. I didn't know what was happening to me.

I finally went to my GP, who I've been seeing for years and years, and I said, "I think I'm dying and I'm terrified. You've got to help me." He was the first doctor to take blood to be tested. And he called me up the next day and said to get over to his office right away. My rheumatoid factor was sky-high; he didn't know how I was walking at all. I had access to the best doctors in New York, and he was the one who found the RA. But I was lucky—it only took me a year to get diagnosed. Many women I know take three to five times as long to find out what's wrong with them.

Kathleen Turner
(diagnosed at age 42)

Unlike the charismatic actress Kathleen Turner, rheumatoid arthritis (RA) may not have much stage presence in the beginning. It may come on so gradually that you can't even remember when the aching and stiffness in your joints began. Or it may announce itself loudly, with a sudden outburst of swelling and joint pain. But the character of RA is revealed in its symmetry—the immune system attack on the joint lining usually affects the same joints on both sides of the body.

The Arthritis Foundation (AF) estimates that rheumatoid arthritis affects some 1.5 million Americans, almost three times more women than men. RA usually strikes in the prime of life but can also affect children (as juvenile RA) and the elderly.

Arthritis is derived from the Greek word *arthron*, meaning "joint," and the suffix *itis*, meaning "inflammation." But inflammation itself doesn't start out to be destructive; it is actually the body's defense mechanism. When there's an injury or invasion, the immune system sends specialized white blood cells to the area to destroy anything foreign and repair damage. For example, when you get a cut, the immune system dispatches a repair crew of white blood cells to the scene to destroy harmful bacteria and heal the damaged tissue. The work done by the repair cells initially makes things red and swollen—inflamed. When the repairs are done, the area heals and the redness and inflammation go away. But if an attack becomes constant, the inflammation doesn't cease. And it eventually becomes chronic and destructive.

A joint (the place where two bones meet) is surrounded by a protective capsule. The ends of the bones are covered by a layer of rubbery material called *cartilage*, which acts as a shock absorber and enables the bones to move against each other smoothly (cartilage breaks down from wear and tear in another common form of arthritis, *osteoarthritis*). The joint capsule is lined with a thin layer of tissue called the *synovial membrane*, which produces a clear fluid that lubricates the joint. The synovium also acts as a filter to bring nutritional materials from the blood into the joint and the cartilage, which does not have a blood supply. So the synovium is very important for maintaining function of the joint.

In rheumatoid arthritis, immune cells for reasons still unknown mistakenly attack the synovium, setting off a destructive cascade of events. As white blood cells pour into the synovium, extra fluid is produced and antibodies and inflammatory molecules (*cytokines*) inflame the joint lining. Eventually, this synovitis results in the warmth, redness, swelling, and pain that are the classic symptoms of rheumatoid arthritis.

As the inflammation continues to percolate, synovial cells start to grow and divide abnormally, thickening a membrane that was once just three or four cells thick. As RA progresses, new blood vessels form to feed the growing mass of abnormal synovial cells and immune cells, which form a sheet (*pannus*) that

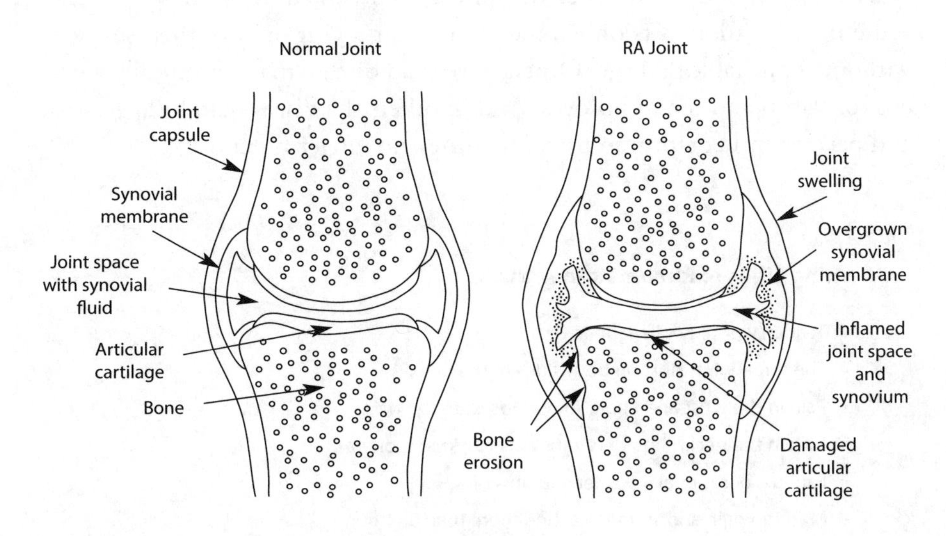

How RA Affects Joints

spreads over the cartilage in the joint. This tissue begins to eat into the cartilage and also erodes and destroys the bone adjacent to the cartilage. This weakens the muscles, ligaments, and tendons that help support and stabilize the joint. When the support system is damaged, it can lead to pain, stiffness, and deformity.

This damage can begin during the first year or two of the disease, long before symptoms start to appear, and by the time RA is diagnosed the disease may have already become destructive. That's one reason that early diagnosis and treatment are so critical.

In women, RA often starts in the fingers of both hands and progresses to the wrist joints and beyond, or it can begin in the feet (as in Kathleen Turner's case). The disease can affect any joint in the body, including those in the spine. Once it's set off, the inflammatory process takes on a life of its own and can reach beyond the joints. Inflammatory cytokines can cause reduced levels of erythropoietin, a hormone that stimulates the bone marrow to make red blood cells; if fewer red blood cells are produced, the result is anemia. Antibodies and inflammation in the eyes, mucous membranes, and salivary glands frequently cause dry eyes and mouth (*Sjögren's syndrome*). Inflammation may also affect the blood vessels (*vasculitis*) as well as the lining of the lungs (*pleuritis*) and the sac around the heart (*pericarditis*).

The inflammatory process of RA differs from woman to woman. In some, acute inflammation lasts only a few months or a year or two, then subsides without appreciable damage. Others have mild disease that periodically worsens (or flares) and then improves. And in others the disease can be aggressive and permanently deform joints so that they no longer function.

Warning Signs of Rheumatoid Arthritis

- Tender, warm, swollen joints
- The same joints hurt on both sides of the body
- Pain in the wrist and finger joints closest to the palm
- Pain in the neck, shoulders, elbows, hips, knees, or feet
- Fatigue, occasional fever, feeling unwell
- Morning pain and stiffness lasting more than an hour

For many women, RA improves during pregnancy and worsens in the postpartum period (initially leading many scientists to believe female hormones and/or glucocorticoids play a protective role in the disease since hormones such as estrogen and progesterone increase dramatically during pregnancy but fall postpartum). RA can become chronic and severe, causing serious joint damage and disability. But in recent years new drugs have been developed to block specific inflammatory molecules, slowing or even stopping the damage caused by rheumatoid arthritis.

What Causes Rheumatoid Arthritis?

RA appears to be caused by a combination of genetic vulnerability, environmental triggers (possibly infections), hormonal influences, and perhaps joint injury.

A number of genes are associated with RA, and they're found in healthy people and in women with other autoimmune diseases. The genes encode human leukocyte antigens (HLAs), which are proteins that contain instructions for the cell to be labeled self or nonself. Women with rheumatoid arthritis may have the genes encoding the particular HLA *allele* (form of the gene) DR4, which may cause healthy tissues to be labeled as foreign. Different versions of the HLA-DR4 genes are associated with an increased risk of rheumatoid arthritis (and other autoimmune diseases that cluster with it, such as thyroid disease). "DR4 also predisposes to developing more severe disease. We don't quite understand why and how that occurs, but if you acquire rheumatoid arthritis, and you have this DR4 molecule, you may develop more severe disease," explains William P. Arend, MD, Distinguished Professor Emeritus/Division of Rheumatology at the University of Colorado, Denver School of Medicine. Other genes linked to RA regulate the inflammatory cytokines like *tumor necrosis factor (TNF)* and *interleukin-1 (IL-1)*, leading to overproduction of these molecules, he adds.

But genes alone don't tell the story; some women with rheumatoid arthritis have no known RA-linked genes, while some who have these genes never develop RA. Even among identical twins (who share identical genes), if one twin has rheumatoid arthritis the other doesn't automatically develop it; the *concordance* (mutual occurrence) rate among identical twins is only about 12 to 15 percent.

Genetically vulnerable people need to encounter other factors, a combination of several "hits" required to set a disease in motion, says Dr. Arend. Those "hits" could include viral or bacterial infections, such as Epstein-Barr virus (EBV), which causes infectious mononucleosis, or *Chlamydia trachomatis (C. trachomatis)*, the most common sexually transmitted infection in the United States. A 2013 study found evidence of a past chlamydial infection in the joints of almost a third of people with reactive arthritis.[1]

According to the National Institute of Arthritis and Musculoskeletal and Skin Diseases (NIAMS), *reactive arthritis* is an autoimmune joint inflammation caused by an infection in other areas of the body (including urinary tract infections). It may occur more often in people carrying a specific gene (HLA-B27). Symptoms of pain and joint swelling may appear two to four weeks after an infection and may last only a few weeks or months. However, reactive arthritis may return in a more serious form.

An estimated 2.86 million cases of *C. trachomatis* are reported annually. The study found that dual antibiotic treatment not only eliminated the bacterium from joints but also improved arthritis.[1]

Food-borne gastrointestinal infections can also trigger reactive arthritis, including *Salmonella*, *Shigella*, *Yersinia*, and *Campylobacter*, caused by eating contaminated food, such as meats or cold cuts that are not refrigerated properly.

Other suspect bacteria include *Escherichia coli (E. coli)*, responsible for urinary tract infections; *Helicobacter pylori*, which causes gastrointestinal ulcers; and *Borrelia burgdorferi*, the corkscrew-shaped bacterium carried by ticks that causes Lyme disease. Lyme disease triggers inflammation around the body with joint pain and can cause an arthritis similar to RA (it's often misdiagnosed as rheumatoid arthritis).

New research suggests that even the normal bacteria that live in our digestive system may provoke an autoimmune reaction that leads to RA.[2]

As we mentioned in Chapter 1, the structure of a virus or bacteria (or proteins they carry) and the structure of some cells and proteins in the body may appear similar, and immune cells react to both, a case of "molecular mimicry." Studies show that T cells from the joints of patients with RA react to proteins on the Epstein-Barr virus.

While recent population studies have also turned up links between RA and some environmental toxins, such as pesticides, your biggest risk may come from tobacco smoke.

Smoking is an established risk factor for RA, and your risk rises each year with every cigarette smoked—even if you're only an "occasional" smoker.[3] Compared to never smoking, the risk of RA more than doubles with long-term heavy smoking.[4] Not only does tobacco smoke contain toxins such as nicotine, hydrocarbons, and carbon monoxide that may themselves trigger an immune attack, but exposure to these toxins may compound your genetic risk.

In recent years, researchers have come to label some foods as "inflammatory" and suggest that some may *increase* the risk of RA, among them, coffee. Is coffee a *real* risk? It's worth examining because the issue keeps percolating in the popular media.

The debate was first stirred up in 2000, when Swedish researchers reported that people who drank four or more cups of coffee a day were more likely to have rheumatoid factor (a marker for RA) in their blood and an increased risk of rheumatoid arthritis.[5] In contrast, an update from the Iowa Women's Health Study in 2002 found that those who drank four or more cups of *decaffeinated* coffee a day were more than twice as likely to develop RA as women who drank regular coffee.[6] Adding to the controversy: among the 31,336 women in the study, those ages 55 to 69 who drank three or more cups of *tea* each day had a 60 percent *reduction* in their risk of RA. Researchers from Harvard reported the next year that they found *no* association between coffee (decaf or regular) or tea and RA risk.[7] These were all population studies, which cannot prove cause and effect. So there's simply no *definitive* evidence. The Arthritis Foundation does *not* tell people to avoid coffee, just to consume it in moderation.[8]

On the other hand, some foods may help dampen inflammation and improve RA. Notably, the omega-3 fatty acids, found in cold-water fish such as salmon, mackerel, and sardines, have been shown to relieve symptoms of RA (see page 45). In general, experts recommend an overall healthy and balanced diet.

Being overweight or obese may also increase the risk of RA, especially in younger women, according to a study of more than 200,000 American women.[9] Previous studies have also suggested that overweight and obese people with RA may experience higher disease activity and pain, and may even respond less well to medications.

Then there's the question of hormones. The fact that rheumatoid arthritis improves in many women during pregnancy (when estrogen levels are very high) and worsens after delivery (when estrogen levels drop) has led some researchers to believe there's a hormonal factor in RA. As we've mentioned, estrogen can influence the activity of immune cells in a number of ways. However, the peak onset of rheumatoid arthritis is between ages 40 and 60, when estrogen levels are declining. So it's still unclear what role estrogen may actually play.

Kathleen's story continues:

I was about two years into the RA, and I kept on working despite the pain.

I had no choice. If I didn't keep working my career would be over. I was offered a play, Indiscretions, *and I thought I'd be able to do it because the character was a diabetic, and the first and the third acts took place in her bedroom . . . I figured I'd be lying around a lot. It didn't turn out that way.*

In the second act of the play, there was a three-story spiral staircase that went up to a catwalk. . . . We would sit up there until we heard the cues and start back down. By the time I got up to the catwalk I was sobbing every night—the pain was so terrible. So I kept tissues, powder, and a lipstick and a mirror up there so I could fix my face before I went back down. I only missed a few performances in the run. I didn't make my disease public at the time . . . because we didn't know at this point how much I was going to recover and if I was going to recover. And people don't understand rheumatoid arthritis. I was put on a whole cocktail of drugs, and that was almost worse than the RA. I was on Plaquenil, I was on gold salts, I was on methotrexate, I was on prednisone, large doses of prednisone. It blew up my body, blew up my face. And the press had a field day—they decided that I had a drinking problem because I was so puffy. And I didn't even care if people thought I had an alcohol problem. I mean, they hire drunks, they hire repeat drug offenders every day in this business. But I knew they wouldn't hire me if they knew I had this disease.

Symptoms of Rheumatoid Arthritis

The first symptoms of RA may be swelling and pain in the joints along with morning stiffness. In 90 percent of people, the first areas affected by rheumatoid arthritis are the hands and feet. The disease often affects the wrists and finger joints closest to the palm, as well as joints in the jaw, neck, shoulders, elbows, hips, knees, ankles, and toes. Any joint in the body can be a target except the low back, which is rarely involved.

Inflammation can cause body-wide symptoms such as low-grade fever, flu-like body aches, and a general feeling of not being well (doctors call it *malaise*). You may also lose your appetite, lose weight, and feel like you have no energy. A majority of RA patients experience fatigue.[10] However, fatigue in RA is different from just feeling tired; fatigue often means you can't function at all. It's unclear whether fatigue is related to inflammation.[11] It may also be a symptom of anemia, which often accompanies RA. Inflammation can affect the tear-producing glands in the eyes and saliva-producing glands in the mouth, so you may experience dry eyes and dry mouth. You can have muscle pain and stiffness after sitting or lying in one position for a long time. Depression is also common.

At first, these symptoms may not add up to much. There are other medical conditions, both rheumatic and nonrheumatic, that can look a lot like rheumatoid arthritis, especially in the early stages, such as lupus and hypothyroidism. In fact, any infection that produces joint aches can look like rheumatoid arthritis. Often a woman will complain of joint pain to her doctor, and all that can be seen is puffiness of the hands, with none of the obvious redness or warmth that typically characterizes RA.

"The reason the patient comes in is usually that they are feeling pain. Maybe it's not rheumatologic, but it has to be taken seriously and investigated," stresses Yusuf Yazici, MD, an assistant professor of medicine at the New York University School of Medicine and the NYU Hospital for Joint Diseases. Some studies find that almost one-quarter of RA patients may already have developed bone erosions by the time they see a rheumatologist. "We know now that it's important to diagnose and treat RA as early as possible to prevent joint damage and disability," he says.

About one-quarter of women with RA develop raised, firm lumps called *rheumatoid nodules.* "Rheumatoid nodules are actually abnormal accumulations of cells, much like the synovial cells that we see accumulating within the joint, but they commonly occur just under the skin. Nodules often appear in an area where there's repeated pressure, such as on the elbows where you lean them on a table, or the finger joints. Because rheumatoid arthritis is a systemic disease, nodules can show up in other places, such as the eye, the heart, and the lungs. They can be very destructive, very damaging, interrupting whatever is in their path of growth. And they can be disfiguring and disconcerting."

Up to half of RA patients can develop inflammation in the linings of the chest and lungs (*pleurisy*), causing pain on taking a deep breath and breathlessness; rheumatoid nodules can also appear in the lung tissue itself, not just the lining. Inflammation can also affect the sac around the heart (*pericarditis*), producing fever, chest pain, a dry cough, and difficulty breathing. Blood vessels can also be inflamed (*vasculitis*); a common sign is tiny broken blood vessels in the cuticle area.

You may first notice the symptoms of RA during the winter, and symptoms often feel worse during the cold months and improve in warm weather.

While RA develops gradually in about 50 percent of women, with symptoms coming and going for months, a more continuous pattern eventually emerges. "It sort of locks in, and then there is a clear day-in, day-out pattern in which people are quite stiff for a long time when they wake up in the morning. The joints are swollen and red, and there's pain when the joint is moved. If this persists for a number of days or weeks, it should be a signal that a woman needs to see a doctor," emphasizes John H. Klippel, MD, former president and medical director of the Arthritis Foundation. "This disease needs to be diagnosed very quickly and treatment needs to be started quickly. So that increases the importance of having women recognize the signs and symptoms."

Kathleen's story continues:

My disease took an incredible toll on my personal life. Making love was almost impossible. Just being touched hurt so bad. It's not like a muscle ache or something where you can lie down and relieve the pain on that part of your body . . . it feels like you've broken a wrist and never set it. And you're living with this and that's what it feels like. . . . And you're depressed, you feel sick all the time, and you feel tired all the time. There's a huge fatigue factor in this disease. My daughter was about three and a half, four years old, and it was hard for me to even play with her. She'd stand on the stairs and say, "Mommy, catch me," and I'd have to scream, "Don't jump—I can't catch you!" One of the worst days, I remember, I had gotten out of the shower and I was sitting on the edge of the tub and I had this big plastic bottle of body lotion and I couldn't squeeze it to get any lotion out. And it was full. And I started to sob, I just started to cry . . . and Rachel walks in and says, "Mommy, what's wrong?" and I said, "I can't do this." And she said, "Oh, I can." And she took the bottle from me and squirted it all over my body like ketchup—which was wonderful and funny, but at the same time it was so terribly sad because I couldn't do what a four-year-old could do.

My husband was wonderfully supportive . . . he and I had a code when we would go out for dinner or something, and if I had to get up to go to the bathroom or we would have to leave, he would come around to my chair and he would pull my chair back, and in the guise of this great courtesy, would get his hands under my arms so that he could just lift me out of the chair because I couldn't get myself up.

Diagnosing Rheumatoid Arthritis

Rheumatoid arthritis can be difficult to diagnose in its early stages. For some, the full range of symptoms develops over a long period of time; in the early stages of RA only a few symptoms may be present. Symptoms can also vary widely from woman to woman; some have more severe symptoms, while others have only slight problems. Symptoms of RA can also mimic other types of arthritis and autoimmune diseases, such as lupus. So those conditions must first be ruled out.

The first thing your doctor will do is take a medical history, asking you to describe your symptoms, when they began, and how they may have changed or progressed over time. You'll be asked about the amount of joint pain you experience, how long you feel stiff in the morning, and how long episodes of fatigue last. The doctor will examine your joints for the classic signs of RA, including redness, swelling, and warmth; assess how flexible your joints are; and test your reflexes and muscle strength.

No single test can definitively diagnose RA, but together the tests can help confirm a diagnosis.

Diagnostic criteria set by the American College of Rheumatology (ACR) and the European League Against Rheumatism (EULAR) can help distinguish rheumatoid arthritis from other causes of chronic joint problems.[12]

They include:

- Morning stiffness lasting at least an hour
- Arthritis in three or more joint areas, with soft-tissue swelling
- Arthritis of the joints of the hand (including the wrist or knuckles)
- Symmetric involvement of joints
- Rheumatoid nodules
- Erosions, bone loss, or other changes seen on an x-ray
- A positive blood test for rheumatoid factor (RF) or antibodies to *cyclic citrullinated peptides (anti-CCP).*

You need to meet four of these seven criteria, and the first four must have been present for at least six weeks. Together with the results of a series of blood tests, they can add up to a diagnosis of rheumatoid arthritis.

Tests You May Need and What They Mean

Rheumatoid factor (RF) is an antibody found in the blood of most patients with rheumatoid arthritis. Not every woman with RA tests positive for rheumatoid factor—especially early in the disease, when it's detected in only 50 percent of patients. Eventually the test is positive in around 80 percent of people with RA. If you test negative, you're said to be seronegative. But RF can also be present in women with other conditions such as lupus and *Sjögren's syndrome*. So a positive test for RF can support a diagnosis of RA, but by itself it isn't enough to diagnose the disease.[13]

Antibodies to cyclic citrullinated peptides (anti-CCPs) are found in 60 to 70 percent of people with RA. Peptides are microscopic pieces of proteins. Antibodies to CCPs can be found in people who do not have RF and may be present even before the earliest signs of RA appear. If the test is positive, there's a better than 95 percent chance that you have RA, according to the ACR. Anti-CCP levels can also be a predictor of future joint damage and show how well you're responding to treatment.[14]

Erythrocyte sedimentation rate (ESR or SED rate) gauges how fast red blood cells settle at the bottom of a tube of whole blood within a one-hour period. Any inflammation in the body (such as the flu or a severe infection) increases plasma proteins, such as the clotting factor fibrinogen, which makes red blood cells clump together. These clumps of cells settle faster than single cells. In healthy people, red blood cells fall at a rate of about 20 millimeters per hour; in women with inflammation, the SED rate speeds up to about 100 millimeters an hour. An elevated SED rate is a nonspecific sign of inflammation and is seen in rheumatoid arthritis and other autoimmune inflammatory conditions.

C-reactive protein (**CRP**) is another marker of inflammation and may be more sensitive than ESR. Your ESR can be normal while CRP can be elevated. CRP is normally around 10 mg/L, but in RA it can range from 40 to 200 mg/L.

Antinuclear antibodies (**ANAs**), autoantibodies that react against the nuclear material of cells, are found in the blood of more than 95 percent of women with systemic lupus erythematosus (SLE) and a majority of women with Sjögren's syndrome, but less than half of women with RA. So a positive ANA may be helpful in distinguishing RA from lupus but, again, keep in mind that the ANA is not specific for lupus.

A **complete blood cell count** (**CBC**) is a standard part of any medical workup. Using laser technology, a machine counts each type of blood cell one by one: red blood cells (RBCs), white blood cells (WBCs), and *platelets* (cells needed for blood clotting) are differentiated by their size. A CBC can detect anemia (low levels of red blood cells), which often occurs in RA. Your hemoglobin level reflects the oxygen-carrying capacity of red cells; the hematocrit (which is three times the level of the hemoglobin) tells how many red blood cells you have in a given volume of blood. Hemoglobin levels can vary from woman to woman, but the normal range is between 12 and 16 grams of hemoglobin per deciliter of blood (g/dL); a hematocrit ranges from 35 to 47. Either (or both) can diagnose anemia. (Reference ranges vary from lab to lab.) Keep in mind that menstruating females often have lower hemoglobin levels than postmenopausal women do.

A CBC also measures the number of key white blood cells, like neutrophils, that destroy invading bacteria and viruses by releasing granules of toxic chemicals. In RA, these cells are overactive and multiply. For example, in some RA patients, neutrophils may be depleted (neutropenia), a disorder called Felty's syndrome that poses an increased risk of infection.

Other blood tests are done as part of an initial workup to assess organ dysfunction due to coexisting diseases. These tests include liver and kidney enzymes that indicate organ damage. This is important because some medications used to treat RA can be toxic to the liver or kidneys and can't be used if these organs are impaired.

X-rays (doctors call them *radiographs* or *plain films*) are used to determine the degree of joint destruction. An x-ray can show damage to the bones, loss of cartilage, and distortion of the joints, as can magnetic resonance imaging (MRI) and ultrasound. Baseline radiographs are done to provide a reference to assess any future progression of the disease and to help judge the effectiveness of disease-modifying agents. In the early stages of the disease, bone damage will not be evident on an x-ray. In fact, the joints may appear normal except for signs of soft-tissue swelling and some thinning of the bone around the joints. But there can be a rapid progression to the signs considered the hallmark of RA seen on x-rays, MRIs, or ultrasound (sonograms)—the start of bone erosion in areas close to the joint. Sonograms can be done right in your doctor's examining room.

Kathleen's story continues:

I went to see a doctor in Boston who was horrified by the mixture of drugs I was taking, and the first thing he said was, "We have to get you off these drugs." And he told me to get into a pool, as much as I could as long as I could every day, and just try to swim. So I joined a club in midtown and I started to try to swim. My hands were OK enough that I could hold onto a kickboard, and my hips weren't affected very much, so I was able to kick straight-legged, and I went back and forth, back and forth, as long as I could stand it. The pain was unbelievable. One day I was able to let go of the kickboard and do a sort of half breaststroke, and that was a great triumph. This was about four years in. One day I got my whole arm to do a stroke, and I stood there in this pool sobbing and yelling, and the poor lifeguard dove in and he grabs me, and I said, "No, no, you don't understand—I just moved my arm!" From then on I said to myself, "OK! I'm getting better."

When the new drugs came out I was in rehearsal for a one-woman show called Tallulah! and my knees blew up. . . . They were extremely painful, so my doctor gave me a new biological drug. I remember it was a Saturday and I injected the medication, and put my legs up and watched over the next four or five hours as my knee swelling went down, and I thought, "Oh

God, I've got something really good here." . . . I'm in remission and I know I'm incredibly lucky.

Treating Rheumatoid Arthritis

In the past 25 years, new medications given early on in the course of disease have made a major difference in the lives of RA patients, boosting life expectancy by a decade to age 86.7,[15] a normal lifespan for most women. Researchers say one of the factors that has led to the decline in RA-related deaths is the use of new medications that reduce inflammation, notably "biological" drugs.

Treatment usually involves combinations of drugs to attack the disease on several fronts, not only to control symptoms but also to lower disease activity, ideally to put RA into remission and prevent future joint damage. This treatment strategy is called "treat to target."

Diagnostic and lab tests can help determine a target (see pages 32 to 33), but how you feel and how you function every day are just as important, if not more so, in treatment decisions you and your rheumatologist will make together.

"The most important outcome for our patient is maintaining function," says NYU's Dr. Yusuf Yazici. "But to maintain function, we need to control their pain, the inflammation in the joints, we need to control the swelling. So all our treatments are geared towards making sure the patient at least maintains the function they have, and if we can reverse the disease, sometimes we can improve their function also."

The choice of medication takes into consideration a number of factors: whether you have established or "early" RA (symptoms for less than 6 months), how active your disease is, how severe your symptoms are, the proven effectiveness of a drug in similar cases, how a drug is given, how much it costs (including the cost of monitoring its use, such as lab tests), how long it will take to work, and its side effects and risks. Some treatments can contribute to premature cardiovascular disease or cause osteoporosis (see pages 55 to 58). If you want to have children, this may restrict your choices, since some medications cause birth defects; you may have to modify your treatment regimen during pregnancy and breastfeeding (see pages 50 to 51).

Ideally, your treatment target should be remission or low disease activity. This is determined by the number of painful and swollen joints (joint counts), the amount of erosion on x-rays, levels of inflammatory blood markers such as C-reactive protein (CRP), and scores on clinical assessment tools you doctor may use. These may include the Disease Activity Score in 28 joints (DAS28), the Clinical Disease Activity Index (CDAI), and the Routine Assessment of Patient Index Data 3 (RAPID3). For example, on the widely used DAS28, remission is defined as a score below 2.6 and low disease activity a score at or above 2.6 to below 3.2. Also taken into consideration are instruments such as the Health Assessment Questionnaire (HAQ), which asks about pain and difficulty in everyday functioning like bathing or getting in and out of bed. These are terms you may see in your medical file.

To help select the right medications and to monitor your progress, your rheumatologist may refer to guidelines from the American College of Rheumatology (ACR) and/or the European League Against Rheumatism (EULAR). You can read the latest ACR Treatment Guidelines at www.rheumatology.org, under Rheumatoid Arthritis, "Clinical Practice Guidelines" and the EULAR guidelines at www.EULAR.org, under "Recommendations for Management." These are guidelines only – not hard and fast rules. Ultimately, your rheumatologist will rely on his or her judgement and your input. And your input is critical.

Analgesic (Pain) Medications

Nonsteroidal anti-inflammatory drugs (NSAIDs) are among the drugs your rheumatologist will likely reach for first to treat joint pain and swelling. They include aspirin and aspirin-like drugs such as over-the-counter *ibuprofen (Motrin, Advil)* and *naproxen (Aleve)*, prescription-only *naproxen (Naprosyn, Anaprox)*, *naproxen sodium (Naprelan)*, and *diclofenac sodium (Voltaren)*.

NSAIDs have both painkilling and anti-inflammatory properties, but they can also raise heart risk and cause gastrointestinal symptoms such as upset stomach or, in some cases, bleeding ulcers.

That's because they work by blocking enzymes in the body called *cyclooxygenase-1 (COX-1) and cyclooxygenase-2 (COX-2)*. While the COX-2 enzyme is related to inflammation, COX-1 protects the lining of the stomach and helps platelets to form clots. Because most NSAIDs block both COX enzymes, they can erode the stomach lining and lead to bleeding, especially among women using corticosteroids and women over age 75 who may have a thinned stomach lining. These complications can be minimized by taking NSAIDs with meals and using acid reducers like *omeprazole (Prilosec, Nexium)* or *cimetidine (Tagamet)*, or a prostaglandin such as *misoprostol (Cytotec)*.

However, recent research suggests prescription-strength Nexium (40 mg) can lead to bone thinning, so discuss its use with your rheumatologist.

NSAIDs that only block the COX-2 enzyme have a slightly reduced risk of serious gastrointestinal side effects (such as bleeding ulcers), but studies show around the same incidence of minor GI problems as the nonselective drugs. COX-2 inhibitors are also much more expensive. Prescription selective COX-2 inhibitors include celecoxib (Celebrex) and meloxicam (Mobic), a less selective COX-2 inhibitor.

Because COX-2 inhibitors don't have the blood-thinning properties of aspirin, they do not lower the risk of blood clots and heart attack (and may potentially increase it). This is a special concern for women, since RA can lead to early heart disease (see pages 55 to 57). If you already have heart disease and need antiplatelet therapy, the ACR recommends using low-dose aspirin (81 mg a day).

Nonaspirin NSAIDs in general can raise your risk of heart attack and other cardiovascular problems—even as early as the first week you take them, according to the FDA.[16]

The American College of Gastroenterology (ACG) and EULAR, among others, recommend that NSAIDs be used at the lowest possible dose for the shortest amount of time—and PPIs (or *misoprostol*) used for gastroprotection, even with COX-2 selective inhibitors.[17]

Disease-Modifying Antirheumatic Drugs (DMARDs)

Disease-modifying antirheumatic drugs (DMARDs) can literally alter the course of RA, preventing damage and destruction of the joints, bones, and cartilage. While many of these drugs work in nonspecific ways to modulate the immune system, newer DMARDs known as biological agents target specific cytokines.

The standard of care is now treatment with DMARDs[18] as soon as a diagnosis of RA is made, says Vivian P. Bykerk, MD, director of the Inflammatory

Arthritis Center of Excellence at the Hospital for Special Surgery in NYC and an associate professor of medicine at the Weill Cornell Medical College.

Early treatment can often slow the disease process and arrest further bone and joint destruction, improving function and reducing disability in RA, says Dr. Bykerk.

The DMARD most commonly used for early and established RA is *methotrexate (Trexall)*, often called MTX for short. MTX is the "anchor" drug used to treat RA, alone or in combination with other therapies.

"In RA, it works by inhibiting adenosine, interfering with the production of inflammatory cells and chemical mediators of inflammation with the net result of less inflammatory infiltrates in the joint," explains Dr. Bykerk. "This lessens swelling, stiffness, pain, and disease-related damage."

Because it's both very effective and well tolerated, MTX is strongly recommended as "first-line" therapy in RA, the medication physicians should prescribe first.

The effective dose of MTX used to treat RA is 20 to 25 mg per week taken as either pills or subcutaneous injections under the skin. As is the case for nearly all medications, MTX can be associated with some side effects. These can include temporary mild nausea or diarrhea. It can cause irritation of liver cells, so it is generally recommend to not drink alcohol when starting MTX. It also cannot be used during pregnancy.

About 3 percent of people using MTX for RA report hair thinning, which may require dose reduction. Lung side effects are extremely rare. Most rheumatologists recommend taking supplements of the B vitamin folic acid to protect against side effects. MTX's anti-inflammatory and immunosuppressant properties take effect fairly quickly.

"Initial treatment with methotrexate is associated with lower disease activity in the first three months, although full benefits may take as long as six months," observes Dr. Bykerk.

MTX may enhance the effects of other DMARDs. The antimalarial *hydroxychloroquine (Plaquenil)* and sulfasalazine (Azulfidine), a sulfa drug that has anti-inflammatory properties, are added to MTX in "double" or "triple conventional DMARD therapy."[18] Sulfasalazine is an oral medication that requires some periodic monitoring with lab tests to detect low levels of white blood cells (*leukopenia*). In some cases, a corticosteroid (such as prednisone) may be added to DMARD monotherapy.

Biologicals such as *etanercept (Enbrel)*, *infliximab (Remicade)*, and adalimumab (Humira), may also be used with MTX.

Older DMARDs—such as *azathioprine (Imuran)*, *D-penicillamine (Cuprimine, Depen)*, *minocycline (Minocin)*, and *cyclosporine (Neoral)*—are now used less frequently.

Leflunomide (Arava) is an oral DMARD that suppresses immune responses and also affects rapidly growing cells. It may take 4 to 12 weeks to start relieving symptoms. Side effects include an increased risk of infections; it can be toxic to the liver, and it also causes birth defects."In patients new to DMARDs, regardless of disease activity, methotrexate is preferred over double or triple therapy. However, the ACR strongly recommends this approach in patients who start out with low disease activity," says Jasvinder Singh, MD, MPH, lead author of the 2015 ACR treatment guidelines for RA. "If patients do not show a good response to methotrexate, with and/or without a corticosteroid, we will move on to combination DMARD therapy and or a biologic," adds Dr. Singh, a professor of medicine at the University of Alabama, Birmingham. Some patients do start out with methotrexate alone, and in other cases, MTX will be combined with one or more DMARDs plus a corticosteroid, depending on the judgement of their physician, says Dr. Bykerk.

Recent studies do show that many early RA patients who start out on combination therapy achieve low disease activity or sustained remission earlier than patients treated with methotrexate alone.[19]

"Some patients need triple therapy, others don't. But sustained remission is the goal for all our early RA patients. We'd like to get them down to zero swollen joints," says Dr. Bykerk. "Sustained remission is important because that means better function."

Biological Agents

Biological RA drugs suppress specific inflammatory cytokines, chief among them *tumor necrosis factor alpha (TNFα)*, the cytokine that causes damage in most cases of RA. Some anti-TNF drugs have been used for more than a decade and have proven highly effective, especially when combined with other DMARDs.

The first TNFα blockers were infliximab and etanercept. Infliximab is a monoclonal antibody, a molecular "smart bomb" that targets TNFα and inactivates it. (The names of drugs in this category have the suffix *-mab*, short for monoclonal antibody.)

Etanercept is a protein that inhibits TNFα and prevents it from locking onto receptors on cells. Both drugs prevent TNFα from promoting inflammation, and both have been shown to dramatically slow the progression of RA and stop joint erosion.

Both of these TNFα blockers are often given with methotrexate. Infliximab is given intravenously every four to eight weeks, and MTX is taken orally once a week. This drug combination could start to produce benefits in a few days, or it may take up to four months. Etanercept is given by self-injection into the skin (subcutaneous) twice a week; it can also take a few days to four months to take effect.

Adalimumab (Humira) is a fully human antibody (infliximab is an antibody that's partly human and partly mouse, a chimeric antibody). It works by binding up excessive molecules of TNF and removing them from the body. Adalimumab is administered by subcutaneous self-injection once every two weeks. Clinical trials showed that the drug produced improvement in almost 70 percent of patients.

Certolizumab pegol (Cimzia) is a newer anti-TNFα agent, a "PEGylated Fab' fragment of a humanized TNF inhibitor monoclonal antibody," to be precise. Injections of this drug are given in a stepwise fashion, with a higher dose for the first month, then a lower dose injected every other week. In some women with RA it can be given as a maintenance drug every month. As with other TNFα blockers, it carries a risk of infections.[20]

Golimumab (Simponi) is another newer TNF blocker, in this case an injectable, man-made protein that binds to TNFα. It can be used with MTX to treat moderate to severe RA. It's available in a pen-shaped auto-injector.[21]

Anakinra (Kineret) is a selective blocker of *interleukin-1 (IL-1)*, another inflammatory cytokine elevated in RA. It's a version of a body's natural molecule called the IL-1 receptor antagonist. In a normal joint this molecule prevents IL-1 from binding to cells; in RA there's not enough of this antagonist molecule, so inflammation caused by IL-1 can lead to cartilage and bone erosion. By preventing IL-1 from locking onto cells, anakinra prevents joint damage. It's also given by subcutaneous injection. A newer anti-interleukin agent is *tocilizumab (Actemra)*, a humanized monoclonal antibody that blocks the receptor for IL-6.[22]

Tofacitinib (Xeljanz) is a synthetic DMARD that disrupts the signaling of Janus kinases (JAKs) and is used when people don't respond well to MTX or are intolerant of the drug. Tofacitinib is an oral medication taken as one tablet twice a day. It can be used alone or in combination with MTX or nonbiologic DMARDs in moderate to severe RA.[23]

Abatacept (Orencia) has a unique mode of action as a selective costimulation molecule. It's a man-made fusion protein that attaches to the surface of antigen-presenting cells (APCs) and prevents them from signaling T cells to fully activate them. Abatacept is a "second-line" drug used when RA does not respond to one or more DMARDs, including MTX. It can enhance the effectiveness of other DMARDs.

These drugs also carry a high risk of serious bacterial, viral, or fungal infections and have been linked to malignancies, such as lymphoma. They can also be quite expensive compared to older DMARDs, costing thousands of dollars a year.

Rituximab (Rituxan) is an intravenous anticancer drug used in combination with methotrexate to help people whose RA has not responded to TNFα blockers and other treatments. Rituximab selectively targets the antibody-producing B cells that that contribute to the disease process in RA, reducing the number of B cells. It is given in two infusions, 15 days apart, and this cycle may be repeated after six months.

In the treat-to-target approach, it's recommended that various combinations of DMARDs and biologicals are given in specific sequences to bring RA into remission or at least reduce disease activity down to the lowest possible level.[18]

For example, if you're diagnosed with early RA (symptoms for fewer than six months), you might be prescribed methotrexate and possibly short-term, low-dose glucocorticoids. If you reach remission or low disease activity within six months, this treatment may be continued. If your treatment doesn't hit the target, produces adverse side effects, or you have moderate or high disease activity, you might then be started on double or triple therapy or one of the biological DMARDs in combination with MTX. Again, you'll be monitored to see if the target is reached in six months. If treatment doesn't prove effective, your rheumatologist might switch biologics or add a second one.

If you have established RA, the sequence may be similar except that if remission is reached, your rheumatologist may consider tapering down the dose of medication, explains Dr. Singh. If you don't reach remission, tofacitinib is now among the medications that may be added to MTX, instead of a TNFα blocker.

Depending on the treatment target, clinical trials show that between 31 and 82 percent of patients reach their target within six months using a treat-to-target treatment strategy.[24]

There are different ways of measuring disease activity and defining remission that use multiple factors including physical exams that evaluate the number of swollen joints—and the information you give your doctor at each visit about symptoms and how you're doing (often with questionnaires like the HAQ), along with lab tests and x-rays. Without this information, there's no way to make the best treatment decisions. "We measure and ask, 'is your disease under control or is it not under control?' It's no more complicated than that," stresses Dr. Singh.

But again, your input is vital. Under ACR guidelines, all treatment decisions must be *shared* decisions with patients.

Corticosteroid Drugs

Corticosteroids (glucocorticoids) are synthetic versions of steroid hormones normally produced in small amounts by your adrenal glands. Not to be confused with the anabolic steroids used by bodybuilders, these are drugs that reduce inflammation and suppress immune activity.

Low-dose glucocorticoids (less than 10 milligrams of prednisone a day) can reduce the symptoms of RA very quickly, sometimes within a matter of days. They are also used to dampen disease flares. Recent studies show that low-dose corticosteroids may even slow the rate of bone damage, so they may have disease-modifying potential. They're often given with DMARDs. The most commonly prescribed corticosteroid for treating RA is prednisone (Deltasone, Orasone), but others may be used as well. These include methylprednisolone (Medrol), prednisolone (Prelone), and dexamethasone (Decadron). They are given as oral medication or as an injection into a joint or even muscle. Corticosteroid injections can relieve pain, especially early in the disease, and can be used for disease flares in one or two joints. The benefits can be dramatic—but temporary.

Because of the side effects of systemic corticosteroids, especially in doses equivalent to more than 10 milligrams a day of prednisone, their use must be closely monitored. Side effects include weight gain (especially around the abdomen), a round face (so-called "moon face"), increased fat on the upper back ("buffalo hump"), increased appetite, acne, increased facial hair, easy bruising, bone thinning (osteoporosis, see pages 57 to 58), and bone death. So if you're taking these drugs you also need to take calcium supplements, vitamin D, and drugs that prevent or slow bone loss (see page 58).

Corticosteroids can also cause high blood pressure, cataracts, an increased risk of diabetes and infections, and sleep disturbances.

Prednisone and other glucocorticoids can also cause extreme psychological side effects, including depression, anxiety, hyperactivity, and outbursts of anger. So if you're on steroid medications, you'll need to be prepared. Anything you can do to help manage anger and stress—such as yoga, meditation, and regular exercise—will be important while you're taking steroids. Some women may be helped by psychological counseling to deal with the effects of these drugs as well as their RA. While taking prednisone can cause physical and emotional stress, you should never stop it on your own. Prednisone and other glucocorticoids should be tapered slowly under a doctor's supervision.

What's Next for RA Treatment?

The next generation of TNFα blockers, including drugs considered *biosimilars* (for example biosimilars to infliximab) are currently in clinical trials, as well as blockers of other members of the interleukin "superfamily" of cytokines (like *IL-17*), and new JAK inhibitors (such as *decernotinib*).

Since there are multiple processes in RA, there are multiple targets to aim at, and it's likely that some of the new agents in development will be used together. Affecting a single element in RA, while it may slow the disease and the destruction it causes, does not eliminate the disease itself.

But what if a dysfunctional immune system could be replaced with a normal one? That's the idea behind stem cell transplantation. In this still experimental approach, the immune system is destroyed with high doses of chemotherapy drugs and then reconstituted with stem cells, "pluripotent" cells that have the potential to grow into any kind of cell, including white blood cells. These cells can be harvested from the blood, the placenta or umbilical cord, or an HLA-matched donor. Some therapies inject stem cells into the joint itself in an effort to regrow damaged tissue. Gene therapy, where genes are coaxed into producing antagonists to inflammatory cytokines, is also being tested.

Surgery

Joint replacement is the most frequently performed surgery for rheumatoid arthritis, and just about any joint can now be replaced with artificial parts made of metal and ceramic. New materials and cements to fix the new joint in place have increased the longevity of artificial joints. However, some artificial joints don't function as well as normal joints, and even the best materials can become worn and need to be replaced.

Because RA can damage or rupture tendons, the tissues that attach muscle to bone, tendon reconstruction is sometimes required. Done most often on the hands, the surgery attaches an intact tendon to a damaged one, helping to restore some hand function, particularly if done before a tendon is completely ruptured.

Synovectomy involves the removal of inflamed synovial tissue and is usually done as part of tendon reconstruction. Other procedures include *carpal tunnel release*, *arthroplasty*, and *joint fusion*. Studies are also under way to investigate the possible use of cartilage regeneration in RA.

Nondrug Therapies

Exercise is important for maintaining healthy and strong muscles to support the joints, preserve mobility, and maintain flexibility. It can also help you sleep and reduce pain. In addition, exercise has documented effects for boosting mood. Special exercise programs can be designed just for you by a physical therapist. But just as important as keeping active is balancing activity with rest. You may need more rest when your disease is active and fatigue starts to take a toll. Rest helps to reduce active joint inflammation and pain and fight fatigue. It's usually more helpful to take short rest breaks than to spend long periods of time in bed, since that can promote stiffness. (These strategies are also helpful for dealing with fatigue in other autoimmune diseases.)

Studies suggest that cognitive behavioral therapy (CBT), which helps reframe how you think and react to events, may also help you overcome fatigue.

Splints and assistive devices can help you function better and reduce stress on your joints. Splints are used mostly on wrists, hands, ankles, and feet to support the joint and reduce pain. They are often custom made by a doctor or a physical or occupational therapist. Self-help devices such as zipper pullers or long-handled shoehorns, special toothbrushes, and jar openers can help make everyday activities easier.

You may have read about the use of "complementary" therapies in RA like acupuncture, fish oil, anti-inflammatory herbs, tai chi exercises, and *Ayurvedic* medicine, the 5,000-year-old traditional herbal medicine of India. Many patients turn to such therapies hoping to avoid or lessen the side effects of medications.

The most evidence so far is for fish oil (omega-3 fats) and a handful of herbs used alongside RA drugs.

Fish oil contains the omega-3 polyunsaturated fats (PUFAs) *eicosapentaenoic acid (EPA)* and *docosahexaenoic acid (DHA)*, which have anti-inflammatory properties that have been shown to relieve joint pain, swelling, and morning stiffness in RA. One recent randomized trial showed that fish oil produced additional benefits when used with conventional medications like methotrexate.[25]

A 2013 survey of more than a dozen herbs and supplements by the British National Health Service (NHS) scored fish oil the highest for effectiveness and safety.[26] However, because fish oil has some anticoagulant properties, you'll need to talk to your doctor before taking it.

A number of herbs are touted as having anti-inflammatory properties in RA, including *evening primrose oil, borage seed oil,* and the plant extract *Tripterygium wilfordii Hook F (TwHF, thunder god vine)*, approved in China for treating RA. Some small studies in China and the United States have suggested that TwHF may be as effective as methotrexate or other DMARDs as short-term therapy.[27, 28] However, these studies involved pharmaceutical grade "standardized" extracts of TwHF (20–60 mg), which are not available in the United States, and Chinese researchers caution that the extract can affect fertility and cause gastrointestinal side effects.

Supplements can interact with your medications, so consult your rheumatologist before buying anything at the health food store or talking to a naturopath or herbalist.

Acupuncture, a popular component of traditional Chinese medicine, involves placing very thin needles at specific spots along the body (*acupoints*) to stimulate the flow of energy (or *qi*) to treat pain and other conditions. Acupoints correspond with key nerve endings, and some RA patients report relief of pain and swelling with acupuncture. However, well-done clinical studies (some using "sham therapy" of needling at acupoints as a control) have had mixed results. If you want to try it, find a certified acupuncturist.

The good news is that research is ongoing in this area, and the "integrative" care of RA is increasing, with a growing number of centers offering complementary therapies alongside conventional treatments.

One of the best sources of information is the National Center for Complementary and Alternative Medicine (NCCAM) at the National Institutes of Health (http://nccam.nih.gov/health/RA/getthefacts.htm). For more, see Appendix A.

Rheumatoid Arthritis Clusters

Many other autoimmune diseases can cluster with rheumatoid arthritis, particularly thyroid disease, which, in the case of Hashimoto's thyroiditis, can compound the fatigue of RA. A recent study found that the risk of hypothyroidism may be increased in RA right from the start, especially among young women.

- Sjögren's syndrome
- Raynaud's phenomenon
- Thyroid disease (underactive or overactive thyroid)
- Psoriatic arthritis (which can be mistaken for RA)
- Giant cell arthritis
- Pericarditis and endocarditis
- Autoimmune primary ovarian insufficiency

Stress reduction is another important component in managing RA. While stress doesn't cause the disease, it can certainly make it harder to live with and even increase disease activity. So learning stress management techniques, such as meditation or taking part in psychological support groups, can go a long way toward giving you more control over your life. Don't smoke to alleviate stress.

The Female Factor

Rheumatoid arthritis is almost three times more common in women than in men. Scientists have been exploring the role of estrogen and other steroid hormones in the body to see whether high or low levels of one or another hormone may make a woman more vulnerable to rheumatoid arthritis.

The observation dating back to 1938 that rheumatoid arthritis improves during pregnancy in 70 percent of women led to speculation that higher levels of estrogen (or certain estrogens) may somehow be protective. But studies using estrogen to improve symptoms have not proven benefit. The improvement during pregnancy (and subsequent worsening during the postpartum period) may not be due to estrogen at all, says David Pisetsky, MD, PhD, professor of medicine at Duke University Medical Center and president of the United States Bone and Joint Initiative. "The initial observation that a hormone produced during pregnancy might be protective actually led to the discovery of cortisol, corticosteroids. So we may be dealing with a steroid effect, but probably not from estrogen. And corticosteroids are anti-inflammatories," comments Dr. Pisetsky.

"There is research to find out which women will get this effect. One very interesting paper suggested that the more genetically different the mother and father, the more steroids, or immunosuppression, the body would produce. And the more similar the mother and the father were genetically, the fewer steroids, or immunosuppression, would be produced," remarks Dr. Pisetsky.

Human leukocyte antigens (HLAs), the molecules that help define what's self and nonself) shared by a woman and her unborn child may not only alter the activity of the mother's immune system during pregnancy, but shared HLAs may also increase—or decrease—the risk of developing RA.

Research by J. Lee Nelson, MD, of the immunogenetics program at the Fred Hutchinson Cancer Research Center in Seattle, showed that greater differences in the genetic makeup between the mother and her fetus were associated with a greater chance of disease remission in RA.[29] The exact mechanism for this is unclear, Dr. Nelson says, but is the subject of ongoing investigation.

It has also been suggested that the immune effects of pregnancy may somehow protect against RA itself (or at least delay its onset). Studies show a twofold increased risk of developing RA in women who have never had a child. On the other hand, a recent study by Dr. Nelson and her colleagues suggest that pregnancy *outcomes*, such as having a very low birthweight baby or a preterm birth, may somehow increase the risk of future RA.[30] This may reflect common risk factors for pregnancy complications and for RA, such as preeclampsia and gestational hypertension and preterm delivery, they speculate. Greater fetal microchimerism may also be linked to adverse pregnancy outcomes, thus influencing the subsequent risk of RA. Alternatively, it may reflect common risk factors for RA and for pregnancy complications, such as preterm delivery, they add.

Over the years, it has been suggested that oral contraceptives may be protective, possibly cutting the risk of RA in half when used for as little as six months. Studies show women using birth control pills at RA onset tend to have milder disease, but a number of randomized controlled trials to assess postmenopausal hormone therapy on the severity and progression of RA have had mixed results.

All of the research into sex-related factors in rheumatoid arthritis is speculative, but it could one day lead to specific prevention or treatment strategies for women.

Kathleen's story continues:
We had always wanted another child. But they told me that I'd have to go off the medications if I were to get pregnant. They told me my symptoms would probably improve while I was pregnant, but that afterward most women with RA not only go back to a fully active state but also usually get worse. So we're talking about my choice of having another child or being able to walk, and move, and work. And to me the choice was very clear. That was the choice I was presented with—to put off childbearing until I had this disease under control. And by then, I was in my middle forties. We did try again and were not successful. And then I was 45 and I was trying in-vitro, and the drugs almost put me back in an active state. It was a real risk taking them, but we really wanted another child. So that's part of the cost of this disease.

How RA Can Affect You Over Your Lifetime

As Kathleen Turner found, rheumatoid arthritis (and the drugs used to treat it) can profoundly affect a woman's life during her childbearing years.

Menstruation and Fertility

Women with inflammatory arthritis, such as RA, often have reduced fertility ("reduced ovarian reserves"),[31] and studies find at least one-third may having trouble conceiving.

The medications you take to control your RA can also affect the menstrual cycle and your ability to become pregnant.

Recent studies show that higher doses of glucocorticoids can reduce the "pulses" of *luteinizing hormone (LH)* from the pituitary gland needed to trigger ovulation. Prednisone may also affect the function of the endometrium, where a fertilized egg is implanted.[32]

NSAIDs like celecoxib may also interfere with ovulation, implantation, and formation of the placenta by dampening prostaglandins.[33]

Cyclophosphamide may cause infertility, especially if taken for periods of greater than one year and if a woman is over age 35. Methotrexate is absolutely contraindicated in women trying to conceive. Contraception is advised for women taking this drug. Because of the potential for birth defects, some drugs may need a "washout" period before trying to conceive.

With Arava, contraception is required while taking the drug (for men who are taking the drug as well). If you want to become pregnant and have taken the drug within the past two years, you (and/or your partner) must undergo a specific drug elimination procedure. You'll be given 8 grams of cholestyramine three times a day for 11 consecutive days, and then blood levels of Arava will be measured with two blood tests 14 days apart until they are below a specific level (0.02 milligrams per liter of blood).

"We stop drugs that are likely to cause trouble like methotrexate. How long the washout period should be can become a guess. For methotrexate, most people would say three to six months for a washout period," remarks Dr. Pisetsky.

Women with RA are more likely to have had fertility treatments, but the effects of those drugs in women with RA have not been well studied. The high doses of hormones needed to stimulate the production of multiple eggs by the ovary may make RA symptoms worse.

Pregnancy and Breastfeeding

As we mentioned before, your symptoms will likely improve during pregnancy but could recur within the first eight weeks after delivery. After six to eight months, you'll return to whatever level of disease severity you had before you became pregnant.

The major issue when you contemplate pregnancy is the effect of medications. The U.S. Food and Drug Administration (FDA) classifies drugs according to whether studies or case reports show risks to the fetus, such as birth defects, and whether those risks outweigh the benefits to the mother. Some drugs demonstrate no risks, while others cannot be used during pregnancy because they've been shown to cause harm. For many newer drugs, such as biological agents, animal studies have not shown harm to a fetus, but there are no data at all or no well-controlled studies of pregnant women—or animal studies have shown adverse effects, but well-done human studies have not.

Then there are medications that may have demonstrated adverse effects in animal studies, but there are no well-controlled studies in humans—or there have been neither animal nor human studies of the drug. Finally, there are drugs that have shown risks to the fetus in studies of pregnant women, but sometimes the benefits of a drug may outweigh the risks for a particular woman. As you can see, prescribing drugs in these categories during pregnancy must be individualized.

Drugs that you take during pregnancy, including those considered safe, may cross the placenta, and many pass into breast milk. According to rheumatologists, the most sensitive time during pregnancy for any drug effects is the first trimester, when the embryo is growing into a fetus. This is the period where birth defects are likely to occur. The third trimester, since it is closest to delivery, carries different risks.

In general, experts say NSAIDs appear safe during most of pregnancy, but physicians try to avoid their use too close to delivery since they inhibit hormones called prostaglandins, which affect uterine contractions and can prolong labor. Corticosteroids are generally considered safe at any time during pregnancy but carry a slight risk of infections.

Azathioprine can cause fetal harm and should not be given during pregnancy unless the benefits strongly outweigh the risks. However, it should be emphasized that women taking azathioprine after organ transplants who have become pregnant have had successful pregnancies. Still, its use is not recommended in nursing mothers. Methotrexate should never be used during pregnancy.

A recent study from Italy suggests that TNFα inhibitors can be considered safe in the "peri-conception" period, making them a possible choice for women hoping to become pregnant. However, the Italian researchers caution that reports of anti-TNFα exposure during the second or third trimesters are "still limited" and they urge caution. Experience with abatacept, tocilizumab, anakinra and rituximab in pregnancy is insufficient, they add.[34] A review of many hundreds of pregnancies in inflammatory arthritis suggest that exposure to anti-TNF therapies at the time of conception or during the first trimester do not result in an increased risk of adverse pregnancy or fetal outcomes.[35]

For Remicade, Azulfidine, penicillamine, and Enbrel, no harmful effects have been seen on a developing fetus, but since risk can't be completely ruled out, the FDA advises that they should be given to pregnant women *only* if clearly needed. Remicade is usually not detectable in breast milk, but sulfa drugs like Azulfidine *are* excreted in breast milk and can cause liver toxicity in infants.

Data are extremely limited about pregnancy outcomes of women exposed to newer biologic DMARDs, including anakinra, abatacept, and tocilizumab. Manufacturers' guidelines suggest abatacept be discontinued for at least 14 weeks prior to conception and between 3 months (tocilizumab) and 12 months (rituximab) prior to pregnancy for other biologics.

You'll need to discuss the use of these drugs with your physician. Carefully read every package insert that comes with any medication, and always ask questions.

Menopause and Beyond

The peak years for a diagnosis of RA are those just before and after menopause, and opinions are divided over whether menopause itself affects the disease.

"The age of diagnosis seems to be creeping up," remarks Dr. Bykerk, with many women now diagnosed around age 53. "Women in early menopause are also more often seropositive" for rheumatoid factor and anti-CCPs, she adds.

While some studies find that RA diagnosed after menopause may progress at a faster rate, recent research suggests that earlier menopause may be linked to milder disease, such as rheumatoid-factor negative RA.[36] "Hormonal changes may influence pathways that are distinct from those leading to severe, progressive disease," Swedish researchers wrote in a study published in *Arthritis Research & Therapy* in 2012.

One study from Sweden found a strikingly decreased risk of more severe anti–cyclic citrullinated peptide antibody (ACPA) positive RA among current users of hormones ages 50 to 70, but not for ACPA-negative RA.[37]

Many rheumatologists focus on treating RA and leave the management of menopausal symptoms up to a woman and her gynecologist.

The ACR says hormone therapy (HT, or hormone replacement therapy, HRT) may be considered for postmenopausal women with severe hot flashes and other symptoms in whom there are no contraindications.

Estrogen therapy is generally considered safe for women with RA, and there have been some hints over the years that ET can even make RA a little better. However, given the increased risk of cardiovascular disease in RA, postmenopausal hormones should be approached cautiously.

Women, including those with RA, who are candidates for and wish to take postmenopausal hormones should take the lowest possible dose for the shortest possible period, advises the North American Menopause Society (NAMS).[38]

Hormone therapy needs to be individualized, depending on the drugs you're taking. For example, it's known that corticosteroids interact with estrogen. They may lessen the effectiveness of estrogen and often cause bleeding. This is because drugs like prednisone may interfere with estrogen receptors and can cause fluctuations in estrogen. So instead of the steady effects of your regular daily dose you get ups and downs that may cause you to bleed or spot.

Short-term estrogen replacement therapy (less than five years) has not been shown to increase the risk of breast cancer. Women with an intact uterus need to take progestin along with the estrogen to prevent precancerous overgrowth of the uterine lining (*endometrium*), such as *micronized progesterone (Prometrium)*.

Use of postmenopausal hormones has declined since 2002, when results first emerged from the Women's Health Initiative (WHI). The WHI, a major prevention trial of a combined estrogen/progestin drug (*Prempro*) among 16,608 healthy women aged 50 to 79, was stopped after five years because of an increased rate of heart attacks, strokes, deep vein clots, and invasive breast cancer among women taking this drug. There were fewer cases of colorectal cancer and bone fractures among women on HT, but the WHI Data Safety and Monitoring Board (DSMB) concluded that the health risks of HT outweighed the benefits and stopped the study. However, the actual risks were small. According to the WHI data, over one year, 10,000 women taking Prempro might experience seven more coronary heart disease events, eight more breast cancers, eight more strokes, and eight more pulmonary emboli (but six fewer colorectal cancers and five fewer hip fractures), compared to women not taking hormones.[39]

The estrogen-only arm of the WHI was continued, with no increased risk of breast cancer seen among that group (all of whom had had hysterectomies).

On the strength of the WHI and other recent studies, the U.S. Preventive Services Task Force recommends that estrogen or estrogen/progestin not be used to prevent heart disease and other chronic conditions, and women should explore other therapies to prevent bone loss.[40] Experts stress that the main indication for hormone therapy is to ease menopausal symptoms.

Menopausal symptoms like hot flashes may get better, but there may be absolutely no difference in your RA. "Physicians do say that in their experience estrogen is helpful. But you can never be sure that it's really doing something for the disease, or whether it's improving a woman's sense of well-being, helping her mood, or lessening her pain perception, and so on," comments Duke University's Dr. Pisetsky.

If you can't (or don't want to) take systemic oral estrogens, estrogen is available in patches (such as *Climara*) that are changed once or twice a week. Estrogen from transdermal patches is believed to have less cardiovascular risk. Local estrogen treatments include creams (*Estrace*) and tablet suppositories (*Vagifem*) that gradually release estrogen into vaginal tissues to prevent drying and thinning (atrophic vaginitis). Local estrogen therapy may also help with vaginal dryness in women who have Sjögren's syndrome secondary to their RA (see Chapter 6).

According to NAMS, nonhormonal therapies for menopausal symptoms include the herbs black cohosh (*Cimicifuga racemosa*, sold in health food stores and under the brand name *Remifemin*) and red clover (sold as *Promensil*). Both have been tested in clinical trials, but not specifically in women with autoimmune disease. Red clover contains plant estrogens, or phytoestrogens, and some studies suggest that it can relieve hot flashes, night sweats, irritability, insomnia, vaginal dryness, and mood disturbances, without any estrogenic effects on the breasts or uterine lining. Do not use black cohosh if you're also taking blood pressure medication. Red clover can interfere with blood thinners like aspirin, so do not use it if you have antiphospholipid antibodies or a bleeding disorder.

Soy protein contains phytoestrogens called isoflavones. Some short-term studies suggest that they can relieve hot flashes, but most studies find little or no effect. Soy advocates recommend 20 to 50 grams a day from soy milk, soybeans, meat substitutes, or tofu.

Some studies suggest that fish oil capsules may help hot flashes but, again, because of its blood-thinning effects, you need to talk to your doctor before using it.

B vitamins, especially vitamin B_6 (200 mg a day), seem to help some women with the emotional symptoms of menopause, including mood swings and anxiety.

Wild yams grow on vines all over North America and contain *diosgenin*, a precursor to natural progesterone (used to make some prescription progestins). Creams containing progesterone made from diosgenin are said to help relieve hot flashes and other menopausal symptoms. According to the North American Menopause Society (NAMS), no adequate clinical trial data confirm these claims. If you want to try wild yam progesterone creams, do so only with your doctor's supervision.

Evening primrose oil (EPO) is made from the seeds of a North American wildflower that, true to its name, opens in the evening. EPO is rich in essential fatty acids, including linoleic acid. Some studies suggest that EPO may help lessen hot flashes and lower blood pressure and cholesterol, as well as relieve joint pain in RA. Side effects include inflammation, blood clots, nausea, and some immunosuppression, according to NAMS. EPO is best taken as capsules; the accepted dose is 2 to 3 grams a day (make sure it is "standardized to 8 percent gamma-linoleic acid"). Keep EPO refrigerated to prevent it from becoming rancid. It cannot be used with anticoagulants.

Cardiovascular Disease

The risk of cardiovascular disease (CVD) is two to three times greater among women with rheumatoid arthritis. There are several reasons for this.

While RA principally affects your joints, systemic inflammation can affect other organs—including the heart and blood vessels—and the risk may rise with more severe disease. Inflammation is reflected in blood markers such as C-reactive protein (CRP), considered an independent risk factor for CVD. Inflammation even in early RA may accelerate *atherosclerosis*, narrowing of the arteries by fatty plaques.[41]

People with RA also have a greater prevalence of traditional CVD risk factors, notably smoking, high blood pressure, obesity, insulin resistance, and elevated cholesterol. And heart risk can be impacted by medications used to treat RA, such as corticosteroids, NSAIDs, and some DMARDs. There's also the issue of physical inactivity due to disability.

Among traditional risk factors are higher levels of harmful blood fats like *low-density lipoprotein (LDL)* cholesterol, which is more prone to accumulate in plaques. One recent study showed that thickening of the inside of the arteries with cholesterol-laden plaques was worse in people with rheumatoid arthritis and that their cholesterol levels were higher, compared to people the same age without the disease.[42]

The risk of CVD increases for all women after menopause, and women with RA are no exception. An update from the Women's Health Initiative found that the risk was 1.5 to 2.5 times higher among postmenopausal women. While traditional cardiovascular risk factors played a strong role, inflammation and joint pain severity were also associated with increased risk.[43]

However, younger women with RA still face heart risks, notes Susan Manzi, MD, MPH, professor of medicine at Temple University and chair of the Department of Medicine of the West Penn Allegheny Health System.

Dr. Manzi notes that mortality ratios for women with RA aged 15 to 49 show an increased risk of death from heart attack and congestive heart failure as high as three times that of healthy women. According to Dr. Manzi, inflammation in RA (as measured by CRP) not only speeds up the development of plaque, "but it also makes the plaque more vulnerable to rupture, leading to clot formation and blockage of the blood vessel."

Recent research suggests that biologic therapy may lower the risk of CVD while reducing overall disease activity.[29] Indeed, improvements in managing cardiovascular disease have contributed to the decline in deaths from RA.

The ACR and EULAR recommended that people with RA be screened regularly and treated for cardiovascular risk factors like high blood pressure and elevated cholesterol.[44]

Current U.S. federal guidelines recommend keeping LDL at an "optimal" level of 100 milligrams per deciliter of blood (mg/dl) or below, and recommend lifestyle changes and drug therapy when LDL tops 130 mg/dl in people at higher risk for coronary heart disease. Low levels of high-density lipoprotein (HDL) cholesterol are also a risk factor, since HDL helps remove LDL from the bloodstream. Under the guidelines, low HDL for women is under 40 mg/dl.[45] However, treatment of elevated cholesterol is no longer based on hitting specific numbers but on reducing an individual's risk.[46] Just having RA or other inflammatory conditions is considered a risk factor for coronary heart disease.

As for blood pressure, stay below the normal level of 120 millimeters of mercury (mm Hg) for systolic pressure (the higher number, measured while the heart is beating) and 80 mm Hg diastolic (blood pressure between beats). According to the National Heart, Lung, and Blood Institute and the American Heart Association, your risk rises when pressure is between 120/80 and 139/89 mm Hg. High blood pressure (hypertension) is any reading above 140/90 mm Hg.

So make sure your doctor—whether it's your internist or rheumatologist—assesses your blood pressure at every visit. Each year your doctor should order blood tests to measure levels of LDL and HDL cholesterol, *triglycerides* (another harmful blood fat), and blood glucose (if it's elevated, that's a sign your body isn't using insulin properly—a red flag for type 2 diabetes, an independent risk factor for coronary disease). A thorough physical exam should include an electrocardiogram (ECG).

Making lifestyle changes can also help. These include avoiding obesity, getting 30 to 60 minutes of moderate exercise most (if not all) days of the week, eating a diet rich in fruits, vegetables, whole grains, healthy oils, and low-fat dairy products, while limiting calories from saturated fat, and avoiding trans fats. You may need advice from a nutritionist to help you work out a heart-healthy diet that you can follow.

Your RA medications may even help lower your risk of cardiovascular disease.

A recent review found that biologic therapies reduced CVD risk for RA patients, presumably by lowering inflammation.[47] In one study of more than 200 patients, biologic therapies moved women from the high and moderate heart risk categories to low risk within 24 months, lowering total cholesterol and LDL and increasing HDL.[48]

Osteoporosis

Bone loss is a threat for any woman with RA, indeed any woman with an autoimmune disease who takes corticosteroids or other drugs that thin the bones. Postmenopausal women are already at increased risk for osteoporosis, and steroid treatment increases the risk even further; bone loss can begin as early as six months after starting steroids. Osteoporosis risk is doubled among women with RA, and it may not all be related to corticosteroids.

One study from Norway measured bone mineral density (BMD) in the hip and spine of almost 400 women with RA aged 50 to 70 and compared them with healthy women in the same age groups from the United States and Europe. The researchers found that over 31 percent of the RA patients had reduced BMD in the hip, and 19 percent had bone loss in the upper spine. Current use of steroids was one factor predicting lower BMD, but rheumatoid factor predicted lower bone mass in the top of the thigh bone in the hip (which may reflect bone erosion in that joint).

Corticosteroids cause bone loss because they interfere with calcium absorption. Even low-dose prednisone (10 milligrams a day) taken long term can cause significant bone thinning, so rheumatologists look for ways to minimize these effects (such as giving other drugs with corticosteroids that allow lower doses to be used, or steroid-sparing drugs). Often the only way to stave off osteoporosis is with drugs that reduce bone loss.

According to the ACR guidelines for preventing steroid-induced osteoporosis, bisphosphonates should be given to premenopausal women on long-term (over three months) corticosteroid treatment and to postmenopausal women when they begin steroid therapy. Bisphosphonates slow the resorption of bone and have been shown to reduce both hip and spinal fractures. For women on long-term therapy, bone mineral density (BMD) scans should be done every one to two years.[49]

The bisphosphonates approved for treating osteoporosis are *alendronate (Fosamax)* and *risedronate (Actonel)*, available in daily and weekly oral preparations; *ibandronate (Boniva)* given in monthly or quarterly injections; *zoledronic acid (Reclast)*, and *parathyroid hormone (Teriparatide)*, both given as a yearly injection.

In addition, ACR guidelines recommend that women take 1,500 milligrams a day of elemental calcium (in diet and supplements), plus 400 to 800 IU of vitamin D (which aids calcium absorption). Women who can't take bisphosphonates should be given calcitonin (*Miacalcin, Fortical*), an antiresorptive agent in nasal spray form.

> *I've always had this sense from doctors and other people that because this is not life threatening, because you're not going to necessarily die from this disease, it's not important. It's just some kind of inconvenience, just creaky joints. But it's lifestyle threatening . . . your sex life, your parenting, your work. Everything is affected by this disease. The most important thing is to know you can fight it—that you can fight it and you can pretty much beat it. There's so much that can be done to alleviate this disease and to fight it and to feel that you're not this victim, that you're not helpless in the face of this disease.*
>
> Kathleen Turner

Notes

1. Zeidler H, Hudson AP. New insights into Chlamydia and arthritis. Promise of a cure? *Ann Rheum Dis.* 2013. doi:10.1136/annrheumdis-2013-204110. Epub ahead of print.
2. Scher JU, Sczenak A, Longman RS, et al. Expansion of intestinal *Prevotella copri* correlates with enhanced susceptibility to arthritis. *eLife.* 2013. doi:10.7554/eLife.01202.
3. Sugiyama D, Nishimura K, Tamaki K, et al. Impact of smoking as a risk factor for developing rheumatoid arthritis: a meta-analysis of observational studies. *Ann Rheum Dis.* 2010;69:70–81.
4. Di Giuseppe D, Discacciati A, Orsini N, Wolk A. Cigarette smoking and risk of rheumatoid arthritis: a dose-response meta-analysis. *Arthritis Res Ther.* 2014;16:R61.

5. Heliövaara M, Aho K, Knekt P, et al. Coffee consumption, rheumatoid factor, and the risk of rheumatoid arthritis. *Ann Rheum Dis.* 2000;59:631–635. doi:10.1136/ard.59.8.631.
6. Mikuls TR, Cerhan JR, Criswell LA, et al. Coffee, tea, and caffeine consumption and risk of rheumatoid arthritis: results from the Iowa Women's Health Study. *Arthritis Rheum.* 2002;46(1):83–91. doi:10.1002/1529-0131(200201)46:1<83::AID-ART10042>3.0.CO;2-D.
7. Karlson EW, Mandl LA, Aweh GN, Grodstein F. Coffee consumption and risk of rheumatoid arthritis. *Arthritis Rheum.* 2003;48(11):3055–60.
8. Wilder, S. Coffee offers health benefits. http://www.arthritis.org/living-with-arthritis/arthritis-diet/healthy-eating/benefits-of-coffee.php.
9. Lu B, Hiraki L, Sparks JA, et al. Being overweight or obese and risk of developing rheumatoid arthritis among women: a prospective cohort study. *Ann Rheum Dis.* 2014. pii:annrheumdis-2014-205459. doi:10.1136/annrheumdis-2014-205459. Epub ahead of print.
10. Repping-Wuts H, Van Riel P, Van Achterberg T. Editorial: Fatigue in patients with rheumatoid arthritis: what is known and what is needed? *Rheumatology.* 2009;48(3):207–209. doi:10.1093/rheumatology/ken399.
11. Minnock P, McKee G, Bresnihan B, FitzGerald O, Veale D. How much is fatigue explained by standard clinical characteristics of disease activity in patients with inflammatory arthritis: a longitudinal study. *Arthritis Care Res.* 2014;66(11):1597–1603. doi:10.1002/acr.22387.
12. Aletaha D, Neogi T, Silman AJ, et al. 2010 Rheumatoid Arthritis Classification Criteria. An American College of Rheumatology/European League Against Rheumatism collaborative initiative. *Arthritis Rheum.* 2010;62(9):2569–2581. doi 10.1002/art.27584.
13. Neilsen SF, Bojesen SE, Schnohr P, Nordestgaard BG. Elevated rheumatoid factor and long term risk of rheumatoid arthritis: a prospective cohort study. *BMJ.* 2012;345:e5244. doi:10.1136/bmj.e5244.
14. Bizzaro N, Bartolini E, Morozzi G, et al. Anti-cyclic citrullinated peptide antibody titer predicts time to rheumatoid arthritis onset in patients with undifferentiated arthritis: results from a 2-year prospective study. *Arthritis Res Ther.* 2013;15:R16. doi:10.1186/ar4148.
15. British Society for Rheumatology 2014, Annual Meeting (BSR 2014), Abstract #034: Norton S, et al. Excess mortality in rheumatoid arthritis: gains in life expectancy over 25 years. 2014;53(suppl 1):i69–i70. *Rheumatology* 2014 Abstracts. doi:10.1093/rheumatology/keu097.006.
16. FDA Drug Safety Communication: FDA strengthens warning that non-aspirin nonsteroidal anti-inflammatory drugs (NSAIDs) can cause heart attacks or strokes. July 9, 2015. http://www.fda.gov/Drugs/DrugSafety/ucm451800.htm.
17. Sostres C, Gargallo CJ, Lanas A. Nonsteroidal anti-inflammatory drugs and upper and lower gastrointestinal mucosal damage. *Arthritis Res Ther.* 2013;15(suppl 3):S3.
18. Singh JA, Saag KG, Bridges SL, et al. 2015 American College of Rheumatology guideline for the treatment of rheumatoid arthritis. *Arthritis Care Res.* 2015. doi:10.1002/acr.22783.

Published online ahead of print. http://www.rheumatology.org/Portals/0/Files/ACR%20 2015%20RA%20Guideline.pdf.

19. Kuijper T, Luime J, de Jong P, et al. Tapering DMARDS in the TREACH trial—flare rates, sustained remission and radiological progression. *EULAR 2015*; Rome: Abstract OP0030.
20. U.S. Food and Drug Administration (FDA). Medication Guide. CIMZIA® (certolizumab pegol). http://www.fda.gov/downloads/Drugs/DrugSafety/ucm088571.pdf.
21. U.S. Food and Drug Administration (FDA). Medication Guide. SIMPONI® (golimumab). http://www.fda.gov/downloads/Drugs/DrugSafety/ucm088571.pdf.
22. U.S. Food and Drug Administration (FDA). Medication Guide. ACTEMRA® (tocilizumab). http://www.fda.gov/downloads/Drugs/DrugSafety/UCM197463.pdf.
23. U.S. Food and Drug Administration (FDA). Medication Guide. XELJANZ® (tofacitinib). http://www.fda.gov/downloads/Drugs/DrugSafety/UCM330702.pdf.
24. Solomon DH, Bitton A, Katz JN, Radner H, Brown EM, Fraenkel L. Treat to target in rheumatoid arthriti: fact, fiction, or hypothesis? *Arthritis Rheumatol.* 2014;66(4): 775–782. doi:10.1002/art.38323.
25. Proudman SM, James MJ, Spargo LD, et al. Fish oil in recent onset rheumatoid arthritis: a randomised, double-blind controlled trial within algorithm-based drug use. *Ann Rheum Dis.* 2015;74:89–95. doi:10.1136/annrheumdis-2013-204145. Published online September 30, 2013.
26. UK: National Health Service: alternative medicine for rheumatoid arthritis. 2013. http://www.arthritisresearchuk.org/arthritis-information/complementary-and-alternative-medicines/complementary-therapies/herbal-medicine.aspx#sthash.yAqf4DSc.dpuf.
27. Lv Q-w, Zhang X, Shi Q, et al. Comparison of *Tripterygium wilfordii* Hook F with methotrexate in the treatment of active rheumatoid arthritis (TRIFRA): a randomised, controlled clinical trial. *Ann Rheum Dis.* 2014. doi:10.1136/annrheumdis-2013-204807. Published online April 14, 2014.
28. Goldbach-Mansky R, Wilson M, Fleischmann R, et al. Comparison of *Tripterygium wilfordii* Hook F versus sulfasalazine in the treatment of rheumatoid arthritis: a randomized trial. *Ann Int Med.* 2009;151(4):229–240, W49–51.
29. Nelson JL, Hughes KA, Smith AG, Nisperos BB, Branchaud AB, Hansen JA. Maternal-fetal disparity in HLA class II alloantigens and the pregnancy-induced amelioration of rheumatoid arthritis. *N Engl J Med.* 1993;329:466–471.
30. Ma KK, Nelson JL, Dugowson CE, Gammill HS. Adverse pregnancy outcomes and risk of subsequent rheumatoid arthritis. *Arthritis Rheum.* 2014;66(3):508–512. doi:10.1002/art.38247.
31. Henes M, Froeschlin J, Taran FA, et al. Ovarian reserve alterations in premenopausal women with chronic inflammatory rheumatic diseases: impact of rheumatoid arthritis, Behçet's disease and spondyloarthritis on anti-Müllerian hormone levels. *Rheumatology.* 2015;54(9):1709–1712. doi:10.1093/rheumatology/kev124. First published online: May 8, 2015.

32. Brower J, Hazes JMW, Lavel JSE, Dolhain RJEM. Fertility in women with rheumatoid arthritis: influence of disease activity and medication. *Ann Rheum Dis.* 2015;74(10):1836–1841. First published online: May 15, 2014. doi:10.1136/annrheumdis-2014-205383.
33. de Steenwinkel FD, Hokken-Koelega AC, de Man YA, et al. Circulating maternal cytokines influence fetal growth in pregnant women with rheumatoid arthritis. *Ann Rheum Dis.* 2012;72:1995–2001.
34. Bazzani C, Scrivo R, Andreoli L, et al. Prospectively-followed pregnancies in patients with inflammatory arthritis taking biological drugs: an Italian multicentre study. *Clin Exp Rheumatol.* 2015;33(5):688–693. Epub 2015 Aug 25.
35. Hyrich KL, Verstappen SMM. Biologic therapies and pregnancy: the story so far. *Rheumatology.* 2014;53(8):1377–1385. doi:10.1093/rheumatology/ket409.
36. Pikwer M, Nisson JA, Bergström U, Jacobsson LTH, Turesson C. Early menopause and severity of rheumatoid arthritis in women older than 45 years. *Arthritis Res Ther.* 2012;14:R190. doi:10.1186/ar4021.
37. Saevarsdottir S, Klareskog L, Alfredsson L, et al. Postmenopausal hormone therapy and the risk of rheumatoid arthritis: results from the Swedish EIRA Study. American College of Rheumatology (ACR) Abstract: #117, presented October 27, 3013.
38. North American Menopause Society (NAMS). http://www.menopause.org/for-women/expert-answers-to-frequently-asked-questions-about-menopause/menopause-faqs-understanding-the-symptoms.
39. Women's Health Initiative (WHI), Fred Hutchinson Cancer Center. https://www.whi.org/.
40. Moyer VA, on behalf of the U.S. Preventive Services Task Force. Menopausal hormone therapy for the primary prevention of chronic conditions: U.S. Preventive Services Task Force Recommendation Statement. *Ann Intern Med.* 2013;158(1):47–54. doi:10.7326/0003-4819-158-1-201301010-005531.
41. Ajeganova S, Andersson MLE, Frostegård J, Hafström I. Disease factors in early rheumatoid arthritis are associated with differential risks for cardiovascular events and mortality depending on age at onset: a 10-year observational cohort study. *J Rheum.* 2013;40(12): 1958–1966. doi:10.3899/jrheum.130365.
42. Choy E, Ganeshalingam K, Semb AG, et al. Cardiovascular risk in rheumatoid arthritis: recent advances in the understanding of the pivotal role of inflammation, risk predictors and the impact of treatment. *Rheumatology*. 2014;53(12):2143–2154. Published online June 5, 2014. doi:10.1093/rheumatology/keu224.
43. Mackey RH, Kuller LH, Deane KD, et al. Rheumatoid arthritis, anti-CCP positivity, and cardiovascular disease risk in the Women's Health Initiative. *Arthritis Rheum.* 2015;67(9):2311–2322. Online 28 May 2015. doi:10.1002/art.39198.
44. Peters MJ, Symmons DP, McCarey D, et al. EULAR evidence-based recommendations for cardiovascular risk management in patients with rheumatoid arthritis and other forms of inflammatory arthritis. *Ann Rheum Dis.* 2010;69(2):325–331.
45. National Institutes of Health. Third report of the National Cholesterol Education Program (NCEP) expert panel on detection, evaluation, and treatment of high blood

cholesterol in adults (adult treatment panel III). http://www.nhlbi.nih.gov/guidelines/cholesterol/atp3full.pdf. Accessed December 6, 2013.
46. Stone NJ, Robinson J, Lichtenstein AH, et al. 2013 ACC/AHA guideline on the treatment of blood cholesterol to reduce atherosclerotic cardiovascular risk in adults: a report of the American College of Cardiology/American Heart Association Task Force on Practice Guidelines. *Circulation.* 2014;129(25 suppl 2):S1–S45. doi:10.1161/01.cir.0000437738.63853.7a.
47. Tam LS, Kitas GD, González-Gay MA. Can suppression of inflammation by anti-TNF prevent progression of subclinical atherosclerosis in inflammatory arthritis? *Rheumatology (Oxford)*. 2014. doi:10.1093/rheumatology/ket454. Epub 2014 Feb 5.
48. Khraishi M, Aslanov R, Doyle K. Effect of biologic disease modifiers on cardiovascular risk of patients with rheumatoid arthritis—2 years prospective cohort study. ACR Abstract: #382.
49. Grossman JM, Gordin R, Ranganath VK, et al. American College of Rheumatology 2010 recommendations for the prevention and treatment of glucocorticoid-induced osteoporosis. *Arthritis Care Res.* 2010;62(11):1515–1526. doi:10.1002/acr.20295.

3

The Shadow of the Wolf—Systemic Lupus Erythematosus

I probably started developing lupus when I was in high school. I remember I had all these weird symptoms my sophomore year. I had red splotches on the bottoms of my hands and the soles of my feet; I thought they were blisters and would actually poke them with a pin. Then I started getting swollen joints, and I was terribly stiff. I remember one time I was at the beach with my friends, and I couldn't even lift myself off the blanket. My parents got worried and took me to a big hospital, and I was told I had juvenile rheumatoid arthritis. I was put on prednisone for a year. It made my face look all puffy and really wrecked my self-esteem, but the symptoms went away. I basically forgot about it until I went away to college and started feeling ill. I had fevers, I was fatigued, I had difficulty concentrating. At first I thought it was stress.

But then my joints started to feel swollen and painful. And no one seemed to know what was wrong with me. I'm trying to cope with college life, I wanted to keep my grades up, and here I was constantly seeing doctors, getting tests. It still took them a while to finally tell me I had lupus. Eventually, it affected my kidneys, my intestines, and my brain. Now when I think back, I think this disease was sort of shadowing me for years.

Deanna, 33

Lupus means "wolf" in Latin, and as it did with Deanna, it can stalk you silently over a period of years or strike suddenly without warning, snarling and scratching the skin of the face and vital organs. Systemic lupus erythematosus, or SLE, is a leading cause of kidney disease in younger women, especially those who are African American, and it can lead to premature cardiovascular disease (hardening of the arteries and heart attacks). In recent years, there has been a troubling rise in deaths from lupus, especially among middle-aged black women. However, in most cases lupus is a chronic disease that can be managed with medication. Many women—like Deanna, who's now married and teaching full-time—live active lives. Importantly, it can be a complicated disease since it affects many different organs, sometimes requiring multiple medications, some of which can put you at risk for other health problems, such as osteoporosis.

Lupus emerges most often between ages 15 and 40, affecting 10 times as many women as men.[1] More African American, Latina, Asian, Native American, and Alaskan native women are affected than Caucasians, with a rate two to three times greater among black women, or about 1 in 500.[1, 2] Exact prevalence figures vary. According to the National Institutes of Health, between 350,000 and 500,000 people may be affected. Other data estimate the number of lupus patients in the United States at 250,000.

Unlike other autoimmune diseases that target a single organ, like thyroid disease, lupus can affect just about any organ or tissue in the body—including the joints, the kidneys, the heart, the blood, the lungs, and even the nervous system. Some forms of lupus are limited to the skin, like *discoid lupus* (which can occur by itself or as part of the systemic disease). Ten percent of women initially diagnosed with discoid lupus may eventually develop systemic disease.

As with other autoimmune diseases, lupus can be challenging to diagnose because the signs (what the doctor can see) and symptoms (what you may experience) can occur separately over time. So it may be months or even years before enough symptoms are present to clearly meet the classification criteria for lupus (see pages 70 to 71). A survey conducted by the Lupus Foundation of America found that half of lupus patients had symptoms for five years before obtaining a diagnosis, consulting three or more doctors before being correctly diagnosed.

Lupus often mimics other diseases. It may be initially diagnosed as rheumatoid arthritis because the first problems seen can be joint pain and stiffness of the hands, wrists, and knees. Fatigue and depression may be mistaken for chronic fatigue syndrome or major depression. Pain and color changes of the fingers in cold weather, called *Raynaud's phenomenon*, can occur in lupus but are common in scleroderma. Dry eyes and mouth suggest Sjögren's syndrome. In fact, as many as a third of women with lupus may have other autoimmune diseases. Symptoms of a second disease may often be attributed to lupus, resulting in a delay in diagnosis. Arthritis is the most common symptom, seen in around 84 percent of women with lupus.

Warning Signs of Lupus

- Achy but not swollen joints (arthralgia)
- Painful and swollen joints, which can be warm and red (arthritis)
- Fevers
- Extreme or prolonged fatigue
- Unexplained rashes on the face, neck, or scalp
- A butterfly-shaped rash across the cheeks and nose
- Anemia
- Pain on deep breathing or when lying down (possible inflammation in the lining of the lungs or heart)
- Skin rashes after sun exposure
- Hair loss
- Raynaud's phenomenon
- Depression
- Painless ulcers in the mouth or nose
- Seizures

What Causes Lupus?

The precise cause of lupus is not known. In SLE, antibodies attack healthy cells—even specific parts of those cells. These include antibodies to components of the cell nucleus, the yolk-like structure in the center of each cell that contains your DNA. Various forms of *antinuclear antibodies (ANAs)* can be associated with skin rashes or damage the kidneys. Other antibodies attack proteins on the cell surface resulting in low white blood cell, platelet, or red blood cell counts. Some autoantibodies result in an increased risk of clotting.

The B cells that produce autoantibodies and directly (as in the case of platelets) or indirectly (as in the case of the kidney) cause inflammation and damage in autoimmune diseases need to be activated by helper T cells. In lupus these B and T cells may be hyperactive, and the regulatory mechanisms that keep this imbalance in check may not be working properly.

A "suicide program," *apoptosis*, is built into every cell and is necessary to eliminate defective cells, cancer cells, cells produced because of too-rapid growth in certain tissues, and lymphocytes that are no longer needed once a particular immune response has ended. This suicide program can be activated by genes within a cell, damage to DNA (such as sun damage from ultraviolet light that can lead to skin cancer), signals sent to cells by cytokines, or even by an infection.

During apoptosis, the contents of the dying cells are spilled out into the bloodstream to be gobbled up by neutrophils or macrophages and eliminated by the body. In lupus, these clearance systems may not be working properly. So the debris from these dying cells—which contain fragments of the cell nuclei—may cause the body to produce those antinuclear autoantibodies, which then attack healthy tissues, explains Bevra H. Hahn, MD, professor of medicine at the University of California, Los Angeles, a noted lupus researcher.

At the same time, the problems of cell suicide programming that promote autoreactivity may also be exaggerated as T cells that inappropriately react with self are not properly regulated. In lupus there may be a genetic predisposition. A person could be born with a defect in a gene that controls apoptosis or other regulatory aspects relating to keeping the immune system in check. In some women genetically destined to get lupus, self-reactive cells may escape destruction during fetal development and produce autoantibodies later in life. An anti-suicide molecule called *B cell activating factor (BAFF)*, also called B-lymphocyte stimulator (BLyS), interferes with apoptosis and enhances the proliferation and survival of autoimmune B cells. The first new treatment approved for lupus in 50 years, *belimumab (Benlysta)*, blocks the effects of BLyS and reduces abnormal B cells (see pages 77 to 78).

Immune complexes also play a major role in lupus. These latticelike structures are formed when antibodies bind to their targets and build up in tiny blood vessels. Accumulation of immune complexes causes blood vessel inflammation and even blockage, and blood clots (caused by *lupus anticoagulant antibodies*) can also block off vessels supplying vital organs.

Proteins called *complement* normally dissolve immune complexes or prevent them from growing too large. Women with lupus may have genetic defects in the complement system, producing too little complement to keep up with rapidly forming immune complexes, or it gets used up too quickly. "Lupus seems to be a problem of regulation that allows increased rates of cell death in circulating lymphocytes, decreased clearance of cellular debris, sustained production of autoantibodies, and the increased formation of immune complexes, which cause organ damage," concludes Dr. Hahn. Simply put: lupus both clogs and corrodes aspects of the body's plumbing system—be it in blood vessels or other tissues. When complement is activated by autoantibodies, the resulting protein fragments of complement can also cause inflammation in organs.

The genes that control these processes may be among many that contribute to lupus. So far, around 35 genes have been linked to lupus, many of them involving complement.[3] The strongest genetic risk factor for lupus is a gene called *C1q*, which encodes a complement protein. Among other things, this protein coats apoptotic cells and helps them to be cleared before antigens on their surface are recognized and targeted by the immune system. When C1q is completely absent (which is rare), the risk of lupus can be as high as 90 percent.[4] Genetic mutations have also been found in complement receptors 2 and 3, the latter associated with lupus nephritis. Another problem may lie with the receptor for the $Fc\gamma$ (gamma) gene, which clears immune complexes.

The genetic defects that contribute to lupus appear to run in families. The chance of two sisters having lupus is 2 to 10 percent, but if they are identical twins (who share the same genes), the chances of both having lupus increases to 25 percent or more. Several centers around the country are collecting and studying genetic data from thousands of lupus patients and family members, and new discoveries are being made all the time.

But genes alone are not enough. An environmental trigger like a drug or a virus could also play a role in triggering lupus in genetically vulnerable women. A virus that inhibits normal cell death could allow infected cells to multiply. Since 1971, studies have implicated *Epstein-Barr virus (EBV)*, which infects B cells and is periodically reactivated.[5] This reactivation could be a source of chronic immune system stimulation and, in theory, could cause increased production of lupus autoantibodies (and possibly disease flares), says Dr. Hahn.

One study by researchers at the Oklahoma Medical Research Foundation and Case Western Reserve University in Cleveland, Ohio, looked at 196 lupus patients and compared them to 392 healthy people matched for age and sex; all but one of the lupus patients had been exposed to EBV at some point, compared to 94 percent of the control group.

In rare cases, lupus can be triggered by drugs, including antibiotics like minocycline, often used to treat chronic acne; procainamide, prescribed for irregular heartbeats; hydralazine, used to treat hypertension; and isoniazid, used to treat tuberculosis. In these cases, the disease usually disappears when the drug is stopped. Environmental toxins may also be triggers.

Then there are hormones. Some studies have suggested that women with SLE have abnormalities processing estrogen and testosterone. Although estrogen is the main female sex hormone, women also produce male hormones, *androgens*, including testosterone. Androgens play a variety of roles in the body, affecting bone density, muscle strength, energy, well-being, sex drive (libido), and possibly immune system function. Women with lupus are also thought to have low levels of testosterone. (For more, see page 80).

Deanna's story continues:

I chiefly remember how difficult it was for me my first two years of college.

I was under enormous pressure. Keeping my grades up was very important to me, but it was a struggle just to get out of bed some days. I had a lot of joint pain; I had headaches. At this point I was running back and forth to hospitals, getting all kinds of tests done. It was so hard for me to concentrate on anything. I usually grasp things pretty quickly, but even the simplest things would take me hours to absorb. I know now that I was experiencing a lupus flare. But my doctors still hadn't figured out what was wrong. I also developed skin lesions on my buttocks—raised red marks, like scabs. I had every test you could think of. It was very stressful. First they said I had vasculitis and that I needed to take steroids. So I found myself back on prednisone and I had the side effects again, the moon face, the hair loss, the weight loss . . . at one point, I was down to ninety pounds. I took steroids my entire sophomore year, but they didn't help. I was getting progressively worse. And I started experiencing blurry vision in my right eye. It was very frightening. I just figured I was stressed out with all the tests and the medication. Then they did more tests and said I had optic neuritis, my blood pressure was up, and they found blood and protein in my urine. The lupus had moved into my kidneys. Only then was I finally diagnosed with lupus.

Symptoms of Lupus

Any one of the warning signs we've listed may herald lupus, but the disease can show itself differently in each woman. It often begins with vague joint pains and fever. You may almost feel like you have the flu—achy and feverish, with swollen glands and fatigue. For some women, like Deanna, there are memory and concentration problems, dubbed a lupus "fog."

Approximately half of women with lupus will have skin rashes, including a classic *malar* or "butterfly" rash. This is a raised, red rash that spreads across the bridge of the nose (the body of the butterfly) and across the cheeks (the wings). Lupus actually got its name from the rash; some people thought it made the face look like it was mauled by a wolf (*erythema* means "red skin"). This rash is quite different from acne, but may be confused with rosacea. In acne, you can see redness and pimples anywhere on the face; the lupus rash does not extend into the folds alongside the nose and mouth. Discoid lupus usually has plugged follicles, patchy hair loss, and scaly lesions. In *subacute cutaneous lupus erythematosus*, you develop a very sun-sensitive, red rash.

In fact, a rash or other skin problem is often the first clue that a woman may have lupus. Sensitivity to the ultraviolet rays of the sun (*photosensitivity*) can also produce or worsen skin rashes (sunscreen is a must when you have lupus).

Fatigue is a common symptom of many autoimmune diseases; around 90 percent of women with SLE may experience fatigue.[6] In lupus, fatigue may be due to *anemia* (a lowered red blood cell count), difficulty breathing, or muscle weakness. You may also have lower white blood cell counts (*leukopenia* and/or *lymphopenia*), which make you more susceptible to infections, or a low platelet count (*thrombocytopenia*) that causes unexplained black-and-blue marks and increases the risk of bleeding after something as routine as brushing your teeth. More than three-quarters of women with lupus may also have depression.[3] This may be partly due to fatigue or feeling unwell. Migraine headaches may also be a problem.

You may have arthritis, with tender, swollen, and painful joints. Hair loss (*alopecia*) may accompany a lupus flare. If your kidneys are affected, you may see some fluid retention, most commonly as swollen ankles and at times swelling up to the knees. The kidneys are responsible for filtering waste products from the body and excreting them; when the kidneys aren't functioning well, it affects the balance of fluid and salt in the body. When the kidneys' filtering system is damaged, it can cause too much protein to leak into the urine (*proteinuria*). Blood pressure may also be elevated.

Ethnicity and race may affect how severe your lupus is. According the Lupus Foundation of America, Latinas, African Americans, and Asians are three times more likely to develop lupus, and studies suggest they are more likely than Caucasians to have disease worsening and organ impairment.[7]

Diagnosing Lupus

To be classified as having SLE, a woman needs to have 4 of the 11 criteria set by the American College of Rheumatology (ACR). Those four criteria need to be present at some point in time, but need not occur together. (Note: These criteria were originally intended for patients who wished to enter into clinical trials.)

- Malar rash (the classic raised, red rash that looks like a butterfly over the nose and cheeks)
- Discoid rash (red, raised patches with scaling and plugged follicles)
- Photosensitivity (an unusual reaction in the skin after being in the sun)
- Oral or nasal ulcers (usually painless ulcers, in the mouth or nose, most often the upper palate)
- Arthritis (tenderness, pain, and swelling in two or more joints)
- Serositis (fluid around the lining of the lungs or heart; this can be called pleurisy if it affects the lungs, pericarditis if it affects the heart)
- Kidney disorder (proteinuria)

- Brain disorder (psychosis or seizures)
- Blood cell disorder (hemolytic anemia, lymphopenia, leukopenia, or thrombocytopenia)
- A positive test for antinuclear antibodies (ANAs)
- Evidence of other autoantibodies (like anti-dsDNA antibodies, anti-SM antibodies, or antiphospholipid antibodies) including a false-positive venereal disease research laboratory test (VDRL)

Some doctors may diagnose SLE even if only three of these criteria are positive. ANAs can be positive in healthy women. A positive ANA is not specific for lupus, although it's the reason most patients are referred to a rheumatologist.

In contrast, the autoantibodies to double-stranded DNA (*anti-dsDNA antibodies*) are very specific and with rare exceptions signify lupus. If two of the symptoms listed are present, a diagnosis of lupus is uncertain until more symptoms develop or other more specific blood tests produce positive results.

In the last several years another set of classification criteria have been published. These are quite similar to the ACR criteria.[8] Under the 2012 Systemic Lupus International Collaborating Clinics Classification Criteria (SLICC), you need to have four criteria, with at least one being considered immunologic. However there is one important change. In the past, a patient might not be considered to have systemic lupus erythematosus if she only had kidney involvement and a positive ANA. With the new criteria, other symptoms do not have to be present and kidney involvement alone is sufficient if the biopsy is read as consistent with lupus.

Tests You May Need and What They Mean

Blood tests are an integral part of the workup for lupus. They can help to pin down a diagnosis since your symptoms may overlap with other diseases.

A complete blood count (**CBC**) is a standard blood test in any diagnostic workup, measuring white blood cells, red blood cells, and platelets. In a lupus workup, it can flag problems such as *leukopenia* (a total white blood cell count below 4,000 cells per cubic millimeter) or *lymphopenia* (fewer than 1,500 lymphocytes per cubic millimeter) or *thrombocytopenia* (fewer than 100,000 platelets per cubic millimeter). Because white blood cell counts can fluctuate in healthy women, it's important that leukopenia and lymphopenia be detected on two or more occasions to satisfy the ACR classification. A CBC can also detect *hemolytic anemia* (a condition in which autoantibodies react against targets on red blood cells and destroy them, resulting in low red cell counts).

Antinuclear antibodies (ANAs) will be positive in more than 95 percent of women with SLE. However, since the test can be positive in other autoimmune conditions, the results have to be considered along with a woman's medical history and any clinical signs and symptoms of lupus that may be present. Since discoid lupus does not usually involve internal organs, the ANA test may be negative (or show very low levels of antibodies).

ANA test results include a *titer* (or quantity) of the antibody. This is a number based on how many times an individual's blood must be diluted to get a sample free of antinuclear antibodies. So a titer of 1:640 shows a greater concentration of antinuclear antibodies than a titer of 1:320 or 1:160. As it turns out, the ANA titer doesn't really indicate whether the disease is active or severe or what organs are affected. Once the ANA is found to be positive, it's not that useful to repeat. Patients in extended remission can actually have no detectable ANAs, but others may always retain these antibodies, even in remission.

Antibodies to double-stranded DNA (anti dsDNA) target DNA, which contains the genetic instructions in every cell. A positive anti-dsDNA test is considered highly specific for lupus. If this test is positive, you have a very strong chance of having SLE. Anti-dsDNA antibodies are found in 30 to 80 percent of women with lupus.

Antibodies that target DNA may sound pretty dangerous. Yet these antibodies rarely cross into the cell itself, but rather bind to DNA when it's released from the cell and an immune complex is formed. Anti-dsDNA antibodies are usually associated with kidney disease, and that is why women with these antibodies need to have urine samples tested several times a year to check for protein (it's done with a simple urine dipstick but is often quantitated by collecting urine over 24 hours). These antibodies also appear to track lupus activity; they can come and go with disease flares.

Anti-SSA/Ro and anti-SSB/La antibodies are antibodies directed against normal cellular components called Ro, or Sjögren's syndrome A (SSA), and La, or Sjögren's syndrome B (SSB). SSA and SSB are detected in approximately 40 percent and 15 percent, respectively, in individuals with SLE. Common clinical features associated with these antibodies are skin rashes worsened by sun exposure, and dry eyes and mouth (these antibodies are detected in 75 percent of women with Sjögren's syndrome). It's important to know about antibodies to Ro and La when planning a pregnancy, since some women with anti-Ro and anti-La antibodies can have children with heart problems and transient skin rashes (pages 89 to 92).

Anti-Smith antibodies (anti-SM) are present in around 25 percent of women with SLE. They are also directed against nuclear material in the cell (they're related to and coexist with anti-ribonucleoprotein antibodies, anti-RNP). Anti-Smith antibodies are specific to lupus and are among the criteria for a diagnosis. Anti-SM antibodies are believed to occur more frequently in African American and Asian women than in Caucasians.

Anti-Ro, anti-La, and anti-SM antibodies are usually detected using a test called an *enzyme-linked immunoabsorbent assay (ELISA)*, in which serum (the clear part of blood not containing any cells and devoid of clotting factors) is analyzed. An ELISA is capable of detecting very small quantities of these antibodies.

Antiphospholipid antibodies (aPLs) are increased in a third of women with SLE, as well as in women with antiphospholipid syndrome. *Antiphospholipid antibodies* can cause damage to blood vessels and act against proteins in blood to promote clotting problems in the veins (leg clots, lung clots) or the arteries (heart attack, stroke). There are several types of antiphospholipid antibodies, each of which can be related to an increased risk of clotting anywhere in the body and/or low platelet counts. These antibodies are also associated with miscarriages, since they can cause blood clots in the placenta.

There are four basic types of antiphospholipid antibodies (aPLs), and each is detected by a different test. These are *anticardiolipin antibodies* (*aCL*, which come in three types, IgG, IgA, and IgM), *anti-beta2glycoprotein I* (*B2GPI*, which also come in the same three types as the aCL), the *lupus anticoagulant* (*LAC*, which is a funny name since it does not cause bleeding but rather clotting), and a *false positive test for syphilis* (see next paragraph). As many as half of patients who test positive for LAC have lupus; up to 47 percent of lupus patients have elevated aCLs. The LAC may be the most highly associated with blood clots and poor pregnancy outcomes. IgG autoantibodies of high titer are also more worrisome than lower titers.

The venereal disease research laboratory test (VDRL) is actually a test for syphilis, but a positive VDRL does not mean you have syphilis. The antiphospholipid antibody in a lupus patient recognizes a similar structure on the syphilis bacteria (another case of molecular mimicry). So a positive VDRL signals the presence of that antibody. In the overwhelming majority of patients, when tested against more specific components of syphilis bacteria, the test is negative (so lupus patients have a false positive VDRL).

Complement levels are used to gauge lupus activity, usually by measuring two specific components of complement, C3 and C4. Again, it's helpful to think of complement as the bullets of a gun. When levels are low, it may mean the complement "bullets" have been fired and caused tissue damage. In some cases, women may be born with a low C4, and it may be hard to tell whether that stems from an inherited deficiency or actual disease activity. It's like a bank account: it can be low because you didn't deposit enough money or because you withdrew too much (as in the case of active lupus). Your doctor may measure these levels at all visits to see if they predict disease flares.

Skin biopsy is done if you have a rash (often a sign of *discoid lupus*). A small biopsy of skin will be taken from the rash area to look for markers of inflammation.

A urine dipstick test for protein in the urine is simple, but extremely important. Excessive protein in the urine means the kidney is losing protein. To more accurately measure the quantity of protein lost, it may be necessary to collect urine over a period of 24 hours. A microscopic examination of the urine may reveal abnormalities, such as red blood cell or white blood cell casts (abnormal elements derived from red and/or white cells), and kidney *glomerular* cells. A kidney biopsy may be done if urine or blood tests indicate evidence of kidney disease.

I was diagnosed with lupus when I was 23—that was more than 30 years ago. Back then, very little was really known about lupus. I was passed around from one doctor to another. I was told I had multiple sclerosis, I had a malignant brain tumor, I had rheumatoid arthritis, it was a psychosomatic illness . . . just about any illness you can think of, depending on what symptom I was having at the time. I was having seizures. And I went through a lot of torturous tests because they thought I had a brain tumor. I was sent to a rheumatologist, a neurologist, and a neurosurgeon, and I was even sent to a psychiatrist, who said a lot of it was all in my head. Unfortunately, I went home and I tried to convince myself that my symptoms were imaginary. But of course that was the wrong thing to do; nothing was imaginary.

My symptoms just kept getting worse . . . I went from specialist to specialist, and no one tried to put together a whole picture. I was finally diagnosed through a kidney biopsy in 1967. I remember when they told me I had lupus, they said I wouldn't live a year. Well, I'm still here. I've had heart trouble, and the lupus has affected my lungs and my kidneys. . . . I also have back problems and I have some trouble getting around these days. But I don't let anything drag me down. And I was fortunate to finally find a doctor who knew something about lupus, and who was aggressive in treating it. I credit my longevity to aggressive doctors, to good treatments, and to God.

JANE, 63

What's a Lupus Flare?

The most important thing to keep in mind is that lupus is a fluctuating disease; you can experience periods of remission in which the disease is quiet, and flares, in which the disease is active, like the swings of a pendulum. The pattern varies from one person to the next. However, a lupus flare does not necessarily mean that your disease is progressing or that permanent damage to the internal organs is occurring. Flares can have a number of triggers, including emotional stress, exposure to sunlight, infections, and certain medications.

The stress connection is very real. One 2001 study from Germany looked at blood levels of cytokines after acute psychological stress in women with lupus, rheumatoid arthritis, and healthy women and found stress-induced increases in *interferon gamma* and *interleukin 4 (IL-4)* in the women with SLE and RA, suggesting that changes in cytokine patterns may be responsible for flares.[9]

In most cases, lupus flares involve physical changes that may be accompanied by abnormalities in the blood analysis. So your doctor will assess lupus activity by taking a history, performing a physical exam, and drawing blood for testing. The degree of activity can actually be measured, and there are several scoring systems developed for this purpose. One such "score sheet" is the *SLEDAI (SLE Disease Activity Index).* This is a list of various physical findings and blood tests. The SLEDAI score literally adds up the number of problems; the more points, the more disease activity. This scoring system is generally used for clinical trials, but some physicians do use the system for keeping track of disease. While keeping score is not the point, it may be helpful to understand just how sick you are by reviewing how the SLEDAI score sheet is used (and you may find it useful for tracking your own symptoms). Many of the symptoms are the same as those in the ACR diagnostic classification (pages 70 to 71).

A mild flare (in some cases a three point or more change in the score) is likely to consist of any one of the following: a new or recurrent facial rash, hair loss, photosensitivity, mouth or nose ulcers, and unexplained fevers. Increased fatigue can be part of a lupus flare, but the SLEDAI doesn't factor it in, although other lupus activity score sheets do. A moderate flare might include joint swelling and pain in more than two joints, pleuritis, or pericarditis. A severe flare (SLEDAI scores greater than 12) generally indicates more internal organ involvement, such as the kidneys or brain, and almost always requires treatment with high doses of glucocorticoids. But the degree of a problem also varies. Depending on the degree of activity, flares are treated differently.

On the other hand, disease progression (and any potential damage) is assessed using the SLE damage index, which records damage or permanent injury to a particular organ that has occurred after the diagnosis of lupus. The damage may be due to lupus itself or may have been caused by treatments. For example, cataracts are a side effect of glucocorticoids, not lupus per se. The purpose of a damage index is to have an assessment of the total health status of a patient over time. Like the SLEDAI, the damage index is generally used only in clinical studies and academic centers where lupus is being researched.

While the SLEDAI and damage index are useful, a careful physical examination and the appropriate lab tests will usually provide all the information your rheumatologist needs. Even without scales and scoring, physicians must assess lupus from at least two perspectives—how sick a patient is or how active her disease is at the time of a visit, and how the lupus has affected a patient's health in general over time. It's hoped that early treatment, where necessary, can prevent permanent damage to organs or tissues.

You can take preventive measures to reduce the risk of flares. Learning stress-reduction techniques can help you minimize stress-induced flares. Getting regular exercise should help combat fatigue and muscle weakness. If you're photosensitive, avoiding excessive sun exposure and using sunscreen when you're out in the sun will usually prevent rashes. If you smoke, stop smoking. Not only can it trigger flares and skin damage, but it's the number one risk factor for heart and blood vessel disease—and cardiovascular disease follows lupus like a shadow.

Living with the unpredictability of lupus flares can be challenging. Which symptoms are the hardest, and who does best? An ongoing study of 400 patients with SLE, run by the University of Texas-Houston Health Science Center and the University of Alabama at Birmingham, found that fatigue and pain were the two most difficult symptoms for patients. But women who were able to cope with their disease from the time they were first diagnosed did much better. Because stress can also play a major role in lupus flares, learning stress-reduction exercises can be very beneficial, as can joining a support group where women can learn more effective coping strategies to help manage both the physical and emotional effects of their disease.

Treating Lupus

Belimumab (Benlysta), the first new drug for treating lupus since 1955, was approved by the FDA in 2011. Approval was based on two large randomized clinical trials of approximately 800 patients each around the world, which showed that belimumab, a monoclonal antibody to circulating BLyS, is effective for managing SLE.[10]

It's thought that too much BLyS is produced in lupus and that this may accelerate autoimmune B cell proliferation and survival. While belimumab has shown benefits in SLE, it seems to work best in women with skin and joint problems and may help those who cannot lower their steroid dose without having a flare. It has also been shown to improve lupus-related fatigue.

Belimumab is very well tolerated and has an excellent safety profile. It does not cause infections to any greater degree than other currently used lupus medications. In rare cases, side effects include nausea, diarrhea, fever, hypersensitivity, and infusion-site reactions.

Belimumab is an intravenous drug given monthly to treat patients whose lupus is active and who are not doing well on conventional lupus medications. However, conventional lupus treatments are tried before belimumab is considered.

In general lupus treatments are aimed at reducing symptoms, decreasing the number and severity of flares, stopping progression of the disease, and minimizing permanent organ damage.

Pain medications, most frequently *nonsteroidal anti-inflammatory drugs (NSAIDs)*, are given to reduce muscle and joint pain and inflammation. NSAIDs include aspirin, *ibuprofen (Motrin)*, *naproxen (Naprosyn)*, and *nabumetone (Relafen)*. However, these drugs can cause gastrointestinal problems, including bleeding. They can also affect kidney function and cause liver abnormalities, so they must be used with caution even though some can be purchased without a doctor's prescription.

Some NSAIDs, called *COX-2 inhibitors*, are less likely to cause serious GI bleeding. They include *celecoxib (Celebrex)* and *meloxicam (Mobic)*, a partially selective COX-2 inhibitor. There's a special precaution, however. *Selective COX-2 inhibitors* do not have the anticlotting properties of aspirin (and therefore don't reduce the risk of a heart attack), so it's important that women who take these drugs first be checked for antiphospholipid antibodies, which may add to the risk of clotting. Celecoxib also contains sulfa, and this may be a problem because lupus patients have a tendency to be allergic to sulfa.

Glucocorticoids (corticosteroids) are used to reduce inflammation and suppress immune activity. Among the most commonly prescribed are *prednisone (Deltasone, Orasone)* and *methylprednisolone (Medrol)*.

Corticosteroids have a number of major side effects (see pages 42 to 43). The biggest risk for side effects occurs when higher doses of steroids are taken for long periods of time. Of particular concern, a large study from Johns Hopkins finds that the risk of developing cataracts more than doubles for SLE patients who have been on 10 mg/day of prednisone (or its equivalent) for 3 to 10 years.[11] While the risk of cataracts with prednisone is well known, this is the first indication of know how long it takes (and at what dose) for the problem to emerge. Adding to the risk: high blood pressure and elevated disease activity.

Corticosteroids are extremely effective in treating lupus and may be needed for weeks in cases of life-threatening complications. However, prolonged use can also lead to a shutdown of the adrenal glands. To get the adrenal glands working again, steroids must be slowly tapered.

Antimalarials are drugs originally used to treat malaria that suppress the inflammation leading to skin rashes, joint pain, hair loss, and fatigue in lupus. They include *chloroquine (Aralen)*, *hydroxychloroquine (Plaquenil)*, and *quinacrine* (*Atabrine*, which must be ordered from a compounding pharmacy not your usual commercial drug store). Hydroxychloroquine is the most commonly prescribed. The side effects include rare nausea, diarrhea, and bad taste in the mouth, most of which can be avoided by taking the drug just before bedtime. In very rare cases a patient may have an allergic rash.

The most serious side effect of these drugs is eye damage (retinal deposit of the drug). This effect is rare and is related to long-term use of the drug and not even at all likely until after five years at the very least. Patients have taken this drug for over two decades with no eye toxicity. It is important to see an eye doctor once per year. Keep in mind that it may take months to see a benefit from antimalarials, so patience is important.

Recent studies suggest that hydroxychloroquine may also have protective effects on bone mass, preventing bone loss at the hip and spine, areas vulnerable to fracture. They may even protect against blood clotting, high lipids, and diabetes. It is also thought that the drug may prevent worsening of lupus. It's generally considered a drug to be taken by all patients with lupus and to be continued as long as there are no signs of eye problems. All other drugs can be added to hydroxychloroquine, and stopping the drug can result in lupus flares.

Immunomodulating drugs belong to a class of drugs called *cytotoxic (cell-killing)* drugs that can help suppress the immune system by reducing populations of immune cells. These drugs include *azathioprine (Imuran)*, *cyclophosphamide (Cytoxan)*, and *mycophenolate mofetil (CellCept)* and are used when steroids are unable to be tapered and when there's more serious kidney or other organ involvement. Methotrexate is often used to treat arthritic symptoms just as in RA.

Side effects include anemia, a low white blood cell count, and an increased risk of infection. There are suggestions these drugs may increase the risk of cancer (but this has not been proven). Cyclophosphamide can also cause sterility (premature menopause), especially in women who begin the drug after the age of 35.

The anticancer drug *rituximab (Rituxan)*, which targets a protein on the surface of B cells and helps deplete their numbers, is still being tested in SLE and is sometimes used to treat low platelets and lupus nephritis that is not responsive to other immunosuppressive agents.

Anticoagulants are prescribed for women with clotting abnormalities to prevent blood clots in leg veins (*deep vein thrombosis*) or in the lungs or coronary arteries. Low-dose aspirin (81 mg) prevents platelets from sticking together to form clots. The oldest of the anticoagulant drugs, *warfarin (Coumadin)*, interferes with some of the proteins that regulate clotting that depend on vitamin K. *Heparin*, usually used as low-molecular-weight heparins (*Lovenox*), affects another clotting mechanism. It's important to remember that blood thinners must be monitored carefully to avoid bleeding episodes.

Intravenous immunoglobulin (IVIG) may be used to raise platelet counts in women with thrombocytopenia (see pages 370 to 373).

Dehydroepiandrosterone (DHEA) is an *androgen,* or male hormone, normally produced by the adrenal glands and converted by the body into estrogen and testosterone. Some scientists believe that women with lupus have low levels of androgens (which have anti-inflammatory properties). DHEA may be helpful if you have mild lupus, especially skin rashes, hair loss, and joint pain. It does not appear to be effective for more serious manifestations of lupus, such as kidney disease. DHEA is usually well tolerated with only minor side effects, including mild acne.

A pharmaceutical preparation of DHEA (*prasterone, Aslera*) has been tested in lupus patients and has yet to be approved by the FDA. But a systematic review of recent studies concludes that while some evidence suggests DHEA may improve disease activity and health-related quality of life in severe or active SLE, it has little or no effect in mild to moderate cases.[12]

While DHEA is available in health food stores as a dietary supplement, these are not standardized or regulated, and some may be ineffective. Because of its anti-inflammatory properties, DHEA may allow you to reduce the amount of prednisone you're taking. But don't take it without a physician's supervision.

What's Next?

Future treatments, including newer biologicals, are currently in clinical trials and are hoped to have a more specific effect on the immune abnormalities of lupus, not just global immunosuppression.

Another drug that blocks B cell activation and survival through BLyS, *blisibimod*, both in membrane and soluble forms, has produced mixed results in clinical trials, enabling some women to reduce corticosteroids, and seems to work best in severe lupus.[13] As this book went to press, blisibimod was still being tested.

Atacicept, an agent that inhibits BLyS and another B cell activating factor dubbed APRIL, so far has been unsuccessful in dampening lupus flares.[14] Another B cell drug, *epratuzimab*, is also under investigation, along with *anifrolumab*, an experimental anti-interferon alpha receptor monoclonal antibody. Recent studies found that epratuzimab was disappointing because it did not meet its efficacy endpoints.

Studies also suggest that low doses of *thalidomide (Thalomid)* may help improve rashes in women with cutaneous lupus who have failed other therapies. Thalidomide has some anti-inflammatory effects, but it has potentially severe side effects and has not been shown to produce remission in discoid lupus.[15] Side effects include a cessation of menstrual periods, weight gain, drowsiness, and blood clots in women who have risk factors for clots. The drug can also cause irreversible nerve damage, so nerve conduction tests must be done at baseline and periodically during treatment. It has not yet been approved for treating lupus, and because of its devastating effects on a developing fetus thalidomide cannot be used by women who wish to become pregnant.

Lupus Clusters

A recent survey by the Lupus Foundation of America found that a third of patients had another autoimmune disease in addition to their lupus. Among the most common are:

- Thyroid disease
- Sjögren's syndrome
- Raynaud's phenomenon
- Antiphospholipid syndrome

Deanna's story continues:

The high doses of steroids I was on made my muscles very weak, and I was in physical therapy to try to get my strength back. There was a period when I couldn't even lift myself off the toilet. I was emotionally a mess from the steroids. I would have temper tantrums. I had an inflamed esophagus, so I had difficulty swallowing food. But the joint pain got better. When my doctor told me I had lupus nephritis, he said I probably would not be able to go back to school. . . . That made me furious. . . . I was determined to get better. Eventually, they reduced the steroids. My face was going back to normal, my hair was growing in again, and my self-esteem was coming back.

I had to go back to college that fall on crutches at first . . . but I worked even harder in school. I felt I had a lot to make up for. I graduated summa cum laude. Highest honors. I couldn't control the lupus, but I could try to control everything else. I graduated from college, taught for a while, and eventually got my master's degree.

The Female Factor

Ninety percent of patients with lupus are women, and numerous studies suggest a role for estrogen in the disease. Unlike rheumatoid arthritis, which gets better during pregnancy when estrogen levels are high (but that's not the whole story), lupus can sometimes flare during or after pregnancy. Some studies suggest that women with lupus may have an abnormality in the way their bodies process naturally occurring estrogens, while others find that women with SLE may metabolize testosterone at a faster rate than men, so high levels of estrogen may go unopposed by androgens. Male hormones may play a protective role in lupus; women with low levels of androgens may be more vulnerable to SLE. Genes have also been discovered that may interact with estrogen to heighten women's responses to inflammation in SLE. These genes, called *toll-like receptors (TLRs)*, may stimulate greater immune system signaling.[16]

Prolactin (produced during lactation) is another hormone that may play a role. It not only stimulates the flow of mother's milk, but it's also produced by immune cells and can act as a cytokine. In this role, prolactin triggers the release of other cytokines and stimulates immune reactions. About 20 percent of lupus patients have higher prolactin levels than the body would normally produce.

There are also studies that suggest a role for microchimerism in lupus, where cells from the fetus get into the mother's bloodstream and may trigger a reaction by the immune system (see pages 13 to 15). However, it may be the maternal cells that get into the fetal circulation and persist into adult life that increase the risk of lupus and neonatal lupus, suggest researchers at the Fred Hutchinson Cancer Research Center and the University of Washington. These cells could travel to certain sites in the body and provoke immune reactions. The researchers noted that biopsies of heart muscle have found maternal cells in babies with neonatal lupus, and that studies also show that lupus can be created in mice by injecting parental cells. However, this area of research is still very much in its preliminary stages.

How Lupus Can Affect You Over Your Lifetime

Lupus can affect women in many ways during their reproductive years, especially during and after pregnancy.

Lupus and Your Menstrual Cycle

You may find that lupus symptoms flare during different times of the menstrual cycle. For some women, flares occur just prior to menses (when estrogens are lowest), while in others, flares occur just before the time of ovulation (when estrogens are highest). It may be the change in hormone levels that triggers a flare, not the absolute level itself. Birth control pills create steady levels of hormones and may help prevent these cyclic flares (although not proven).

Menstrual periods can stop during times of severe disease activity. One Brazilian study found that disease activity was a major factor associated with menstrual disturbances. The study, which included 36 SLE patients ages 18 to 39 years, determined half of the women had menstrual dysfunction, with increased menstrual flow being the most frequent.[17] About 11 percent had elevations in follicle-stimulating hormone (FSH), with or without menstrual disturbances, suggesting there may have been subclinical ovarian damage. The study found no significant association of low-dose prednisone with menstrual changes. But other studies have shown that women being treated with high-dose steroids do have menstrual cycle irregularities, with a temporary loss of periods being most frequent. Unfortunately, treatment with cyclophosphamide (especially in women older than 35) can result in permanent sterility.

Lupus and Pregnancy

In general, recent studies show lupus patients can do well during pregnancy, with little or no permanent exacerbation of their disease.

Severe flares occur most often among women with prior kidney disease and low platelet counts, problems that can recur during pregnancy and must be carefully monitored for. Minor flares, with fatigue, joint pain, and rashes, may be uncomfortable but usually don't pose a significant threat to mother or baby.

According to the largest study of pregnancy outcomes in SLE, rates of mild to moderate flares were just under 13 percent in the second trimester and less than 10 percent in the third trimester.[18] The eight-year multiethnic PROMISSE study (Predictors of Pregnancy Outcome: BioMarkers in Antiphospholipid Syndrome and Systemic Lupus Erythematosus) looked at 385 patients with stable or mild/moderate SLE, and only 3 percent of women had severe flares.

Poor pregnancy outcomes—including preterm birth (before 36 weeks) due to low blood supply to the fetus (called placental insufficiency), maternal hypertension, preeclampsia (abnormally high blood pressure during pregnancy), low birthweight babies, and fetal death—occurred in only 19 percent of the women.[18] That means the vast majority of the women (89 percent) had uncomplicated pregnancies. Rates of poor pregnancy outcomes were higher among African American and Hispanic women.

Risk factors for poor outcomes include higher disease activity, platelet counts lower than 100K, the need for medications to control high blood pressure, and the presence of the lupus anticoagulant.

There's no question that having SLE does increase your chances of complications. According to a recent analysis of almost 11,000 pregnancies, comparing women with and without SLE, those with lupus had almost double the risk of hypertension, preeclampsia (abnormally high blood pressure during pregnancy), preterm delivery, and stillbirths.[19] The study also found a more than sixteenfold occurrence of nephritis in SLE pregnancies, depending on disease activity.

However, fewer than half the women in this study with SLE received hydroxychloroquine,[19] although studies suggest that it prevents flares in pregnancy. One reason may be that the women in the study saw a rheumatologist infrequently, comments Michelle A. Petri, MD, PhD, professor of medicine and director of the Johns Hopkins Lupus Center in Baltimore, the study's lead author.

As for medical costs, Dr. Petri and her colleagues found that the costs of managing pregnancy in SLE could be as high as $20,000, about double that for a non-lupus pregnancy.

Most important, no matter how well you are doing, it's critical that you be seen frequently by your rheumatologist, as well as by your obstetrician (who should be familiar with taking care of pregnant lupus patients). These doctors should be specialists in high-risk pregnancies (maternal fetal medicine specialists) and should be affiliated with a neonatal intensive care unit in case your baby needs special attention.

Women with SLE-related kidney disease are also more likely to have protein in the urine, or proteinuria, which may signal a lupus flare or preeclampsia. Experimental biomarkers that may predict preeclampsia (and flares) as early as 20 weeks are being researched, and clinical trials are underway in non-SLE patients of *ATryn*, an antithrombin recombinant drug, to treat preeclampsia during the twenty-fourth to twenty-eighth weeks of pregnancy.[20]

Angiogenesis is the process of growing new blood vessels, key to formation of the placenta in pregnancy, and dysregulation of this process may lead to preeclampsia and *placental insufficiency* (insufficient blood supply from the placenta) in SLE.

Recent studies led by Jane E. Salmon, MD, research professor at the Hospital for Joint Diseases in New York, found that levels of several angiogenic factors that interfere with placental development are elevated in women with lupus and antiphospholipid antibodies who go on to have preeclampsia, pregnancy complications, and poor outcomes.[21] According to Dr. Salmon, increases in angiogenic factors detected before 15 weeks of pregnancy could identify women at risk.

Regular monitoring for preeclampsia and other risky conditions in pregnancy is a must. As soon as you know you're pregnant, a baseline measurement of protein in the urine over 24 hours should be done; after that, dipsticks should be done at each obstetrical visit, and 24-hour urine collections should be done each trimester.

Being in remission for six months is the best time to consider having a baby. This usually means being clinically well without major organ involvement such as active kidney, heart, lung, or brain disease, and taking less than 20 milligrams per day of prednisone. Taking greater than 20 milligrams of prednisone, despite feeling well, is not likely to represent a true state of remission. In fact, the definition of remission is quite individual. For example, blood tests may indicate a minor degree of disease activity (slightly low complement levels and slightly elevated anti-dsDNA antibodies), but a woman may have no other signs of a problem. So you needn't always wait for a complete absence of evidence of lupus activity in your blood work before getting pregnant. If you're planning a pregnancy, you also need to make sure that you're not anemic and do not have a very low platelet count or over a gram of protein in your urine. Minor joint or skin involvement is usually not a reason to avoid pregnancy.

Fertility and sterility rates for women with SLE are comparable to those for women who don't have SLE when the disease is in remission. However, your fertility may be depressed during times of severe disease activity.

If women experience problems becoming pregnant, they may need hormonal stimulation to produce multiple eggs for implantation during in vitro fertilization (IVF).

IVF can be successful in women with SLE and antiphospholipid syndrome (APS, see Chapter 11, pages 347 to 362), but hormonal stimulation may increase the risk of flares and complications.

One small study conducted at three lupus centers in New York City found that ovulation induction, ovarian hyperstimulation, and IVF resulted in increased disease activity in around a quarter of women with SLE.[22] The study, associated complications during pregnancy and postpartum, including toxemia, lupus flares, and diabetes; postpartum problems included a flare in kidney disease, cartilage inflammation (*costochondritis*), and depression.

If you make the decision to undergo IVF, it's vital that adhere to your lupus treatments. A study of 34 women with SLE and/or APS who had undergone at least one cycle of IVF found that 92 percent had successful pregnancies. However, 10 percent did have hormone-related flares or clots, partly because of lack of adherence to SLE treatments, researchers told the 2013 ACR meeting.[23] Treatments included hydroxychloroquine, steroids, aspirin, and/or low-molecular-weight heparin.

Tests you'll need if you're pregnant. Once you're pregnant, you will need routine blood tests, such as a comprehensive chemistry to check kidney function, liver function, glucose, complete blood count, and urinalysis. The standard tests to assess lupus activity should also be done, such as measuring complement levels and anti-DNA antibodies.

During your first trimester you'll need several other blood tests. The first set of tests assesses the risk of a spontaneous miscarriage and measures antibodies to phospholipids, which may cause blood clotting in the placenta. One of the tests you'll need is the VDRL (a standard test for syphilis that can also detect anticardiolipin antibodies). A traditional ELISA for direct measurement of anticardiolipin antibodies and antibodies to B2GPI will also be done, along with special clotting tests. One type of clotting test is called a Dilute Russell Viper Venom Time (DRVVT), which checks for the presence of the so-called lupus anticoagulant (which actually promotes clotting, not bleeding).

A second set of antibody tests is done to assess the rare risk of permanent cardiac damage in the developing fetus and/or skin rash and liver disease in early infancy. These are antibodies to SSA/Ro and SSB/La proteins. Of course, a positive test for any of these antibodies does not mean you'll have problems with the pregnancy, but your doctors need to know so they can be prepared.

Also, as a precaution, during each trimester you should be tested for anti-DNA antibodies and complement levels and also have a 24-hour urine collection to test for protein and creatinine. Protein in the urine means the kidneys are leaky—think of a colander in which the holes might be too big and spaghetti can leak out. The creatinine level tells you how well the kidneys are filtering waste products.

Each trimester, sonograms are done to check the baby' growth and amniotic fluid. Later in pregnancy, fetal movements and breathing will be carefully measured. If there are signs of fetal distress, you may need to be hospitalized and may need to consider early delivery. There is a higher rate of premature births in women with lupus. Patients with lupus also have a higher risk of preeclampsia (toxemia of pregnancy, which includes high blood pressure and protein in the urine) than the general population.

Medications during pregnancy and breastfeeding. Keep in mind that all drugs taken during pregnancy could have potential harm to the growing baby since they may cross the placenta. However, certain drugs are necessary even if there are risks, since they're intended to either keep your lupus at bay or prevent a problem in the baby.

In general, low-dose aspirin (81 mg per day) is not likely to cause harm but may be helpful in preventing preeclampsia, and most doctors now recommend it. High-dose NSAIDs are not recommended during pregnancy because they may be associated with high pulmonary pressures in the fetus in some cases in lupus (for more on NSAIDs, see pages 36 to 37). NSAIDs can prolong labor and are generally avoided close to the time of delivery; because of the risk of bleeding, aspirin is also generally stopped when you're close to term.

Prednisone at doses less than 20 milligrams daily is generally not a problem for the fetus, since the placenta inactivates the drug. At higher doses, slightly more active drug is available in fetal circulation, but it still may not be dangerous. Possible side effects of steroids to the fetus include decreased amniotic fluid, decreased growth, and suppression of the adrenal glands.

"The risks and benefits of treatment must be weighed carefully during pregnancy," says Dr. Petri. "Prednisone in particular will increase the risk of both preeclampsia and gestational diabetes, but it is safe for the fetus."

Hydroxychloroquine (Plaquenil) does cross the placenta, although the available literature shows very few problems. Concerns about hydroxycloroquine have declined to such an extent that most rheumatologists with experience in treating pregnant lupus patients suggest staying on the drug. The reason is that there is a risk of a flare if it's discontinued, and this may override any potential harm to the fetus.

Azathioprine (Imuran) can be used during pregnancy. It is most often used when a patient has had previous kidney disease and was being treated with mycophenolate mofetil (MMF, CellCept). MMF is contraindicated in pregnancy. Cytoxan is also contraindicated during pregnancy, as is methotrexate. Low-molecular-weight heparin for treatment of clotting problems is often used to prevent recurrent fetal loss.

Certain antihypertensive drugs are unsafe during pregnancy. These include angiotensin-converting-enzyme (ACE) inhibitors and angiotensin II receptor blockers (ARBs). If blood pressure control is needed, other medications such as Aldomet, beta-blockers, and calcium channel inhibitors may be used.

Drugs can be passed to your baby if you breastfeed. NSAIDs are generally safe, since they do not pass easily into breast milk. However, high doses of NSAIDs can pose a problem, since babies eliminate them more slowly than adults do and they can accumulate in an infant's system. Hydroxychloroquine is excreted in small amounts in breast milk but seems to pose no risk. Lower doses of prednisone appear to be safe.

Using immunosuppressive agents is controversial. Small amounts of azathioprine have been found in breast milk, and some pediatricians advise against its use. Cyclophosphamide and cyclosporine cannot be used if you nurse because they are toxic to an infant.

Maternal autoantibodies can pass to the baby via breast milk but only during the first few days of life, so this is not likely to pose problems. Breastfeeding may increase fatigue, but don't let that stop you. On the other hand, breastfeeding is not for everyone, and if you do not want to, don't feel guilty as babies do quite well on formulas.

Neonatal lupus. During pregnancy, antibodies in the mother s circulation travel across the placenta into the bloodstream of the developing fetus, starting at about 12 to 14 weeks of gestation. The fetus is unable to make antibodies on its own and is dependent on maternal antibodies to fight infection. Mothers with antibodies SSA/Ro and SSB/La can have children with neonatal lupus. Two concerns in neonatal lupus are heart problems and skin rash.

The most concerning heart problem is *congenital heart block*, in which there is a block in the middle of the heart (called the *atrioventricular AV node*) that interrupts the electrical signal coming from the sinus node located at the top of the heart to the bottom of the heart (ventricles). This electrical signal is responsible for normal cardiac rate and rhythm. Blockage of the signal causes the ventricles to contract more slowly, and the overall result is an abnormally slow heartbeat. In congenital heart block, the AV node is damaged by the maternal autoantibodies or other as yet unidentified associated factors. This cardiac dysfunction (slow heartbeat) is most often detected between 18 and 24 weeks of gestation, with the twentieth week probably being the most vulnerable.

A slow fetal heart rate can be identified by routine examination using an amplified stethoscope, an obstetrical sonogram, or a special fetal echocardiogram. In almost all cases, heart block occurs as an isolated problem (there are no structural deformities of the heart itself). Curiously, the presence of these autoantibodies is not associated with heart problems in the mother, only in her offspring. The risk of having a child with heart block is 2 percent if you have antibodies to SSA/Ro and SSB/La. If you have had one baby with heart block, there is about an 18 percent risk of having a second affected child.

The skin rash of neonatal lupus is most commonly noted at about six weeks after delivery but can be detected at birth. The rash often involves the eyelids, face, and scalp. It is generally very red and can have a circular appearance. The skin rash can be triggered by sun exposure, so babies born to women with lupus should not be exposed to the sun without the use of sunscreen during the first months of life.

Liver abnormalities and low white blood cell and platelet counts are extremely rare problems but need to be checked. Most affected children have either heart block or skin rashes, but some do have both. Studies to date suggest that girls may be more prone to the rash than boys, but both sexes are equally susceptible to congenital heart block.

Actually, the term neonatal lupus is misleading. The name came about because the skin rash seen in infants resembled that seen in adults with SLE. While many mothers do have lupus, some mothers of affected children are totally asymptomatic themselves and have only the anti-Ro and/or anti-La antibodies in their blood. It's important to note that just because you may have anti-Ro or anti-La antibodies and your baby has neonatal lupus does not mean you have lupus or Sjögren's syndrome. Even more important to know: a child with heart block or skin rash does not have SLE. The rash, liver, and blood abnormalities are transient and usually disappear by six months of age as the maternal antibodies disappear from the child's circulation. Unfortunately the heart block is permanent.

Helping Mothers at Risk

If you're found to be at risk for having a child with neonatal lupus, it's best to take precautionary steps, whether it's a first pregnancy or you've previously had a baby with heart block or other signs of neonatal lupus.

It's recommended that you have a fetal echocardiogram (a sonogram of the heart that gives a far better picture of the heart structure and function than routine obstetrical ultrasound) between the sixteenth and eighteenth weeks of pregnancy. This should be done every week, if possible, until about the twenty-sixth week. After that, it may not be needed as further research suggests that heart block first occurring after 26 weeks is extremely rare. Just listening with a stethoscope may be sufficient.

Should a problem in the fetal heart be detected, therapies may be needed to treat the inflammation in the heart. However, once established, complete heart block is not likely to be reversed (sometimes the block is not complete, which is better). Most children will eventually need a pacemaker.

In the situation of a mother with known antibodies who has already had a child with heart block, the risk of having a second affected child may be 10 times higher. In studies from the National Research Registry for Neonatal Lupus, the recurrence rate is approximately 18 percent.[24] It is also possible to have one child with heart block and a second child with a rash and vice versa. At this time, no data suggest a benefit to prophylactic therapies, such as plasmapheresis (to filter antibodies from the blood) and/or steroids prior to the detection of a problem, but there are some new considerations, as follows.

If the fetus is diagnosed with heart block, and the block has been present for more than three weeks, the baby is watched and weekly echocardiograms are performed to determine if there are signs that heart function is deteriorating (for example, if fluid builds up around the heart or lungs).

If the heartbeat is second-degree block (incomplete), it is theoretically possible (but not yet proven) that treating the mother with a steroid such as dexamethasone, which can cross the placenta and be available in the fetal circulation, will reverse the block before it progresses to third-degree heart block. Unfortunately, the block is usually complete when it is first detected. If the fetus shows signs of inflammation, such as fluid around the heart or lungs or abdomen, this may be a more serious sign and dexamethasone may be initiated.

A study is underway to see if it's possible to prevent a recurrence of fetal heart block by giving hydroxychloroquine early in pregnancy (before 10 weeks) to women with anti-Ro antibodies. Since hydroxychloroquine can cross the placenta, it's hoped the drug may dampen some of the inflammation triggered by maternal anti-Ro antibodies in the fetal circulation. If the study—Preventive Approach to Congenital Heart Block with Hydroxychloroquine, PATCH for short—shows good results, a nationwide screening and prevention trial may be possible.

What's the outlook for your baby? The prognosis for the child with heart block is generally good. However, heart block is permanent, and in 20 percent of cases the condition is fatal (most often before three months of age). Most children will require pacemakers, probably for life. Pacemakers are commonly implanted within the first three months after birth. In a child whose only manifestation of neonatal lupus is a skin rash, the situation is generally excellent since the rash usually disappears by about six months. In most cases no medications are needed and no scars or marks are left.

Although any child born to a mother with SLE does have a higher risk of developing SLE later in life (approximately one in 10 if it's a girl), no data persuasively indicate that the risk is increased if the child also had neonatal lupus.

Lupus and Estrogen

For both healthy women and women with SLE, there are times when estrogen may be needed. A woman may want birth control, and the best method may be oral contraceptives (OCs). After menopause, women may need the symptom relief that estrogen therapy can bring.

It's been suggested that OCs may even be useful in controlling cyclical disease activity in some patients. The estrogen in oral contraceptives may be useful in preventing steroid-induced osteoporosis and may preserve fertility in women taking cyclophosphamide. For years, the conventional wisdom was that estrogens might provoke lupus flares. However, based on the Safety of Estrogens in Lupus Erythematosus, National Assessment (SELENA) trials, a duo of randomized double-blind placebo-controlled trials, one for hormone therapy and one for oral contraceptives, the OC trial found that birth control pills do not increase the risk of flares in women with stable SLE.[25]

In the HT-SELENA trial, researchers found that one year of HT (0.625 mg of conjugated estrogen daily and 5 mg medroxyprogesterone 12 days each month) increased mild and moderate, but not severe flares in women with inactive or stable-active SLE. In both trials, antiphospholipid/anticardiolipin antibodies and/or a history of blood clots in the leg (deep vein thrombosis) were exclusion criteria.[26] However, even in these women, in the HT trial (351 women) there was one death, one stroke, two cases of deep vein thrombosis, and one case of thrombosis in an arteriovenous graft; in the placebo group, only one patient developed deep vein thrombosis.

Lupus and Menopause

The Women's Health Initiative (WHI), a major clinical trial of one form of combined hormone therapy (*Prempro*) among healthy women, was halted in 2002 because of slight increases in heart attacks, strokes, blood clots, and invasive breast cancers among women taking the drug (although there was a reduced risk of colon cancer and benefit to the bones).

Given the consideration that HT may further increase the already elevated risk of cardiovascular disease (CVD) in women with lupus, the HT arm of the SELENA trial was also stopped early due to DVTs and cardiovascular complications.[26]

Women with a history of DVTs and elevated levels of antiphospholipid antibodies (aPLs), *anticardiolipin antibodies (aCLs)*, the *lupus anticoagulant (LAC)*, and *anti-beta2 glycoprotein I antibodies* should not take postmenopausal hormones. A false positive VDRL may also be a reason for seeking alternatives to estrogen therapy.[27] While there are a number of nonhormonal remedies for menopausal symptoms, among them vitamins E and B, soy, and herbs like black cohosh (see page 54), you should avoid some menopausal remedies. Evening primrose oil promotes clotting and cannot be used by women who have antiphospholipid antibodies, and red clover can interfere with blood thinners used to treat antiphospholipid syndrome and promote bleeding.

Experts also advise women with lupus to be extremely cautious about plant estrogens like soy or black cohosh. Both act like estrogens in the body, binding to the same receptors. Herbal products are not regulated, and their contents can vary quite widely. So don't try herbs or soy as menopausal remedies without first talking it over with your rheumatologist.

Lupus and Your Heart

Women with SLE have an increased risk of cardiovascular disease, and a review of almost two dozen studies found that the risk of CVD among people with lupus has doubled in recent years compared to the general population.[28] The risk may be greater before age 45. One study found that women aged 35 to 44 were actually 50 times more likely to have a heart attack than women of similar age in the general population, but women with SLE aged 45 to 64 had only two to four times the risk.

The natural estrogen present in your body thought to protect women before menopause may actually promote blood clotting in younger women with SLE who have aPLs, high blood pressure, or kidney disease. Immune complexes in the blood may irritate the lining of blood vessels and cause inflammation, promoting atherosclerotic lesions. These fatty plaques narrow the carotid arteries—the major blood vessels supplying the brain—more often in premenopausal women with SLE, says Susan Manzi, MD, MPH, co-director of the Lupus Center of Excellence and chair of the Department of Medicine at West Penn Allegheny Health System in Pittsburgh.

A study by Dr. Manzi and colleagues also found that stiffness in the aorta might be an early marker of atherosclerotic disease. As women become perimenopausal and develop more heart disease risk factors (such as high cholesterol, high blood pressure, and obesity), this process may speed up, adds Dr. Manzi. Having aPLs increases the risk of stroke.

Taking corticosteroids causes abnormalities in blood fats, including cholesterol, and may promote insulin resistance. Cholesterol-lowering drugs may be one way to lower the risk of heart attacks.

Other steps you need to take to protect your heart include keeping your weight under control, getting regular exercise, and following a heart-healthy diet (see page 56). Blood pressure should be monitored carefully, and levels of LDL and HDL cholesterol, triglycerides, and homocysteine should be measured once a year. Your annual physical exam should include an electrocardiogram (ECG).

The Threat of Osteoporosis

Lower than average bone mineral density (BMD), or *osteopenia*, may affect as many as 39 percent of women with SLE, and bone loss (osteoporosis) is seen in upwards of 5 percent of people with SLE.[29]

The use of corticosteroid therapy is a major risk factor for osteoporosis in SLE, but the disease itself may lead to bone loss through abnormalities in bone metabolism, pro-inflammatory cytokines that promote bone resorption, and premature menopause.

Avoidance of sun exposure and low vitamin D also play a role.[30] Without exposure to ultraviolet light, the body cannot produce enough natural vitamin D through the skin.

Pain and fatigue may keep many women from exercise and other activities that help keep bones strong. Age is a major risk factor for bone loss in women, and vertebral compression fractures of the spine (resulting in loss of height and *kyphosis* or "widow's hump") are common in SLE. They may be painless and only show up on x-rays.

Any woman taking corticosteroid therapy for autoimmune disease is at risk for bone loss. The ACR Task Force on Osteoporosis Guidelines recommends oral contraceptives to prevent steroid-induced bone loss in premenopausal women, and antiresorptive bisphosphonate drugs like *alendronate (Fosamax)* for older women and those on long-term glucocorticoid therapy (see pages 57 to 68).[31] The monoclonal antibody drug *denosumab (Prolia, Xgeva)* interferes with a signaling protein to reduce the action of osteoclasts.[32] It can be prescribed for people with impaired kidney function and could be an option for women with lupus nephritis.[27] The antimalarial drug hydroxychloroquine may also help protect against bone loss due to corticosteroids.

Deanna's story continues:

The one important thing is not to let it get you. Make sure you get the proper care, take care of yourself, eat right, and exercise, and you can beat it. I firmly believe that. I've met women in the support groups who let lupus consume them, and their disease just gets worse and worse. I've had kidney problems, intestinal problems; I had bone death because of the steroids I was on, and I have had both hips replaced. But I focused on my work, on living my life no matter what, and that kept me going. I got married last June, and I look at the wedding pictures and outwardly, you'd never know anything was wrong. I look healthy. Sometimes when I don't feel well, my husband will still say, "But you don't look sick." Despite all the problems I've had, I try not to think of myself as being sick. Maybe you can't control the disease, but you can control your attitude. I really believe the power of the mind can be stronger than the disease.

Deanna

Notes

1. Lim SS, Bayakly AR, Helmick CG, et al. The incidence and prevalence of systemic lupus erythematosus, 2002–2004: The Georgia Lupus Registry. *Arthritis Rheumatol.* 2014; 66(2):357–368. doi:10.1002/art.38239.
2. Somers EC, Marder W, Cagnoli P, et al. Population-based incidence and prevalence of systemic lupus erythematosus: the Michigan Lupus Epidemiology and Surveillance program. *Arthritis Rheumatol.* 2014;66(2):369–378. doi:10.1002/art.38238.
3. Sestak AL, Fürnroh BG, Harkley JB, Merrill JT, Namjou B. The genetics of systemic lupus erythematosus and implications for targeted therapy. *Ann Rheum Dis.* 2011;70(suppl):i37-i43. doi:10.1136/ard.2010.138057.
4. Leffler J, Bengtsson AA, Blom AM. The complement system in systemic lupus erythematosus: an update. *Ann Rheum Dis.* 2014;73(9):1601–1603. doi:10.1136/annhhrumdis-2014-205287.
5. Pender MP. CD8+ T-cell deficiency, Epstein-Barr virus infection, vitamin D deficiency, and steps to autoimmunity: a unifying hypothesis. *Autoimmune Dis.* (2012), Article ID 189096, 16 pages http://dx.doi.org/10.1155/2012/189096. doi:10.1155/2012/189096.
6. Fonseca R, Bernardes M, Terroso G, de Sousa M, Figueiredo-Braga M. Silent burdens in disease: fatigue and depression in SLE. *Autoimmune Dis.* Jan 28, 2014. http.dx.doi.org/10.1155/2014/790724.
7. Kroslin KL, Wiginton KL. The impact of race and ethnicity on disease severity in systemic lupus erythematosus. *Ethinic Dis.* 2009;19:301–307. doi.ethn-19-03-10.3d 26/6/09 16:19:56.
8. Petri M, Orbai AM, Alarcon GS, et al. Derivation and validation of the Systemic Lupus International Collaborating Clinics classification criteria for systemic lupus erythematosus. *Arthritis Rheum.* 2012;64(8):2677–2686. doi:10.1002/art.34473.
9. Jacobs R, Pawlak CR, Mikeska, E, et al. Systemic lupus erythematosus and rheumatoid arthritis patients differ from healthy controls in their cytokine patterns after stress exposure. *Rheumatology.* 2001;40:868–875.
10. FDA approves Benlysta to treat lupus. First new lupus drug approved in 56 years. *FDA News Release,* Mar 9, 2011. http://www.fda.gov/NewsEvents/Newsroom/PressAnnouncements/ucm246489.htm.

11. Alderaan K, Sekicki V, Magder LS, Petri M. Risk factors for cataracts in systemic lupus erythematosus (SLE). *Rheumatol Int.* 2015;35(4):701–8. doi:10.1007/s00296-014-3129-5.
12. Crosbie D, Black C, McIntyre L, Royle P, Thomas S. Dehydroepiandrosterone for systemic lupus erythematosus. *Cochrane Database Syst Rev.* 2007:(4), Art. No. CD005114. doi:10.1002/14651858. CD005114.pub2.
13. Furie R, Leon G, Petri MA. A phase 2, randomised, placebo-controlled clinical trial of blisibimod, an inhibitor of B cell activating factor, in patients with moderate-to-severe systemic lupus erythematosus, the PEARL-SC study. *Ann Rheum Dis.* 2014 [published online Apr 19, 2014. doi:10.1136/annrheumdis-2013-205144.
14. Isenberg D, Gordon C, Licu D, et al. Efficacy and safety of atacicept for prevention of flares in patients with moderate-to-severe systemic lupus erythematosus: 52-week data (APRIL-SLE randomized trial). *Ann Rheum Dis.* 2015;74(11):2006–2015. doi:10.1136/annrheumdis-2013-205067.
15. Cortés-Hernández J, Torres-Salido M, Castro-Marrero J, et al. Thalidomide in the treatment of refractory cutaneous lupus erythematosus: prognostic factors of clinical outcome. *Br J Dermatol.* Mar 2012;166(3):616–623. doi:10.1111/j.1365-2133.2011.10693.x.
16. Young NA, Wu LC, Burd CJ, et al. Estrogen modulation of endosome-associated toll-like receptor 8: an IFNα-independent mechanism of sex-bias in systemic lupus erythematosus. *Clin Immuno.* 2014;151(1):66–77. doi:10.1016/j.clim.2014.01.006.
17. Pasoto SG. Menstrual disturbances in patients with systemic lupus erythematosus without alkylating therapy: clinical, hormonal and therapeutic associations. *Lupus.* 2002;11(3):175–180. doi:10.1191/0961203302lu163.
18. Buyon JP, Kim MY, Guerra MM, et al. Predictors of pregnancy outcomes in patients with lupus: a cohort study. *Ann Int Med.* 2015;163(3):153–63. doi:10.7326/M14-2235.
19. Petri MA, Daly P, Pushparajah DS, et al. Pregnancy complications in lupus: data from a large US database. 2013 ACR Abstract: #2534. *Arthritis Rheum.* 2013;65(10-suppl): S1082.
20. http://revobiologics.com/news/revo-biologics-inc-initiates-preserve-1-phase-3-clinical-trial-atryn%C2%AE-early-onset-preeclampsia.
21. Salmon JE, Kim M, Guerra MM, et al. Angiogenic factor dysregulation and risk of adverse pregnancy outcome in lupus pregnancies. 2013 ACR Abstract: #765. *Arthritis Rheum.* 2013;65(10-suppl):S323.
22. Guballa N, Sammaritano L, Schwartzman S, Buyon J, Lockshin MD. Ovulation induction and in vitro fertilization in systemic lupus erythematosus and antiphospholipid syndrome. *Arthritis Rheum.* 2000;43(3):550–556.
23. Costedoat-Chalumeau N, Orquevaux P, Masseau A, et al. In vitro fertilization in systemic lupus erythematosus and antiphospholipid syndrome: a series of 82 cycles. 2013 ACR Abstract: #2554. *Arthritis Rheum.* 2013;65(10-suppl):S1090.
24. Llanos C, Izmirly PM, Margaret Katholi M, et al. Recurrence rates of cardiac manifestations associated with neonatal lupus and maternal/fetal risk factors. *Arthritis Rheum.* 2009;60(10):3091–3097. doi:10.1002/art.24768.

25. Petri M, Kim MY, Kalunian KC, et al. Combined oral contraceptives in women with systemic lupus erythematosus. *N Engl J Med.* 2005;353(24):2250–2258. doi:10.1056/NEJMoa051135.
26. Buyon JP, Petri M, Kim MY, et al. The effect of combined estrogen and progesterone hormone replacement therapy on disease activity in systemic lupus erythematosus: a randomized trial. *Ann Intern Med.* 2005;142(12 pt 1):953–962.
27. Buyon J. Have we reached an estrogen comfort zone? A review of research on prescribing estrogens in systemic lupus erythematosus. *The Rheumatologist,* May 2007. ACR/ARHP. http://www.the-rheumatologist.org/details/article/1304763/have_we_reached_an_estrogen_comfort_zone.html.
28. Schoenfeld SR, Kasturi S, Costenbader KH. The epidemiology of atherosclerotic cardiovascular disease among patients with SLE: a systematic review. *Semin Arthritis Rheum.* 2013;43(1):77–95. doi:http://dx.doi.org/10.1016/j.semarthrit.2012.12.002.
29. Bultink IEM. Osteoporosis and fractures in systemic lupus erythematosus. *Arthritis Care Res.* 2012;64(1):2–8. doi:10.1002/acr.20568.
30. García-Carrasco M, Mendoza-Pinto C, Escárcega RO, et al. Osteoporosis in patients with systemic lupus erythematosus. *IMAJ.* 2009;11:486–491.
31. Grossman JM, Gordon R, Ranganath VK, et al. American College of Rheumatology 2010 recommendations for the prevention and treatment of glucocorticoid-induced osteoporosis. *Arthritis Care Res.* 2010;62(11):1515–1526.
32. Denosumab: mechanism of action. http://www.xgeva.com/hcp/denosumab-mechanism-of-action.html.

4

The Elusive Butterfly Gland—Thyroid Disease

I really had no idea anything was wrong with my thyroid until I literally passed out in the street and had to be taken to the emergency room. The doctors said it was a "thyroid storm." The way they explained it, it was like driving a car with the gas pedal pushed all the way down to the floor. My body was speeding along and just crashed. I had always been a "hyper" person, always active, always fidgety. I had a high pulse rate, I was skinny. But up until I collapsed, I didn't think anything of it. That's just the way I was.

Anne Marie, 36

The thyroid is a butterfly-shaped gland located in the neck, just below your voice box. Although it's small—a little more than two inches wide—the thyroid gland plays a big role in the body. Thyroid hormones influence almost every organ and regulate metabolism, the rate at which the body converts food into energy.

Having thyroid disease is akin to living in a house where the thermostat doesn't work properly—it's either set too high, turning up the heat and making you feel jumpy, or set too low, making you feel cold and tired.

The thyroid is part of the *endocrine system*, a network of glands that secretes hormones right into the blood, rather than piping them in through a network of ducts. The other endocrine glands are the pancreas, the pituitary, the adrenals, the parathyroids, and the ovaries—all of which can be the targets of autoimmune attacks.

The pituitary gland (located in the brain just behind the eyes) is known as the "master gland" because it regulates the other endocrine glands, including the thyroid. The master gland has a master switch, and that's the hypothalamus, a tiny area in the base of the brain connected to the pituitary. Secretion of just the right amount of thyroid hormones is governed by a feedback system between these three structures.

The hypothalamus sends out a hormone called *thyrotropin releasing hormone (TRH)*, which prompts the pituitary to release *thyroid stimulating hormone (TSH)*, triggering the secretion of thyroid hormones by the thyroid gland. There are two thyroid hormones: *thyroxine (T4)* and *triiodothyronine (T3)*. Thyroxine is produced by the follicular cells of the thyroid and converted to T3 by enzymes in various organs (some T3 is produced by the thyroid, too). If thyroid hormones in the bloodstream rise above normal levels, they cause a decrease in TRH and TSH that prompts the thyroid to cut back on the amount of hormones it secretes. If thyroid hormone levels drop below normal, the hypothalamus increases secretion of TRH, which prompts the pituitary to pump out TSH to stimulate the thyroid.

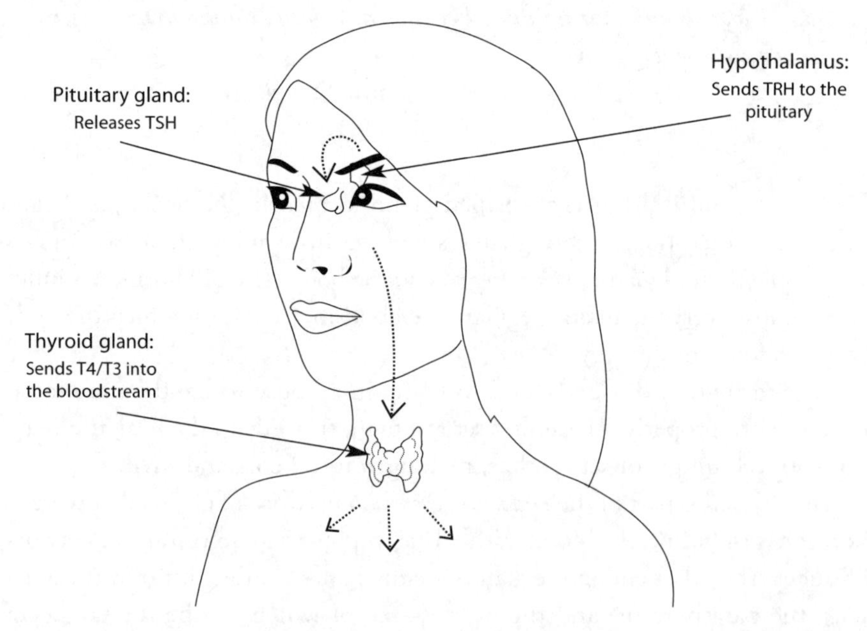

The Thyroid Feedback Loop

This feedback loop is like a thermostat, constantly keeping thyroid hormones at just the right level (this is called *euthyroid*). When the immune system attacks the thyroid, it leads to overproduction or underproduction of thyroid hormones. Either the heat's too high, as excess thyroid hormone speeds up energy use and causes weight loss, hyperactivity, sweating, and nervousness; or the heat's too low, as too little thyroid hormone slows energy use, causing weight gain, fatigue, coldness, and depression.

Thyroid diseases are the most common of all autoimmune diseases, affecting more than 10 million people. *Hashimoto's thyroiditis*, an *under*active thyroid gland, affects 8 to 10 times more women than men.[1] *Graves' disease*, in

Warning Signs of Thyroid Disease

Hashimoto's Thyroiditis (Underactive Thyroid)

- Fatigue
- Intolerance to cold
- Dry skin, dry hair
- Depression
- Unexplained weight gain
- Constipation
- Weakness
- Muscle cramps
- Impaired memory

Graves' Disease (Overactive Thyroid)

- Anxiety, nervousness
- Rapid heartbeat, atrial fibrillation, palpitations
- Trembling hands
- Unexplained weight loss
- Feeling warm, heat intolerance
- Difficulty concentrating
- Muscle weakness
- Brittle or thin hair, hair loss
- Protruding eyes

which the thyroid becomes *over*active, is five times more common in women.[2] Both can lead to infertility and miscarriage, emerge during or after pregnancy and present a threat to an unborn child, and, in older age, be mistaken for signs of aging. Untreated hyperthyroidism can also lead to bone loss, since excess T3 activates bone-eating cells called *osteoclasts*.[3]

What Causes Thyroid Disease?

In Hashimoto's thyroiditis, T cells attack the follicular cells in the thyroid gland, causing inflammation that hampers production of thyroid hormones. Healthy thyroid cells are replaced by lymphocytes and macrophages and, eventually, by scar tissue, so little or no hormones are secreted.[4] Autoantibodies (sometimes called *thyroid autoantibodies*) are directed against the contents of the thyroid cells, either thyroglobulin (TG) or thyroperoxidase (TPO), two proteins needed for the production of thyroid hormones. "Whether these antibodies cause the disease, worsen it, or are simply results of thyroid disease has not been fully established," remarks Noel Rose, MD, PhD, whose initial investigations into the autoimmune basis of thyroid disease in 1956 launched the field of autoimmunity. "Many people have these antibodies with no evidence of clinical disease. So there must be additional factors triggering thyroiditis."

In Graves' disease, antibodies attack receptors for thyroid stimulating hormone on the surface of thyroid follicular cells, triggering overproduction of thyroid hormones.[4] These autoantibodies, *thyrotropin receptor antibodies (TPO)* (also called *thyroid stimulating immunoglobulins* or *thyroid stimulating antibodies*), affect every cell in the thyroid, causing the gland to enlarge as it becomes hyperactive. So Graves' is also called *diffuse toxic goiter*. Antibodies to *thyroglobulin* and *thyroperoxidase* are also found in Graves' disease.

Graves' and Hashimoto's are closely related; women with thyroiditis may eventually develop Graves' and vice versa. "There's a phenomenon we call Hashitoxicosis, where patients with Hashimoto's disease become hyperthyroid because they have the thyroid stimulating antibody as well as the typical thyroid inflammation. And you also have a phenomenon where patients start out hyperthyroid and become hypothyroid," says Dr. Rose, now at the department of pathology at Boston's Brigham and Women's Hospital and a professor at Harvard Medical School. There may be separate autoimmune processes taking place in the thyroid, but one may be clinically dominant over the other, and this may shift over time."

Autoimmune thyroid diseases tend to run in families. It's not uncommon for one family member to have Hashimoto's and another to have Graves' disease. A woman with autoimmune thyroid disease in close relatives may have a five- to tenfold risk of developing thyroid disease. Thyroid diseases frequently occur with other autoimmune diseases (see page 117).

It's still not known just what sets off the process that destroys or overstimulates the thyroid. One possibility is that excess iodine in the diet triggers the autoimmune response. Another theory is that fetal cells that enter a woman's circulation during pregnancy (microchimerism) may play a role in thyroid disease (see page 13). Other factors, such as severe stress or smoking in Graves' disease could be involved.

In some cases, a woman may develop Graves' disease or Hashimoto's during pregnancy or after giving birth (see pages 120 to 121). One report by the American Thyroid Association (ATA) calls pregnancy "a stress test for the thyroid," noting that changes in the gland during this period (and accompanying fluctuations in thyroid hormones) can result in hypothyroidism in women with limited thyroid reserves or who are iodine deficient, and postpartum thyroiditis in women with underlying Hashimoto's who were euthyroid before conceiving.[5] It's thought that the immune system rebound after pregnancy causes production of autoantibodies (or increases levels of previously undetected antibodies), leading to dysfunction of the thyroid.

Symptoms of Hashimoto's Thyroiditis

When your thyroid produces too little thyroid hormone, it not only slows metabolism but also decreases production of body heat. The body tries to conserve heat by diverting blood flow from the skin, which keeps the skin cool and reduces sweating, preventing the loss of body heat. So women with an underactive thyroid often feel cold (even though their body temperature is normal) and look somewhat pale. Skin may become dry, nails and hair may become brittle, and there may even be hair loss on the scalp and elsewhere on the body (including the eyebrows, eyelashes, and pubic hair). Hair loss may be so gradual that you don't even notice it at first.

As the body slows down conversion of food to energy, you may gain weight and feel tired and drowsy. Some of the weight gain comes from fluid accumulation. Muscle contractions in the intestines, which move digested food along for absorption and waste excretion, also slow down, so you may experience hard stools and constipation. An underactive thyroid also leads to elevated cholesterol.

A key symptom of Hashimoto's is depression, and if you have a persistent low mood you should be tested for low thyroid hormones. Depression is also common in women with multiple sclerosis and lupus, as is difficulty concentrating. Clinical depression is a separate illness and does not accompany thyroid disease. However, women being treated with the mood stabilizer lithium for a form of depression called bipolar disorder (manic depression) may develop hypothyroidism.

Nerve problems can also occur in Hashimoto's. You may feel tingling or a pins-and-needles sensation in your hands and feet (which may also occur in MS and other neurological disorders).

Carpal tunnel syndrome can also occur, because of tissue swelling and pressure on the median nerve, which passes through a tunnel-like space in the wrist. Carpal tunnel syndrome causes tingling in the hands and fingers, especially at night. The problem is often blamed on repetitive stress, especially if you work at a computer, but it may in fact be caused by an underactive thyroid. You may also have shortness of breath because of a lowered heart rate, muscle aches or cramps caused by decreased blood flow to the muscles, and slow reflexes. These symptoms may be attributed to a coexisting autoimmune disease.

As Hashimoto's becomes progressively worse, the thyroid can become enlarged, causing a feeling of pressure around the throat when swallowing, so your voice can become hoarse. Menstrual flow can increase and periods may become longer. There may be bleeding between periods and a failure to ovulate, leading to infertility. Women with undiagnosed hypothyroidism are also at risk for miscarriage, premature delivery, stillbirths, and certain birth defects (see pages 118 to 119).

All of these symptoms can come on very gradually. "The reserve of the thyroid is huge. So before you may actually present with symptoms of hypothyroidism, a large proportion of the gland would need to be destroyed," remarks Dr. Rose.

Anne Marie's story continues:

After I collapsed, they tested me for everything under the sun. And it was then that I noticed how much weight I was losing and how much I was eating. I was eating everything and dropping weight so quickly. A pound or so every few days. I weigh 120 now, but eight years ago I maybe weighed 99, 100 pounds. I would feel like I was jumping out of my skin. When I had a "1thyroid storm" I felt a kind of madness, and my pulse was pounding. And I had this stare. My eyes were protruding and I was very self-conscious about it. Now I realize I must have had thyroid symptoms for a long time; they must have started very gradually. After I was told my thyroid was overactive, it all made sense to me. But truthfully, I didn't pay much attention until I had a problem.

Symptoms of Graves' Disease

While Hashimoto's causes a slowing down of body functions, Graves' disease speeds things up. Metabolism increases, causing weight loss. Because the body needs more blood to compensate for increased energy use, the heart must pump faster. So you can have a rapid pulse, palpitations (heightened awareness of a pounding heartbeat in the neck or chest, or a brief episode of rapid heartbeat, even at rest, or a sensation of a skipped heartbeat), sometimes accompanied by shortness of breath.

Excess thyroid hormone can lead to the development of an irregular heartbeat (arrhythmia), including *atrial fibrillation (AF)*, a rapid fluttering of the upper chambers of the heart. AF, which occurs in up to 15 percent of women with an overactive thyroid, can increase the risk of stroke.[6] Because the atria are not pumping properly, blood may stagnate, forming clots that can break off and block blood flow to the brain.

The thyroid "storm" experienced by Anne Marie is very rare—the incidence is thought to be two in one million—but it can be fatal in 11 percent of cases.

As the body produces more heat, sweating increases. If you have an overactive thyroid you may feel warm and flushed and uncomfortable in hot weather or warm environments. The gastrointestinal system speeds up passage of food through the intestines, so bowel movements become more frequent. As metabolism increases, you feel more energetic, even hyperactive, jumpy, or "wired." It can become hard to sit still and concentrate, and you jump from task to task (some women describe this as feeling like their "motor is always running"). You may even talk rapidly. The motor doesn't slow down properly at night, so it may be hard to fall asleep and stay asleep; your mind may still feel like it's racing. Since you don't sleep properly, you can become fatigued.

Muscle weakness is also common, especially in the muscles of the hips, thighs, and shoulders. It can be so bad you may have difficulty raising your arms to brush your hair, climbing stairs, or even getting out of a chair. Changes in the skin and nails also occur. Your nails may grow faster, causing them to get soft and tear easily. Skin feels thin and almost silky, and there may be areas of increased (or decreased) pigmentation. In rare cases, women may develop reddish, lumpy, and thickened skin in front of the shins, just above the ankles (*pretibial myxedema*).[2]

Hair becomes softer and finer and may begin to fall out. Hair loss may be related to another autoimmune disease, alopecia areata, which causes roundish bald spots on the scalp (pages 160 to 166). But more often, it's thinning hair, which can be extensive. Treatment with thyroid hormone usually stops hair loss.

The emotional symptoms of Graves' include irritability and wide mood swings. Small annoyances may set off a major reaction. Or you may act manic, with bursts of energy and intense activity. Since this can also be a sign of bipolar disorder, if no other symptoms of hyperthyroidism are present, an evaluation by a mental health professional may be needed.

The thyroid gland often becomes enlarged in Graves' disease, but may not cause discomfort. In severe cases, where the thyroid grows three to four times its normal size, you may have a feeling of pressure in the neck when swallowing or turning your head.

Menstrual flow may become lighter if you have Graves' disease, and periods may become shorter; some women may stop having periods altogether (page 118).

The hallmark symptom of Graves' disease is eye inflammation and the development of protruding eyes (*Graves' ophthalmopathy*). This occurs in about 50 percent of women with Graves' as the eyes are pushed forward because of swelling and inflammation of muscles around the eye and tissues behind the eyeballs. It can cause major vision loss if it damages the optic nerve. Increased pressure behind the eye hampers normal blood and fluid drainage, causing swelling of the tissues around the eye and aching or pressure. The eyes may also be red and inflamed. Weakened eye muscles can hamper movement of the eyes, leading to double vision or impaired vision. Eyelids may not close completely at night over protruding eyeballs, causing the cornea to become dry and prone to ulcerations. The severity of these problems usually has nothing to do with the degree of hyperthyroidism and may even occur without significant elevation of thyroid hormones.[2]

Symptoms may gradually get better over 6 to 12 months, but there's no way to predict whether eye problems will improve. Inflammation is usually not permanent, and less than 1 percent of women have serious or permanent problems. Most often, problems are mild, requiring artificial tears to prevent dryness; more severe cases may necessitate steroid medications, radiation therapy, or surgery (see pages 114 to 115).

Diagnosing Thyroid Disease

A diagnosis is made by examining the thyroid gland and doing key blood tests. The thyroid becomes enlarged in both Hashimoto's thyroiditis and Graves' disease, but feels different in each. In Hashimoto's, the gland feels hard and rubbery (sometimes pebbly in texture); in Graves' it feels smooth and soft to firm in texture. During your physical examination, your doctor will palpate the thyroid, often while having you slowly swallow a cup of water, and listen with a stethoscope for a sound called a *bruit*, caused by increased blood flow in the thyroid (characteristic of Graves' disease).

Other signs like cold, dry skin or hand tremor and a fast pulse rate, along with clinical symptoms (such as depression or anxiety), will usually point to a specific diagnosis, but blood tests to assess thyroid function are needed to confirm it.

Tests You May Need and What They Mean

A complete blood count (CBC) and metabolic profile are needed to rule out anemia, abnormal liver function, excess calcium in the blood (*hypercalcemia*), and other possible causes of symptoms.

Thyroid stimulating hormone (TSH) levels are the best indicator of thyroid function. TSH is increased in women with hypothyroidism and is low or undetectable in women with hyperthyroidism, says Dr. Rose. The most sensitive test, capable of detecting very low levels of TSH, is called a third generation assay. The normal range for TSH is 0.4 to 5.5 micro international units per milliliter of blood (μ IU/ml), but ideally a young, healthy person should have a TSH below 3.0. A woman with hyperthyroidism usually has a TSH below 0.1 μ IU/ml; in hypothyroidism, TSH is elevated above 5 μ IU/ml.

Total and free thyroxine (T4) are measured separately. A test for total T4 measures all of the circulating thyroxine; a test for free T4 measures only the biologically active thyroxine (the amount that is not bound up by serum-binding proteins and can attach to hormone receptors in cells). The normal reference range for free T4 in nonpregnant women is 0.8 to 2.7 nanograms per deciliter of blood (ng/dl). The normal range for total serum T4 is 4.5 to 12.5 micrograms per deciliter of blood (mcg/dl). A woman with Graves' disease would have a total T4 above 12 mcg/dl; a hypothyroid woman would have a T4 below 5 mcg/dl.

Total triiodothyronine (T3) measures the amount of circulating T3, which can be influenced by factors that change levels of thyroxine-binding globulin, including estrogen. Normal levels of T3 range from 0.4 to 4.2 μ IU/ml. This blood test may only be done if additional information is needed about thyroid function.

Thyroid antibody blood tests look for autoantibodies to components of the thyroid cells (thyroid antibodies), such as antibodies to *thyroglobulin (TG)* and *thyroperoxidase (TPO)*. "More than 80 percent of women with Hashimoto's disease also have antibodies to thyroid peroxidase," says Dr. Rose. "Since they are not overlapping almost all Hashimoto patients have antibodies to one or the other, or both thyroid specific antigens."

Antibodies against the TSH receptor (TRAbs) are found in the blood of almost everyone with untreated Graves'. Serum TRAbs, along with elevated TSH and signs of Graves' ophthalmopathy, can confirm a diagnosis.[2]

Radioactive iodine uptake (RAIU) may normally be ordered if a woman has thyroid nodules or a goiter (and may be done in conjunction with a thyroid scan). The iodine that we take in from food is absorbed by the thyroid gland and is a key building block of thyroid hormones. The test involves giving a small amount of oral radioactive iodine and measuring the amount absorbed by the thyroid gland; the normal range of absorption is 8 to 30 percent after 24 hours.[2] Radioactive iodine will be elevated above 30 percent in women with Graves' disease. It will also be elevated in postpartum thyroiditis, and in women taking replacement thyroid hormone.

A thyroid scan uses a special detector that's able to see how much radioactive iodine has been taken up by the thyroid and how evenly it's dispersed in thyroid cells. If the radioactive iodine is taken up by the entire thyroid, it rules out the possibility that overactive nodules are causing hyperthyroidism. A benign nodule producing too much thyroid hormone will be "hot" on the scan, in contrast to a "cold," hypofunctioning nodule, which can be benign or malignant.[2]

Ultrasound examination of the thyroid may be done if your doctor feels nodules when examining your thyroid. Ultrasound uses sound waves to create pictures of thyroid nodules felt on examination to determine whether they are solid or fluid-filled (it can also show nodules that can't be felt).

Needle aspiration biopsy may be performed if a nodule looks suspicious. In this procedure, a small needle is inserted into the nodule to withdraw a small amount of fluid or cells for analysis. This test is 90 percent accurate in detecting cancer. Most of the time, these nodules turn out to be benign. A recent study found that, during five years of follow-up, cancer was found in only 0.3 percent of thyroid nodules.[7]

Anne Marie's story continues:

After I was diagnosed with Graves' disease, they gave me drugs to slow down my thyroid. I would go through periods of feeling very tired and periods of feeling very awake, hyper-awake. Then they ablated my thyroid with radioactive iodine. You go into a hospital, down to nuclear medicine, and they give you this tablet. It looks like an ordinary pill, but it's radioactive. And it made me feel very strange. It makes you feel like you're sweating out of your pores, you feel lethargic, kind of out of it. At least that's how I felt. I had some thyroid tissue left over after the ablation, and it was very hard to regulate my thyroid. I needed blood tests every few weeks. But I take my thyroid pill religiously every day. Sometimes my numbers are out of whack and they have to give me less, and sometimes they have to up the dose. It's been a long process.

Treating Autoimmune Thyroid Disease

Treating an underactive thyroid is very straightforward: giving replacement thyroid hormones. Graves' disease is easily treated, but several steps may be needed.

Treating Hashimoto's Thyroiditis

Hypothyroidism is treated with synthetic *levothyroxine sodium (synthetic T4)* to normalize levels of thyroid hormone. The goal of treatment is not only euthyroid blood levels of thyroid hormones but also the resolution of signs and symptoms. You want to feel "well." According to 2014 treatment guidelines from the American Thyroid Association (ATA), "steady-state" levels of thyroid hormones in your body are generally reached about six weeks after you start therapy. The goal is to be within the "reference ranges" (average blood levels) of TSH.[8]

It may take some time to find the right dose for you. If the dose isn't high enough, hypothyroid symptoms may persist and your cholesterol may rise. If the dose is too high, you may develop symptoms of an overactive thyroid, as well as heart rhythm problems or even bone loss. This may be more pronounced in older women.[8] So, generally doses are gradually increased until blood levels of TSH are in the normal, euthyroid, range and your symptoms resolve.

One may not always accompany the other, the ATA acknowledges; some women may not notice differences between dose levels while others may not feel "well" on a dose that produces thyroid hormone levels within the normal range. Since symptoms like cold sensitivity and sluggishness and signs such as dry skin can't be measured as hormone levels can, blood tests play a key role in determining your dose.[8] There are also physiological signs such as heart rate, as well as symptoms like depression or anxiety levels, that can be monitored. But you'll have to work closely with your endocrinologist to achieve the best quality of life. Annual physical exams and blood tests are needed to make sure thyroid hormone levels stay in the normal range and symptoms haven't returned.

Hashimoto's goiters may shrink by almost a third over a two-year period with T4 supplementation. Around 10 percent of women may have a spontaneous remission four to eight years after starting treatment. But in some cases thyroid failure is progressive, and levothyroxine doses may need to be increased as the thyroid continues to slow down.

Levothyroxine is sold by prescription under a number of brand names, including *Synthroid*, *Levothroid*, and *Levoxyl*. According to the ATA, if you start on a brand name and are doing well, you should stick to that brand. As for generics, given changing drug formularies within the same insurance company, there's no way to assure that you'll get the same formulation each time. "Bioequivalence is not therapeutic equivalence" and "switching of products could lead to perturbations in serum TSH," the ATA guidelines state. If a change in product is made, thyroid function tests should be rechecked, the treatment guidelines advise.[8]

The ATA also recommends that levothyroxine be taken an hour before breakfast or at bedtime (three hours after any evening snack) to ensure the best absorption. Fiber and soy may impair absorption, as can that morning cup of coffee (another reason to take it at bedtime).[8]

The absorption of levothyroxine be impaired by other drugs, including male hormones (*androgens*); antacids containing *aluminum hydroxide* (such as *Rolaids*); acid reducers called proton pump inhibitors (PPIs) such as Nexium; antidepressants like *fluoxetine (Prozac)*, *amitriptyline (Elavil)*, and *phenelzine sulfate (Nardil)*; blood thinners such as *warfarin (Coumadin)*; insulin; digitalis-type drugs such as *digoxin (Lanoxin)*; iron supplements; *cholestyramine (Colestid, Questran)*; calcium supplements; and multivitamins containing calcium and iron. So take your thyroid hormones separately, the ATA advises.[8]

Postmenopausal women taking hormone therapy (HT) may need higher doses of thyroid hormone (see page 122).

You'll need periodic bone scans after menopause to check for bone loss, and because mild thyroid hormone excess over many years may increase the risk for heart rhythm problems, you may also need periodic electrocardiograms.

Both the ATA and the American Association of Clinical Endocrinologists (AACE) recommend against taking dietary supplements that claim to enhance thyroid function.[9]

Treating Graves' Disease

In Graves' disease, the overactive thyroid gland must be calmed down or destroyed, and then replacement thyroid hormone is given.

Antithyroid drugs, including *propylthiouracil (PTU)* and *methimazole (Tapazole)*, make it harder for the thyroid to use iodine to make thyroid hormone, which lowers secretion of thyroxine. PTU and methimazole are typically used in mild Graves' disease (or when Graves' occurs in children or young adults) and are often prescribed for elderly women who also have heart disease.[10] Women over age 65 who have chest pain or irregular heart rhythms may suffer heart damage if they become more hyperthyroid. PTU is given three times a day, methimazole is given once a day.[10]

Treatment with radioiodine (page 113) may temporarily boost levels of thyroid hormone; giving antithyroid drugs prevents this increase.[10] Between 20 and 30 percent of women with early, mild Graves' disease will experience a prolonged remission after 12 to 18 months of treatment with antithyroid drugs. As many as 40 percent of patients may have a permanent remission.

However, PTU and similar drugs sometimes provoke allergic reactions. About 5 percent of women may develop skin rashes, hives, or, less commonly, fever and joint pain. In some cases, these drugs may cause a decrease in certain white blood cells (neutrophils), which may increase the risk of infections. In rare instances, white cells may actually disappear entirely, causing *agranulocytosis*, which can be fatal if you get a serious infection. If you're taking an antithyroid drug and develop an infection (such as strep throat), call your doctor immediately and ask if you need to get a white blood cell count. If white blood cells have been decreased, stopping the drug can return the neutrophil count to normal. During therapy you should also avoid immunizations with live virus vaccines,[11] as methimazole can lower the body's resistance and may lead to the very infections vaccines are designed to prevent.

These drugs may also cause liver problems. Signs of trouble can include jaundice (skin and white of eyes turn yellow and urine turns darker), joint pain, fever, nausea, and abdominal pain. PTU and MMI can also cause an itchy rash or sore throat (pharyngitis).[10]

If you go into remission, antithyroid drugs will be continued for another year or two. Signs of a remission include a decrease in the size of the thyroid and a near-normal or higher TSH. But neither is a reliable predictor, and more than half of patients will develop a recurrence within five years. You'll need to be monitored by your doctor every three months for the first year of treatment and annually after that.

Radioiodine/radioactive iodine (or iodide) accumulates in the thyroid and damages thyroid cells, reducing the amount of hormone-producing tissue. Radioactive iodine emits two types of radiation: *gamma rays*, which travel through tissue and can be seen with a special detector (as in thyroid scans); and *beta rays,* which travel only a few millimeters and are absorbed by thyroid cells. The beta rays don't kill the thyroid cells but cause enough inflammation and DNA damage to prevent them from producing too much thyroxine and from reproducing. The dose is determined by how much radioactive iodine is absorbed by the thyroid during an uptake test.

Radioactive iodine is given in capsule form (taken with lots of water). Within 24 to 48 hours, most of the radioactive iodine will be taken up by the thyroid, and the remainder is excreted in urine (or decays into a nonradioactive state). The level of radioactivity of the iodide left in the thyroid declines by 50 percent every five to seven days. It's not going to be harmful to family members, but it might be wise to limit contact with infants and pregnant women for the first week after taking the radioisotopes, just to be safe.

Because of increased inflammation (and possibly increased autoantibodies) in the thyroid caused by radioactive iodine, secretion of thyroxine will be greater for a few weeks, and may heighten symptoms, especially in older women and those with heart disease (for that reason, antithyroid drugs are given beforehand). You'll likely begin to improve in three to six months, but there's a chance you may remain hyperthyroid and need a second or third dose.[10] A majority of women become hypothyroid after treatment and need replacement thyroid hormone.

The word *radioactive* may sound scary, but no serious complications from treatment have been seen in 50 years of using the drug. In fact, more than 70 percent of American adults with hyperthyroidism are treated with radioactive iodine, with no increased risk of cancer.

If you plan to become pregnant, you must wait three to six months after treatment before trying to conceive.[10] This is to ensure your baby will not be exposed to radioactive iodine, which can cause developmental problems and destroy the baby's thyroid.

Thyroidectomy, surgical removal of the thyroid, may be advised if you're allergic to antithyroid drugs, don't wish to take radioactive iodine, have a large goiter, or are pregnant.[10] First, hyperthyroid symptoms need to be brought under control with an antithyroid drug or a beta-blocker (which controls the effects of too much thyroid hormone), so that there is not an abrupt increase in hormones. The drugs are usually given a week or two prior to surgery. Surgery cures hyperthyroidism, but you still can become hypothyroid afterward and will need yearly blood tests to measure thyroid function and levothyroxine.

Beta-blockers may be needed if you're undergoing any of these treatments to reduce symptoms until the therapy takes full effect. These drugs—including *propranolol (Inderal)*, *atenolol (Tenormin)*, or *metoprolol (Lopressor)* block the effects of circulating thyroid hormone in the body, helping to slow heart rate and lessen anxiety and nervousness. Patients who can't take beta-blockers include women with asthma and heart failure (which may be worsened by beta-blockers) and people with diabetes who take insulin (because symptoms of low blood sugar may be masked while on these drugs).

Treating Graves' Ophthalmopathy

Most of the time, Graves' ophthalmopathy is a mild problem that does not damage the cornea or impair vision. However, if your lids do not completely close, your eyes can dry out at night. Special adhesive tapes normally used for first aid can be used to tape the lids closed while you sleep, or you can wear an eye patch. Artificial tears can also be used during the day for added lubrication (see pages 184 to 185), side panels for glasses lessen air flow around the eyes to prevent dry eye, and tinted glasses can ease light sensitivity.

Surgery to remove swollen tissue and decrease the opening of the eyes can lessen the appearance of a prominent stare. You'll need to consult an ophthalmologist to determine the type of surgery and its timing.

Corticosteroids are used to reduce inflammation and lessen swelling of tissue around the eye in cases of severe congestive ophthalmopathy. Oral steroids such as *prednisone (Deltasone)* and *methylprednisolone (Medrol)* can be used for short periods of time, or in low doses for longer periods to relieve redness, swelling, and eye pain. Side effects include weight gain, muscle weakness, and, with long-term treatment, an increased risk of osteoporosis, bone fractures, diabetes, high blood pressure, and infection (discussed on pages 42 to 43).

Radiation therapy, which directs low doses of radiation to the area around the eyeball, has been widely used for decades, but the actual benefits of the procedure are still uncertain.[12] In recent years it has been used less frequently and may be done only when corticosteroids are no longer effective.

Corrective eye surgery removes or repairs swollen muscles around the eye that can cause pressure on the optic nerve and double vision. The surgery should be performed by an ophthalmic surgeon only after ophthalmopathy has been stable for three to six months.

Orbital decompression surgery, which enlarges the bony opening around the eyes to provide more space for the eye and eye muscles, is done only when other treatments fail.

Risk factors for Graves' ophthalmopathy include smoking, radioiodine therapy for hyperthyroidism, and hypothyroidism following radioiodine treatment.[10]

The Female Factor

While the ratio of males to females is about equal in juvenile thyroiditis, after puberty it's more common in females, suggesting that female hormones play a role in thyroid disease.

Estrogen and progesterone both exacerbate thyroid inflammation, and thyroiditis can be reversed with testosterone, as shown in experiments with mice bred to have an animal model called *experimental autoimmune thyroiditis (EAT)*. "When the testes were removed in the mice and we gave them estrogen, they became more susceptible to thyroiditis. When we removed the ovaries of the female mice and gave them testosterone, they became less susceptible to thyroiditis," says Dr. Rose.

During pregnancy autoimmune thyroiditis gets better, but in the year after giving birth it worsens. Some studies show that in women with mild thyroid inflammation, the increased immune response after pregnancy (remember, the immune system has modulated its responses to tolerate and protect the growing fetus)[13] tips the balance and may cause thyroid dysfunction (*postpartum thyroiditis*). And up to 25 percent of women may develop a permanent autoimmune hypothyroidism within 10 years after delivery. There's also an increased risk of developing Graves' disease in the postpartum period. However, estrogen is not the whole story. There are other hormonal influences, such as stress hormones, that may come into play.

Fetal cells that enter the maternal circulation during pregnancy may contribute to autoimmune thyroid disease, says Terry F. Davies, MD, the Florence and Theodore Baumritter Professor of Medicine at the Mount Sinai School of Medicine in New York and Director of their Division of Endocrinology and Metabolism at the James J. Peters VA Medical Center. In one study of mice, Dr. Davies's research team found fetal cells in the thyroid glands of mice with EAT during pregnancy and the postpartum period but none in mice without EAT. Dr. Davies and other researchers have also isolated cells containing the male chromosome in thyroid tissue from women undergoing thyroid surgery who had previously given birth to boys.

"The theory is that during pregnancy the fetal cells actually suppress thyroid disease, in the same way that the immune system is suppressed and doesn't attack the fetus. And that may be why the thyroid disease improves during pregnancy," explains Dr. Davies. "Once the placenta and the baby are gone, then the number of fetal cells starts to fall rapidly and their ability to suppress the thyroid disease decreases, and you get a recurrence."

The fetal cells may be attracted to the thyroid by inflammation. "The inflammation would be organ specific. If you start off with thyroid inflammation, thyroiditis, fetal cells may accumulate in the thyroid. If you start out with beta cell destruction in diabetes, then fetal cells may be attracted to the pancreas," he adds.

However, the exact relationship between fetal cells and autoimmune thyroid disease is still unknown, as is the relationship between environmental factors such as stress or infections and female hormones.

It wasn't until years after I was diagnosed with Hashimoto's that I found out I had a strong family history of thyroid disease. My father had a goiter, one of his first cousins had Graves' disease, and another has Hashimoto's. Their children also had thyroid disease; one of them also has lupus. But until I asked questions, no one had ever mentioned it. It wasn't regarded as important, not like if someone had cancer. I got my period late, around age 14, and maybe that was the beginning of it. My mother took me to a gynecologist, who couldn't find anything wrong. Back then, and we're talking maybe 50 years ago, no one even thought to look. Now I know Hashimoto's can occur when you are a teenager.

Lynne, 67

Thyroid Disease Clusters

Hypothyroidism is very common in other autoimmune diseases; up to 30 percent of women with type 1 diabetes may develop thyroid disease after many years.

Among the diseases that cluster with thyroid problems:

- Rheumatoid arthritis
- Myasthenia gravis
- Lupus
- Type 1 (insulin-dependent) diabetes
- Sjögren's syndrome
- Vitiligo
- Alopecia areata
- Pernicious anemia (an inability to absorb vitamin B_2 in the stomach)
- Addison's disease (adrenal insufficiency)
- Primary ovarian insufficiency (formerly called premature ovarian failure)
- Celiac disease
- Primary biliary cirrhosis

How Thyroid Disease Can Affect You Over Your Lifetime

Menstruation and Fertility

Women with Hashimoto's thyroiditis often have heavier periods that last for longer than a week. They may also have bleeding between periods because of a failure to ovulate (*anovulation*). Normally, the ovaries are stimulated to produce an egg in the first part of the menstrual cycle, the follicular phase. After ovulation, in the luteal phase, the uterine lining builds up an extra layer of blood vessels in preparation for a fertilized egg. If pregnancy doesn't occur, the lining is shed as menstrual flow. In Hashimoto's, the normal hormonal feedback between the ovaries, the pituitary, and the hypothalamus is disrupted. So a woman may fail to ovulate, but the uterine lining will continue to be stimulated, so bleeding can occur outside the normal cycle. Anovulation is common in hypothyroidism.

Hashimoto's is also associated with primary ovarian insufficiency (POI), (formerly called premature ovarian failure, see pages 231 to 233). In women with Graves' disease, an increase in metabolism causes a decrease in menstrual flow and a shorter cycle. A woman whose period normally lasted four or five days may see it decrease to two or three days. In severe hyperthyroidism, some women stop having periods altogether.

Taking oral contraceptives containing estrogen can also increase the amount of *serum thyroxine binding globulin*, which makes T4 less available to cells. Women with normal thyroid function will secrete more thyroxine to compensate, but women with Hashimoto's can't produce the extra T4, remarks Dr. Rose. This also occurs during pregnancy, mainly due to increased estrogen levels, and in women taking estrogen therapy (ET) after menopause (see page 122).

Pregnancy

Pregnancy has a number of effects on the thyroid gland due to hormones (especially the pregnancy hormone hCG) and the body's increased metabolic needs.

The thyroid actually expands in size by 10 percent during pregnancy, even in women with sufficient dietary iodine intake. Iodine reserves keep levels stable during pregnancy, but some women may need supplements. Circulating T4, freeT4, and thyroid-binding globulin (TBG) increase between six and eight weeks after conception.[14] As a consequence, women have lower serum TSH concentrations during pregnancy, especially during the first trimester. This is usually temporary and may be related to hCG levels. Serum TSH and the reference range gradually rise in the second and third trimesters. So the "reference ranges" used to judge test results are different during each trimester.[11]

Until the fetal thyroid gland is developed, at approximately 12 weeks' gestation, the mother's thyroid is the only source of thyroid hormone for the baby (transferred through the placenta and amniotic fluid). If you were diagnosed with thyroid disease before you conceived, you'll need to be monitored closely during pregnancy. If you're hypothyroid, you'll probably need to have your thyroid hormone dose increased by an average of 45 percent to normalize TSH. "I recommend that pregnant women with thyroiditis have their TSH checked once every six weeks," says Mount Sinai's Dr. Terry F. Davies.

Women being treated for hypothyroidism usually require a higher dose of levothyroxine early in the first trimester of pregnancy. An extra dose may be recommended as soon as a woman knows she's pregnant.[11]

However, TSH can also *increase* in up to 3 percent of women, so pregnancy can trigger temporary hypothyroidism and, in some cases, Hashimoto's. Hypothyroidism during pregnancy is associated with complications including premature birth, low birthweight babies, possible miscarriage, and even later fertility problems.[11]

Persistently low TSH can lead to gestational hyperthyroidism. Preexisting Graves' may also be diagnosed for the first time during pregnancy.

So if you're thinking of getting pregnant, thyroid hormones must be monitored. The optimal time to conceive is when you're euthyroid.

The U.S. Preventive Services Task Force (USPSTF) and the Endocrine Society recommend that all women who are "high risk" for thyroid disease should be tested for elevated TSH, including women currently taking levothyroxine and women with a goiter or known thyroid antibodies.[15]

The recommendations include not only all women over age 30 with a family history of autoimmune thyroid disease or hypothyroidism, but also women with type 1 diabetes, infertility, or a prior history of preterm delivery. Women who've had prior radiation therapy to the head or neck or prior thyroid surgery should also be tested.

If you're being treated for hypothyroidism, you'll probably need to have your thyroid hormone dose increased by an average of 45 percent to normalize TSH. According to the ATA, you may need testing every four weeks during the first half of pregnancy and at least once during weeks 26 and 32 of your pregnancy. Once you deliver, your dose of levothyroxine will be reduced to your prepregnancy level, with TSH testing done every six weeks.[11]

If you have Graves' disease and are being treated with the antithyroid drug PTU, this will continue during pregnancy. Exposure to methimazole has been associated with birth defects during the first trimester,[16] so switching to PTU is recommended.[11]

Until the fetal thyroid gland is developed, at approximately 12 weeks' gestation, the mother's thyroid is the only source of thyroid hormone for the baby (transferred through the placenta and amniotic fluid). If you were diagnosed with thyroid disease before you conceived you'll need to be monitored closely during pregnancy.

Untreated thyroid disease during pregnancy may negatively affect a child's psychological development. In Graves' disease, thyroid stimulating hormone receptor antibodies can cross the placenta and cause neonatal hyperthyroidism. Women with untreated thyroid deficiency during pregnancy may be up to four times more likely to have children with lower IQ scores, as well as deficits in motor skills, attention, language, and reading abilities, according to a landmark 1999 study from Harvard. In the study, 19 percent of the children born to mothers with undetected hypothyroidism scored 85 or lower on the IQ testing, compared to only 5 percent of children born to women without thyroid disease. (Scores below 85 typically signal that a child will have difficulty in school.)

Radioactive iodine is not given until six weeks after a woman stops breastfeeding, to make sure there's no residual radioactivity concentrated in breast tissue.[10]

Infants can develop a temporary form of *neonatal thyroid disease*, which is related to the transfer across the placenta of antibodies from the mother. It's a rare condition that occurs in 1 to 5 percent of babies born to women with Graves' disease. Research from Japan has found that a subset of women with autoimmune thyroiditis make what are called *TSH inhibiting antibodies*, and these antibodies can cross the placenta, resulting in transient hypothyroidism in the baby. In Graves' disease, stimulating antibodies also cross the placenta, temporarily causing an overactive thyroid in the baby. However, all infants are routinely screened for thyroid problems.

There are no increased instances of birth defects in children born to mothers who took radioactive iodine and waited the recommended six months before becoming pregnant. Women who have trouble conceiving because of hyperthyroidism often have fertility restored after treatment.

Postpartum Thyroid Disease

Some women have antithyroid antibodies in their blood for years, but never develop a problem until after giving birth. Immune function is modulated during pregnancy, and the normal rebound after delivery may elevate levels of antithyroid antibodies during between three and eight months postpartum.[11]

In some women, this may not produce noticeable symptoms. Others may blame their symptoms on normal fatigue, the "baby blues," or postpartum depression. "I think thyroiditis is much more common than is reported, because a lot of postpartum depression may actually be postpartum thyroiditis," remarks Dr. Noel Rose. And postpartum depression can be worsened by thyroiditis.

If the thyroid gland is severely inflamed, it may become overactive, causing a sudden onset of hyperthyroid symptoms. Once the thyroid hormone stored in the gland is depleted, hypothyroidism sets in. In some women, the thyroid may eventually normalize. Symptoms typically last six months or less.[11]

As many as 8 to 10 percent of women may develop thyroid problems after giving birth. Radioactive iodine uptake will be low in women with postpartum thyroid inflammation; in women with Graves' disease there will be an increased uptake of radioactive iodine due to overproduction of thyroid hormone. Before the test, breast-feeding should be discontinued for three to five days, as radioactive iodine can pass into breast milk. Having a prior episode of postpartum thyroiditis increases the risk of recurrence with each pregnancy. Women with recurrent postpartum thyroiditis have a 20 to 30 percent chance of developing permanent hypothyroidism 5 to 10 years afterward. Antithyroid antibodies may help identify women at increased risk.

The hyperthyroid phase of postpartum thyroiditis doesn't usually require treatment, but symptoms such as palpitations and nervousness can be treated with the beta-blocker propranolol.[11] If other symptoms develop, TSH should be tested every four to six weeks.

Hypothyroidism will require replacement thyroid hormone for 6 to 12 months. If you have a goiter, it will usually shrink in response to treatment. Only tiny amounts of thyroid hormone pass into breast milk, so you can continue taking it while breast-feeding.

Hypothyroidism may become permanent after pregnancy in as many as 30 percent of women who have a preexisting problem, says Dr. Rose. So treatment is usually stopped for four to six weeks in order to do blood tests for T4 and TSH to determine whether the hypothyroidism has resolved. Women may need annual thyroid testing to see whether a thyroid problem recurs.

The ATA recommends that women experiencing postpartum depression have their thyroid hormone levels checked, since depression is associated with hypothyroidism.[11]

Menopause

As many as 14 percent of women will develop subclinical hypothyroidism (below clinical cutoffs) in the years just before and after menopause, mostly due to Hashimoto's.

During perimenopause, production of estrogen and progesterone becomes erratic and may disrupt pituitary-thyroid function and even interfere with the action of thyroid hormones. Autoantibody production might also increase. "It's really not clear what is going on. The age, sex, and postpartum distribution suggest that there's some connection between the immune system and the endocrine system," remarks Dr. Rose.

Hypothyroid symptoms, especially depression, may be mistakenly attributed to perimenopause or menopause, he adds. Therefore many experts say routine screening for underactive thyroid may be needed at menopause and afterward.

Menopausal women taking hormones may need an increased dose of levothyroxine. A small but important study in the *New England Journal of Medicine* in 2001 looked at the effects of estrogen therapy on pituitary-thyroid function in 11 postmenopausal women with normal thyroids and 25 women being treated for chronic hypothyroidism. In the normal women, ET produced an increase in thyroxine-binding globulin, prompting an increase in thyroxine production. But in those with hypothyroidism, there was a significant drop in the amount of free thyroxine, requiring an increased dose of medication.

An accompanying editorial suggested that in women taking thyroid hormones, thyroid function should be checked after starting ET and the dose of levothyroxine adjusted accordingly. Conversely, if a woman discontinues ET, her dose of thyroid medication may need to be reduced.

Thyroid Disease in Later Life

Thyroid hormone production and metabolism change during normal aging.[17] Some studies estimate that up to 16 percent of women over the age of 60 have elevated TSH (often with antithyroid antibodies), even if they don't have symptoms of hypothyroidism.[18] One study suggested that 20 percent of these women will develop Hashimoto's. The risk is greatest if TSH is high and antithyroid antibodies are present.

Symptoms may be difficult to recognize in older women. Depression, dry skin, hearing loss, muscle cramps, numbness and weakness of the hands, unsteadiness of gait, anemia, and constipation may simply be blamed on aging. Hyperthyroidism can also be easily overlooked. Few of the classic symptoms, such as an enlarged thyroid, may be present in older women. Additional symptoms may include shortness of breath, palpitations, depression, nervousness, and muscle weakness.[14]

Studies indicate that hypothyroidism in later life can be associated with impaired memory and concentration, as well as problems with language and "executive function," your ability to reason, solve problems, balance your checkbook, and plan things.[13] Trouble is, those are also signs of mild cognitive impairment (MCI), a precursor to Alzheimer's disease, and of Alzheimer's itself. The same is true for late life depression. So experts in geriatric medicine suggest people experiencing memory problems or depression have their thyroid hormones tested as part of a medical workup. Hypothyroidism is treatable—and its cognitive and mood problems are reversible.

The risk of atrial fibrillation (AF) increases with age but is greater among women with Graves', with AF affecting 25 to 40 percent of hyperthyroid women after age 60.[6]

Because AF causes blood to stagnate and form clots leading to strokes, blood thinners (including aspirin) are usually prescribed. Beta-blockers such as propranolol are used to regulate abnormal heart rhythms. ATA guidelines recommend that older women with Grave's disease undergo a cardiac evaluation, including an echocardiogram (ultrasound imaging of the heart), an electrocardiogram (ECG), or Holter monitoring to monitor heart rhythms over time.[10]

The notion of preventing problems normally associated with aging with thyroid hormones remains controversial.

What's not debatable is that treatment of hypothyroidism needs to be adjusted in later life. Levothyroxine is metabolized and excreted more slowly in older women, so smaller doses may be needed. Antithyroid drugs are often used before radioactive iodine treatment in older women, especially if they have other medical problems, such as chest pain (*angina*) or AF.

Radioactive iodine can trigger a temporary rise in thyroid hormone that can cause complications or heart damage. Beta-blockers may also be needed to dampen the effects of excess thyroid hormone before treatment with radioactive iodine.

All patients over age 65 need long-term follow-up with annual blood tests for TSH and T4 because thyroid function may continue to decline as years go by.

Bone Loss

After age 50, one in three women and one in five men may experience a fracture of the spine, hip, or wrist,[19] and the risk rises with hyperthyroidism and other autoimmune disorders (such as RA and lupus) as well as medications used to treat them, particularly corticosteroids like prednisone (see pages 57 to 58).

Thyroid hormones have a direct effect on bone. There are TSH receptors on both types of cells involved in bone growth and remodeling—*osteoclasts*, which break down bone tissue, and *osteoblasts*, which build it back up.[3] One study suggests that when antibodies to these receptors (TRAbs) are elevated, the effect of TSH on bone may be reduced or even blocked, increasing bone breakdown (*resorption*).[20]

This is compounded after menopause, when bone resorption is speeded by the absence of estrogen. The study also suggests bone loss is worsened if Graves' disease arises during the vulnerable period just before and after menopause.[15]

So it's important to detect, treat, and monitor thyroid disease—at every stage of life.

Notes

1. Caturegli P, De Remigis A, Rose N. Hashimoto thyroiditis: clinical and diagnostic criteria. *Autoimmun Rev.* 2014;13:391–397. http://dx.doi.org/10.1016/j.autrev.2014.01.007.
2. Menconi F, Marcocci C, Marinò M. Diagnosis and classification of Graves' disease. *Autoimmun Rev.* 2014;13:398–402. http://dx.doi.org/10.1016/j.autrev.2014.01.013.
3. Tuchendler D, Bolanowski M. The influence of thyroid dysfunction on bone metabolism. *Thyroid Res.* 2014;7:12. doi:10.1186/s13044-014-0012-0.

4. Rose N, Mackay I, eds. *The Autoimmune Diseases.* 5th ed. Academic Press (Elsevier, New York); 2014:557, chap 40. doi: http://dx.doi.org/10.1016/B978-0-12-384929-8.00040-X.
5. Stagnaro-Green A, Abalovich M, Alexander E, et al. The American Thyroid Association Taskforce on thyroid disease during pregnancy and postpartum: guidelines of the American Thyroid Association for the diagnosis and management of thyroid disease during pregnancy and postpartum. *Thyroid.* 2011;21(10):1081–1125.
6. Bielecka-Dabrowal A, Mikhailidis DP, Rysz J, Banach M. The mechanisms of atrial fibrillation in hyperthyroidism. *Thyroid Res.* 2009;2:4. doi:10.1186/1756-6614-2-4.
7. Durante C, Costante G, Lucisano G, et al. Natural history of benign thyroid nodules. *JAMA.* 2015;313(9):927–935.
8. Jonklaas J, Bianco AC, Bauer AJ, et al. Guidelines for the treatment of hypothyroidism: prepared by the American Thyroid Association Task Force on thyroid hormone replacement. *Thyroid.* 2014;24(12):1670–1751. doi:10.1089/thy.2014.0028.
9. Garber JR, Cobin RH, Gharib H, et al. Clinical practice guidelines for hypothyroidism in adults: co-sponsored by the American Association of Clinical Endocrinologists and the American Thyroid Association. *Endocr Pract.* 2012;18(6):989–1028.
10. Bahn RS, Burch HB, Cooper DS, et al. The American Thyroid Association and American Association of Clinical Endocrinologists Taskforce on hyperthyroidism and other causes of thyrotoxicosis. *Thyroid.* 2011;21(6):593–646. doi:10.1089/thy.2010.0417.
11. Recommendations of the Advisory Committee on Immunization Practices (ACIP): use of vaccines and immune globulins in persons with altered immunocompetence. *MMWR.* 1993;42(RR-4):1–18.
12. Bartalena L, Baldeschi L, Dickinson A, Eckstein A, Kendall-Taylor P, Marcocci C. Consensus statement of the European Group on Graves' orbitopathy (EUGOGO) on management of GO. *Eur J Endocrinol.* 2008;158(3):273–285. doi:10.1530/EJE-07-0666.
13. Mor G, Cardenas I. The immune system in pregnancy: a unique complexity. *Am J Reprod Immunol.* 2010;63(6):425–433. doi:10.1111/j.1600-0897.2010.00836.x.
14. Stagnaro-Green A, Abalovich M, Alexander E, et al. Guidelines of the American Thyroid Association for the diagnosis and management of thyroid disease during pregnancy and postpartum. *Thyroid.* 2011;21(10):1081–1125. doi:10.1089/thy.2011.0087.
15. LeFevre ML. Screening for thyroid dysfunction: U.S. Preventive Services Task Force recommendation statement. *Ann Intern Med.* 2015;162(9):641–650. doi:10.7326/M15-0483. Published online Mar 24, 2015. http://www.uspreventiveservicestaskforce.org/Page/Topic/recommendation-summary/thyroid-dysfunction-screening.
16. Yoshihara A, Noh J, Yamaguchi T, Ohye H, et al. Treatment of Graves' disease with antithyroid drugs in the first trimester of pregnancy and the prevalence of congenital malformation. *J Clin Endocrinol Metab.* 2012;97(7):2396–2403. doi:10.1210/jc.2011-2860.
17. Begin ME, Langlois MF, Lorrain D, Cunnane SC. Thyroid function and cognition during aging. *Curr Gerontol Geriatr Res.* 2008, Article ID 474868, 11 pages. http://dx.doi.org/10.1155/2008/474868.

18. Gesing A, Lewiński A, Karbownik-Lewińska M. The thyroid gland and the process of aging; what is new? *Thyroid Res.* 2012;5:16. doi:10.1186/1756-6614-5-16.
19. International Osteoporosis Foundation, Facts and Statistics. http://www.iofbonehealth.org/facts-statistics.
20. Ercolano MA, Drnovsek ML, Silva MC, et al. Negative correlation between bone mineral density and TSH receptor antibodies in long-term euthyroid postmenopausal women with treated Graves' disease. *Thyroid Res.* 2013;6:11. doi:10.1186/1756-6614-6-11.

5

The Body Snatchers—Scleroderma and Autoimmune Skin Disorders

I developed an overwhelming fatigue, and when I got up in the morning my fingers would swell and feel tight when I tried to bend them. Within a few weeks, my feet were so swollen I couldn't put my shoes on, one leg was bigger than the other, and I developed such shortness of breath I couldn't stand. I saw two rheumatologists when I first started having the fatigue and joint stiffness, but the tests were all negative and both doctors said maybe I wasn't handling stress very well. One doctor even said I might be imagining some of my symptoms and suggested that I talk to a therapist. At the time, I was 27 and I was in a difficult master's degree program, putting in 60- to 80-hour weeks.

So at first I thought maybe they were right—maybe it was stress. But when my symptoms got much worse, I knew something was wrong. My skin started to harden all over my body. When I would reach up into the cupboard, the inside of my arm was like webbing. When I tried to smile, the skin on my face would pull. I felt like I had been put into this nightmare body with no way out.

Karen, 40

Some autoimmune disorders profoundly affect the skin, connective tissue, and hair, causing pain, damage, and disability. These "body snatchers" include *scleroderma* (also called *systemic sclerosis, SSc*), which causes skin to

Warning Signs of Scleroderma

- Patches of thick, hard skin
- Extreme sensitivity of the fingers to cold, with pain and color changes (white, blue, and then red)
- Small ulcerations on the fingertips
- Swollen hands or feet
- Joint pain
- Fatigue
- Trouble swallowing
- Chronic heartburn
- Shortness of breath

harden and scar, and *alopecia areata*, which can lead to total hair loss. All told, they affect hundreds of thousands of women, altering their appearance and their lives.

What Causes Scleroderma?

Scleroderma gets its name from two Greek words—*sklero*, meaning "hard," and *derma,* meaning "skin." However, it can affect not only the skin, but also other sites in the body, including the lungs, esophagus, and kidneys.

In scleroderma, the immune system attacks and damages cells that produce collagen, the substance that makes skin elastic and supports other connective tissues (joints, ligaments, and the capsules that surround internal organs). Collagen is a protein normally made in small amounts by specialized cells, called fibroblasts, and deposited on the outside of cells to support and heal tissues. It's constantly being made and broken down. If you cut your finger, a clot forms and collagen is laid down along the injured area to fill in the gap and form a scar; scar formation is an essential part of the healing process. Eventually the collagen is broken down, and the scar may become smaller and skin becomes more normal in appearance. But in scleroderma, fibroblasts start overproducing collagen where there's no injury to be healed, laying down too much of it and replacing normal tissue.

Scleroderma can be localized, affecting only the collagen-producing cells in the skin, or it can be systemic, affecting collagen-making cells and small blood vessels in other areas of the body, interfering with normal function of organs and tissues.

For example, the esophagus and intestines are less able to contract to move food along because blood flow is reduced or collagen accumulation has affected nerves that control motility. In the lungs, lung cells can't swap carbon dioxide for oxygen because scar tissue has formed over the thin membrane where this exchange takes place. Systemic scleroderma can be widespread (diffuse) or limited, affecting just a few areas.

The disease is relatively rare, and estimates vary as to how many people have it. According to the Scleroderma Foundation, as many as 300,000 may be affected, one-third with systemic disease.[1] Around 80 percent of those with scleroderma are women.

The vascular component of scleroderma causes tiny blood vessels in the fingers and other areas of the body to become narrowed. In the kidneys, this can lead to high blood pressure. In the hands, diminished blood supply makes the fingers extremely sensitive to cold, causing *Raynaud's phenomenon*, exaggerated, painful spasms of the blood vessels when exposed to cold accompanied by color changes (see pages 131 and 139).

Raynaud's occurs in 95 percent of people with scleroderma and also appears alongside RA and lupus, and it can occur in otherwise healthy women.

It's not known just what triggers the immune reaction that causes collagen production to run amok, says Maureen D. Mayes, MD, MPH, who heads the National Scleroderma Registry at the University of Texas Health Science Center in Houston. "In scleroderma, small blood vessels initially become 'leaky,' releasing immune substances that activate the skin to make too much collagen. What causes the blood vessel damage in the first place is still unknown."

Also unknown: why some women develop localized scleroderma and others suffer systemic disease, sometimes without any visible signs on the skin.

The presence of specific antibodies may provide clues as to which women develop certain complications. "There are probably a host of genetic factors, and potentially toxins or environmental factors that trigger a reaction in people who are genetically susceptible and prompt the appearance of certain antibodies, which are probably present long before there are any symptoms," remarks Virginia D. Steen, MD, professor of medicine at Georgetown University in Washington, D.C., who has studied the disease for more than 40 years. "For example, we see certain antibodies in Caucasian women who develop pulmonary hypertension, and another antibody in African American women who develop pulmonary hypertension."

There are other ethnic differences. African American women are more likely to develop the disease than Caucasian women, and they develop it at an earlier age, says Dr. Steen. "The average age at diagnosis is 40, but in African American women it tends to be earlier. Black women tend to have more diffuse disease and also have more skin pigment changes than Caucasians."

A 2002 study from Johns Hopkins and the University of Maryland also found that black women have a 60 percent greater risk of dying from scleroderma than white women of the same age with the disease.

Genetics may play a limited role. While Dr. Mayes finds that scleroderma is twice as common in people with a family history, the absolute risk for each family member is actually less than 1 percent.

Symptoms of Systemic Scleroderma

Some women experience joint pain and puffy hands as the first symptoms of scleroderma, but most often they develop extreme sensitivity to cold and Raynaud's phenomenon (see pages 139 to 140).

Normally when we're exposed to the cold, the body tries to slow the loss of heat and preserve normal core temperature by sending less blood to arteries near the surface of the skin and moving more blood deep within the body. To divert blood flow, the tiny blood vessels near the skin's surface (*arterioles*) contract. Everyone has these spasms in blood vessels, causing the hands to feel cold and painful and appear blotchy red. But in Raynaud's the reaction is intensified, and the color changes are more profound—and distinctive.

"A woman may notice her fingertips tingle and turn pale within a few minutes of cold exposure as blood vessels tighten and keep blood from entering her fingers. The fingers then turn a bluish color from the deoxygenated blood. Then, as the fingers warm up and blood vessels relax, they turn very red as blood rushes in. This can be extremely painful with exposure to even slight cold, including an air-conditioned room or the freezer section of grocery stores. Women often put up with it for long periods of time," remarks Dr. Mayes. "But some women may develop little pinpoint-type sores, also called *digital pits*, on their fingertips, because of decreased blood supply. If the decrease in blood supply is more severe, ulcers can develop on the fingertips. They can be quite painful and take weeks to heal. In some cases, the skin on the fingers has already started to become thickened. It's usually at this point that a woman will see a doctor."

It's important to note that up to 5 percent of healthy women have Raynaud's without any other disease (or *primary Raynaud's*). The disorder is classified as *secondary Raynaud's* when it occurs in people with autoimmune disease. Between 85 and 95 percent of women with scleroderma and mixed connective tissue disease, and a third of women with lupus, have secondary Raynaud's.

In women with scleroderma, the inside of the blood vessel wall becomes *fibrotic* because of excess collagen deposits, and the thickening of skin in the surrounding area causes an increased demand for oxygen in the tissues. When cells lining the blood vessels are damaged, they produce a substance called *endothelin*, which acts as a potent vasoconstrictor, causing an increased tendency to spasm. Ulcers can occur as a complication of restricted blood flow (*ischemia*). In severe or prolonged cases, the tips of the fingers may become shorter, and the bone may even become damaged from lack of blood supply.

Raynaud's may initially appear along with puffy hands, but it's the skin thickening that's the primary symptom of scleroderma. Skin thickening in the fingers is called *sclerodactyly* and usually starts from the middle joints out to the fingertips.

The thickened skin isn't red or bumpy—it's smooth and shiny with few wrinkles. The swelling and skin thickening can make the fingers feel stiff, because the joints don't bend normally. The skin covering the finger joints can become so tight and inelastic that the fingers do not extend and are forced to bend inward (*joint contracture*). In severe cases, they may eventually become "frozen" in this position.

At the nail folds, the area where the nail meets the cuticle, the capillaries may be enlarged, show tiny hemorrhages, or may even be missing altogether.

Other skin problems include itching caused by inflammation; pigment changes (darker or lighter patches of skin); ulcerations due to poor circulation, injury, or tearing of tight skin at joints and pressure points; and red spots caused by enlargement (*dilation*) of small blood vessels in the skin (*telangiectasias*), usually on the face and hands.

There may be hair loss in areas of thickened skin, due to both excess collagen around hair follicles and reduced blood supply (hair loss on the scalp can occur, but it's more common in lupus). Later in the illness, tiny calcium deposits can form (*calcinosis*), which feel like firm bumps under the skin; these can become very painful and inflamed, and can become infected.

In the esophagus, the movements that normally push food into the stomach (*peristalsis*) are decreased because of scarring of nerve tissue and reduced blood flow, so you may have an uncomfortable sensation of food sticking in the throat or chest. The valve that's supposed to keep acid in the stomach becomes weakened, allowing acid to back up or *reflux*, leading to chronic heartburn and *gastroesophageal reflux disease (GERD)*. Heartburn doesn't just happen after meals but can occur at other times as well, especially when lying down at night.

This constellation of symptoms in limited systemic scleroderma has been called *CREST*—an acronym for calcinosis, Raynaud's, esophageal problems, sclerodactyly, and telangiectasias. However catchy the acronym, it was an imprecise term and is now used less often. Not every woman will have all of the external symptoms. Some may have internal involvement limited to the esophagus. Some may have limited cutaneous scleroderma with damage in the intestines and lungs.

Excess collagen deposits can also limit contractions of the bowel needed to move food and waste along. As a result, bacteria begin to overgrow in the small intestine, which interferes with the absorption of nutrients and fat, causing diarrhea and weight loss. When the large intestine is affected, it can cause constipation.

Most of the time, the earliest signs of systemic scleroderma may be dismissed as a minor complaint. "Many women say they had symptoms for two or three or even four years and sought help from a physician, but no clear diagnosis was made," comments Dr. Mayes.

It's a different story with diffuse scleroderma. Symptoms may come on suddenly and often do not include Raynaud's. A woman may have swollen hands and feet, swollen and/or painful joints, extreme fatigue, or a sudden, severe rise in blood pressure (due to blood vessel spasm in the kidney, which causes severe headaches, shortness of breath, a stroke, or even kidney failure). A woman may then have progression of thickened skin beyond the hand that spreads up over the arms, legs, and trunk over a short period.

Other organ involvement includes the small intestines and the lungs. In the lungs, excess collagen interferes with the normal exchange of carbon dioxide for oxygen across the thin membrane that separates the tiny capillaries and the air sacs (*alveoli*). It's not clear what triggers the process, but activated immune cells and damaged blood vessels play a role. There's also inflammation in the air sacs, called *alveolitis*, which leads to scarring (*pulmonary fibrosis*) and breathing problems.

Pulmonary fibrosis might also be linked to reflux; there's some speculation that microscopic particles of stomach acid could be inhaled when a patient lies down during sleep. The primary symptoms of lung involvement are a chronic cough and shortness of breath.

In rare cases (about 5 percent of cases), women may have a condition called *scleroderma sine sclerosis*, or scleroderma without skin thickening. "She will have Raynaud's phenomenon, but there's often a long period of time between the onset of Raynaud's and other problems, leading to a delay in diagnosis, because the most visible and characteristic sign, thickening of the skin, is not present," says Dr. Mayes.

Occasionally, diffuse scleroderma can have a very rapid course, progressing quickly to affect the kidneys, lungs, heart, and other organs, and can even be fatal. Fortunately, this is uncommon. Most women with scleroderma have a relatively normal life span.

In localized scleroderma, patches of thickened, pigmented skin are called *morphea*. Localized skin thickening can also appear as a band or line down the face or an arm or leg (*linear scleroderma*), which may extend deep into the skin and muscle. Around 20 percent of women with localized scleroderma may develop joint pain (sometimes before skin changes appear, causing confusion with rheumatoid arthritis). Localized scleroderma may be self-limiting, with symptoms subsiding after a few years.

Karen's story continues:

The third rheumatologist I saw took one look at my hands and said I had scleroderma. He said that some people don't test positive for the antibodies for scleroderma, and to this day I don't test positive. There were times this disease really consumed me. I would lie on the couch far 14 to 16 hours a day. I had no energy at all; it was an effort to get up and walk to the bathroom. And I had been a pretty high-energy person, so this was very disturbing. I would sleep 10 or 11 hours a night and still wake up exhausted. Having a doctor to help me through it made all the difference. You need hope and good medical care.

Diagnosing Scleroderma

A diagnosis of scleroderma can often be made by a physical exam alone, but bloodwork and other diagnostic tests may be needed to assess the extent of the disease.

"Most of the symptoms, like swollen fingers or heartburn, are pretty common, and many women and their doctors may dismiss them. The skin thickening may also be very subtle in the beginning and is not easily detected," says Dr. Mayes. "The difficulty we have is in determining when this constellation of symptoms points to scleroderma."

While Raynaud's phenomenon is often the first sign of scleroderma, it can also occur on its own, and it's fairly common in otherwise healthy women. "In the beginning, it's hard to distinguish between scleroderma and primary Raynaud's phenomenon," says Dr. Mayes. "One of the major indications of secondary Raynaud's is the sores on the tips of the fingers. This does not occur in primary Raynaud's disease."

In 2013, the American College of Rheumatology (ACR) and the European League Against Rheumatism (EULAR) issued new classification criteria for scleroderma to aid diagnosis. Each item on the list is assigned a points value. A total score of 9 points or above is required for a definite diagnosis. Your rheumatologist may use this list during your exam.[2]

The first item on the list is "skin thickening of the fingers of both hands extending *proximal* (near) *to the metacarpal phalangeal* joints." The bones of the fingers are called *phalanges*, and the bones of the palm are the *metacarpals*. The finger joints closest to the palm are the *metacarpophalangeals (MCP)*. Skin thickening in those areas is an automatic 9 points and indicates scleroderma.

The other items on the list:

- Other skin thickening on the fingers, such as puffiness or sclerodactyly = 4 points.
- Fingertip lesions (fingertip ulcers and/or pitting scars) = 3 points.
- Telangiectasias = 2 points
- Abnormalities of the nailfold capillaries = 2 points
- Interstitial lung disease and/or pulmonary hypertension = 2 points
- Raynaud's phenomenon = 3 points
- Autoantibodies (e.g., anticentromere antibodies, see below) = 3 points

Again, if your score adds up to 9, a physical exam alone may lead to a diagnosis. But other tests may be needed to confirm a diagnosis of scleroderma.

Tests You May Need and What They Mean

Antinuclear antibody (ANA) tests using an indirect immunofluorescent method will be positive in 85 to 90 percent of scleroderma patients (and in 99 percent of women with lupus). However, with some of the newer ANA tests, using a different method, 40 percent of women with scleroderma may have a negative test depending on which method is used. A woman with Raynaud's phenomenon and a positive ANA but no other symptoms needs to be followed closely for six-month intervals over a period of two to five years.

Other antibodies, such as *anticentromere antibodies* (associated with limited scleroderma and esophageal problems and pulmonary arterial hypertension), *anti-Scl 70 antibodies (anti-topoisomerase I antibodies)* (associated with systemic sclerosis), and *anti-RNA polymerase III antibodies* (associated with severe diffuse skin disease and high risk of kidney involvement) can be helpful in making the diagnosis as well as giving prognostic information about the course of the disease, but they are not 100 percent specific.

A complete blood count (CBC) will be needed to see whether there is a low red cell count due to anemia (which can be due to many causes) or a low white cell count. Serum creatinine will be tested to help assess kidney function.

Special x-ray tests are performed if a woman is experiencing chronic heartburn to assess potential problems or damage to the gastrointestinal tract.

There are several types of tests: A *barium swallow* involves drinking a small amount of liquid containing barium (which shows up white on the x-ray) to see whether there is scarring or an ulcer in the esophagus.

An x-ray "movie" called a *cine esophagram* may be done to see if there's decreased motion in the esophagus, an ulcer in the lower end of the esophagus, or a stricture. In an *upper GI series,* ingested barium is followed as it moves through the stomach to the small intestine. A small intestine transit study measures the amount of time this takes and can indicate impaired bowel function.

If you have chronic heartburn, *endoscopy* may also be done to check for inflammation or ulcers. This test uses a small tube (*endoscope*) with a fiberoptic device passed through the mouth down into the esophagus and stomach, allowing the doctor to examine the lining.

Pulmonary function tests (PFTs) with diffusing capacity are usually done to assess potential damage to the lungs if a woman has shortness of breath or a dry cough but should also be done at the time of diagnosis of scleroderma as baseline. Pulmonary function testing involves breathing into a machine that measures lung volume and lung flow and the ability to exchange carbon dioxide for oxygen (diffusing capacity) to establish a baseline. "This way if a woman does develop shortness of breath or a dry cough, we can look back on that test and determine whether there's been a change from that," says Dr. Mayes. CAT scans can reveal scar tissue and inflammation in the lungs before it's apparent on chest x-rays.

Based on the results of the skin exam, a diagnosis of limited or diffuse scleroderma can usually be made. A diagnosis of *undifferentiated connective tissue disease (UCTD)* or *undifferentiated autoimmune syndrome (UAS)* is given when a woman does not fully meet the criteria for scleroderma (or lupus or Sjögren's syndrome).

Scleroderma-like Disorders

There are a number of disorders that can resemble scleroderma but are actually quite distinct.

Scleredema causes thickened skin on the upper body (the face, neck, head, and shoulders), sometimes spreading down to the arms or trunk. The disorder can occur in people with long-term diabetes. Women usually will not have Raynaud's, ANAs, or organ involvement.

Eosinophilic fascitis (EF) occurs when white blood cells (eosinophils and leukocytes) attack tissues called *fascia*, which separate muscle from fat. This thin sheet of tissue becomes inflamed, swollen, and tender. The skin overlying the area becomes dimpled (like the skin of an orange), and the underlying tissue will feel hard. EF affects the arms, trunk, and legs but not usually the hands or face (there's little fascia in those areas). The onset of EF is rapid, with skin changes that may be followed in a few weeks by decreased range of motion in the central body, shoulders, and hips and contractures of the elbows and knees. Raynaud's is usually not present, and ANAs will be negative, but there will be marked increases in eosinophils in the blood and fascial tissue (seen on biopsy).

Chronic graft-versus-host disease (GVHD) can cause patches of thickened skin on the arms, trunk, and legs that look like localized scleroderma. GVHD can occur in bone marrow transplant patients but is not reported after organ transplantation. In marrow transplants, high-dose chemotherapy is first given to "kill" the host immune system by destroying the bone marrow, and then a patient is given an infusion of marrow from a matched donor to reconstitute the immune system. However, even with the best matches, the donor marrow cells can react against the recipient and set off a barrage of toxic cytokines; this acute GVHD is treated with immunosuppressants. The reaction can be chronic in some marrow transplant patients. Immunosuppressants can control chronic GVHD, but they may not cure it.

The Female Factor

The vast majority (85 to 90 percent) of those diagnosed with localized and systemic scleroderma are women. But if female hormones play a role, it's only slight, speculates Dr. Mayes. "Scleroderma is different from lupus or rheumatoid arthritis. Pregnancy usually makes symptoms of RA better, but in some cases lupus can worsen. In systemic sclerosis, pregnancy is considered a high-risk period because the disease itself, and not hormones, can cause problems for some women."

One of the intriguing theories of why women are more prone to scleroderma (and other autoimmune diseases) has to do with *microchimerism*, the presence of fetal cells from a past pregnancy that remain in a woman's

Scleroderma Clusters

Among the diseases that may occur with scleroderma is *mixed connective tissue disease (MCTD)*, a combination of scleroderma, lupus, rheumatoid arthritis, and *polymyositis*, a relatively rare inflammation of multiple muscles that leads to muscle weakness, swelling, tenderness, and tissue damage. The unifying feature of MCTD that must be present to make the diagnosis is the presence of antibodies to RNP (however, these antibodies can also be seen in SLE). MCTD is considered an "overlap syndrome" with scleroderma.

Other diseases that cluster with scleroderma include:

- Sjögren's syndrome
- Rheumatoid arthritis
- Lupus

bloodstream for many years (see page 13). It may be that the combination of self and nonself antigens (some from the father, some from the mother) in fetal cells may contribute to a form of graft-versus-host disease.

Studies have found that women with scleroderma have 20 times the number of persistent fetal cells found in other women who'd had children but didn't have scleroderma.

"However, there are many scleroderma patients who have never been pregnant (or are male) that are not explained by this theory. Microchimerism may just be an incidental finding, since it is seen in other diseases and not all scleroderma patients. It may be a risk factor, like genes," remarks Dr. Steen. "We have no strong candidate for what causes scleroderma, whether it's a virus or environmental toxin. In fact, scleroderma could be several diseases which occur differently in women, depending on their genetic makeup."

Karen's story continues:

At first I was put on penicillamine, but I started to develop kidney problems and still had the fatigue. So I was put on low-dose steroids. That calmed the disease down initially. But then my skin turned hard all over my body. It turned hard on my chest, and I couldn't wear a bra. It turned hard on my stomach, my legs, my arms, and my face. When I tried to smile or raise my eyebrows my skin would pull and stretch—it was just terrible. You feel like you've been put into this nightmare and you have to find the inner resources to pull yourself out of it, to try to cope with it. I had almost alligator skin. My doctor finally put me on this drug that's used for transplant patients, cyclosporine. It helped dramatically. Within about three months, my skin was softening all over. I was on the drug for four or five years, when the disease was very active. I got really well on cyclosporine.

I went back to work three days a week. The scarring in my esophagus didn't go away, and the stomach acid backed up, so I took acid-blocking drugs. I also had some kidney damage and developed high blood pressure. I took medication for that and I'm still on steroids. The skin on my hands is still very tight, and they are very curved. But I feel much better and I have a pretty active life again and have plenty of energy for my children.

Treating Scleroderma

While there's no cure for scleroderma, many of the problems created by the disease can be treated individually. We have used current treatment recommendations from EULAR and the EULAR Scleroderma Trials and Research group (EUSTAR).[3]

Raynaud's

Medications used most often to ease symptoms of Raynaud's are vasodilators, usually *calcium channel blockers*, which improve blood flow to the small blood vessels in the fingers (see pages 339 to 140). The first-line treatment is *nifedipine (Procardia)* or *amlodipine (Norvasc)*. Other drugs in this class are *diltiazem (Cardizem, Dilacor, and Tiazac)*, *felodipine (Plendil)*, and *nicardipine (Cardene)*.

"Frequently, scleroderma occurs in young women who are quite thin, and they will have blood pressures of 90/60 and you cannot lower their blood pressure any further. They are going to get dizzy and lightheaded," says Dr. Mayes. "With most women you start at a low dose, and if they become lightheaded, dizzy, or develop headaches, you have to stop or lower the dose of the drugs."

In such cases, alternatives include *pentoxifylline (Trental)*, which helps blood flow more easily through narrow blood vessels and can slightly lower blood pressure, and *dipyridamole (pentoxifylline)* or *clopidogrel bisulfate (Plavix)*, which prevent platelets from forming clots. The latter two drugs do not lower blood pressure, but they can cause an increased risk of bleeding and cannot be used in pregnancy. Doctors generally advise against using pentoxifylline while breast-feeding. Nitroglycerin patches can be used to improve circulation and heal finger ulcers. The antihypertensive *losartan (Cozaar)* may help reduce the frequency and severity of Raynaud's attacks.

Sildenafil (Revatio) and *tadalafil (Adcirca)*, the *phosphodiesterase type V (PDE V) inhibitors* better known as the erectile dysfunction drugs *Viagra* and *Cialis*, also may help relieve Raynaud's by dilating small blood vessels in the fingers.[4]

For healing digital ulcers related to Raynaud's and scleroderma, *intravenous iloprost (Ventavis)*, a synthetic version of *prostacyclin* that inhibits platelets from clumping, dilates blood vessels, and increases blood flow to the fingers. It may also help heal endothelial cells and prevent fibrotic changes in the skin. Moisturizers and lubricants must be used regularly to prevent fissures and infections. If ulcers become infected, topical or systemic antibiotics are used.

Biofeedback training, in which people learn to increase blood flow to the fingers through electronic or thermal feedback, has been touted as an alternative approach to treating Raynaud's. But most studies were small and uncontrolled, and there's no strong evidence to show that it works.

Most important—if you smoke, quit immediately. Nicotine is a potent vasoconstrictor and can make your Raynaud's worse.

Gastroesophageal Reflux Disease (GERD)

In GERD, the esophagus is being affected by a weakening of the valve that keeps acid in the stomach, allowing the acid to "reflux" into the esophagus. Drugs called proton pump inhibitors such as *omeprazole (Prilosec)*, *pantoprazole (Protonix)*, or *lansoprazole (Prevacid)* decrease acid production.

Esomeprazole (Nexium) can heal irritation and erosions caused by acid. It is available in prescription strength (40 mg) and over-the-counter (23.5 mg). Other drugs like *cimetidine (Zantac, Tagamet)* block formation of stomach acid. Prokinetic agents like *metoclopramide (Reglan)* may improve decreased motility of the esophagus or small intestine.

The diarrhea caused by bacterial overgrowth in the small intestine can sometimes be cleared up with a short course of antibiotics. Malabsorption may also be caused by bacterial overgrowth.

Also helpful: eating slowly, chewing food thoroughly, drinking plenty of water (alternating sips of water with bites of food can ease passage of food), not eating within two hours of going to bed, and sleeping with the head of your bed elevated.

Lung Problems

Inflammation of the air sacs of the lungs, called *alveolitis,* often precedes *interstitial lung disease,* which affects the tissues and spaces around the air sacs. Cytoxan is used to treat interstitial lung disease, given orally or in "pulses" (monthly intravenous infusions), and more commonly now, another transplant drug, *mycophenolate mofetil (MMF, CellCept),* is used.

Pulmonary fibrosis, due to *interstitial lung fibrosis,* may also be aggravated by breathing microscopic particles of stomach acid during sleep, and treating GERD may improve symptoms. Other management includes prevention of infections and exercise, along with home oxygen therapy in some cases.

High blood pressure in the lungs (*pulmonary arterial hypertension, PAH*) occurs in about 15 percent of scleroderma patients, as small blood vessels in the lungs become thickened and resistant to blood flow. *Bosentan (Tracleer),* an endothelin receptor antagonist (ERA), is used for treating pulmonary hypertension. The drug, given orally, relaxes the endothelial cells lining blood vessels by blocking a receptor for a protein that acts as a *vasoconstrictor* (*endothelin*). Clinical trials showed improved breathing, exercise potential, and quality of life. An inhaled form of *iloprost* may be used for PAH.

Blood Pressure and Kidney Problems

Patients with early diffuse scleroderma need to monitor their blood pressure regularly to be aware of any increase, which is the first sign of serious kidney problems. If blood pressure begins to rise, a physician must be consulted immediately so *angiotensin-converting enzyme (ACE) inhibitors,* a lifesaving treatment, can be given. These include *captopril (Capoten)* and *enalapril (Vasotec).*

Sildenafil and *tadalafil* can improve exercise capacity and blood flow and are also used to treat PAH. Pulmonary hypertension can also be treated with oxygen and blood thinners.

In severe cases, prostacyclins, including intravenous *epoprostenol (Flolan), and intravenous and subcutaneous treprostinil* may be given in continuous infusions, using a small portable pump. This drug is a form of prostaglandin, a substance that occurs naturally in the body and is involved in many biological functions. Prostacyclins relax blood vessels and increase the blood supply to the lungs. Studies are under way with oral and inhaled prostaglandin preparations to make therapy easier and less expensive.

Skin Thickening

Skin thickening sometimes improves by itself, but so far no drugs have been shown to soften skin. Methotrexate may improve skin in early diffuse disease and shows some positive effects on muscles, joints, and tendons. Physical and occupational therapy are extremely important for patients with diffuse skin thickening in order to maintain as much mobility as possible. Adequate pain control is also necessary so patients can do the difficult and aggressive exercise program.

What's Next?

High-dose chemotherapy with stem cell rescue involves harvesting stem cells (the cells that grow into different kinds of cells, including white blood cells), purifying and freezing them, then destroying a patients' abnormal immune system with high doses of chemotherapy (usually cyclophosphamide). After chemotherapy, the stem cells are defrosted and infused back into the patient to reconstitute the immune system with lymphocytes that hopefully will not be autoreactive. Recent clinical trials are using *autologous peripheral blood hemapoietic stem cells,* stem cells taken from the patient's bloodstream, rather than bone marrow.

Studies so far suggest these transplants pose a tough trade-off—the risk of serious side effects (such as organ failure), dying from the treatment, or the chance of living longer.

One major clinical trial, the Autologous Stem Cell Transplantation International Scleroderma (ASTIS) trial, found that *hemapoietic stem cell transplant (HSCT)* was more effective than intravenous cyclophosphamide, despite causing more deaths in the first two months after treatment and more serious events in the first year.[5] Compared to cyclophosphamide, HSCT led to better long-term survival among 156 people with early diffuse cutaneous disease. The ASTIS results, reported in 2014, also show improved lung function (most of the patients had interstitial lung disease) and skin softening after two years. Around 22 percent of patients relapsed before two years and needed more immunosuppressant therapy.[3]

A small 2011 clinical trial at Northwestern University also found that HSCT improved skin and pulmonary function in scleroderma patients for up to two years, compared to conventional treatment.[6] Other trials are ongoing.

Overall, stem cell transplantation has a relatively high mortality rate (around 5 to 10 percent). So the procedure is usually reserved for people diagnosed within the last four to five years with diffuse cutaneous scleroderma and only mild-to-moderate organ involvement or limited cutaneous disease with progressive internal organ involvement after conventional treatment has failed. "But it's very hard to predict who will do well," comments Dr. Mayes.

There are several new studies looking at promising medications particularly for skin thickening and for lung fibrosis. Patients should strongly consider participating in such trials at scleroderma centers of excellence, which can be identified at the Scleroderma Foundation website or through clinicaltrials.gov.

An experimental oral drug, *selexipag*, has shown some promise for treating PAH. Selexipag is a *selective prostacyclin IP receptor agonist* and dilates blood vessels in the lung. In a recent clinical trial, the drug improved survival and breathing difficulties by 14 percent after four years.[7]

Tracking Your Symptoms

Unlike lupus, where there are assessment scales to track disease activity by the frequency of certain symptoms, in scleroderma there's no gold standard to assess increased disease activity and severity to determine when more aggressive treatment is needed.

The Canadian Scleroderma Research Group, a consortium of rheumatologists, basic scientists, and patient representatives, has been working on a scleroderma activity index for a number of years.[8] Among its findings so far, elevated *C-reactive protein (CRP),* a marker of inflammation, may be correlated with disease activity, severity, poor pulmonary function, and shorter survival. CRP is elevated in one-quarter of systemic sclerosis patients, especially in early disease.[9]

The 51-point modified *Rodnan skin scoring system (mRSS)* for skin thickening is used to monitor disease progression. Higher scores (above 15) on the mRSS indicate more severe skin thickening.

Until a standardized global disease activity scale for scleroderma is developed, Dr. Mayes suggests that several red flags should prompt medical attention:

- **Increasing shortness of breath, muscle weakness, and leg swelling.** "Fatigue tends to be chronic; it will wax and wane. But if a woman can distinguish progressive muscle weakness from fatigue, I think that's a key symptom. Leg swelling can be a symptom of kidney or heart problems."
- **Increased blood pressure.** "During the first five years after a diagnosis, women should keep a careful watch on their blood pressure with weekly blood pressure readings using a home monitor. Their physician can give them instructions on what to do if blood pressure goes over a certain level," says Dr. Mayes.
- **Fingers that turn blue or pale in the cold** and do not return to normal color. "If a woman has a blue or pale finger that does not go back to pink when warmed, that stays cool and discolored for 24 hours, that's something that should prompt physician attention," warns Dr. Mayes. "In this case, we need to try to open up the blood vessels with medication. If caught early, and treated early, we may be able to avoid the development of finger ulcers or irreversible tissue loss."
- **Weight loss and diarrhea** that lasts more than two to three days. This can be a sign of bacterial overgrowth in the gut, which is treatable with a short course of antibiotics. Some women may need to be on intermittent antibiotics. Weight loss can also be caused by an esophageal stricture that interferes with swallowing. A stricture can be dilated using an endoscopic procedure.

Karen's story continues:

It affected me in so many ways. Your sexual life is affected, so you have to make adjustments there. I had always wanted to have kids, but the doctors had advised us not to get pregnant because they really didn't know what the disease was going to do, and I didn't want to take any chances. So we decided to adopt a child. Then I got pregnant. But three months into the pregnancy I went into a hypertensive crisis and was in the intensive care unit for 10 days. I almost lost my life and I lost the baby. But the adoption went through when all this was happening. And this child was really a lifeline. Even when I had to have dialysis, I had to shift my focus to taking care of this baby.

Eventually I got off dialysis, my energy came back, and we decided to adopt a second child, and my two girls are my joy. Still, it's hard sometimes. When I look in the mirror, my face looks so different. This disease changes your whole self-concept. But I have learned to live with this disease; it's part of my life. I focus on the positive aspects of my life, what's important. My husband is an exceptional man, but there were times I thought he should bail out. But he said, "I don't take a vow lightly, and this is not something I'm going to run from." He has been my strength. I couldn't have made it without him.

How Scleroderma Can Affect You Over Your Lifetime

Scleroderma can not only affect a woman's appearance, but treatments can also affect menstruation and fertility and influence the decision whether to become pregnant.

Menstrual and Reproductive Effects

Scleroderma does not appear to flare premenstrually. However, women with scleroderma may have menstrual and ovulation irregularities, and some of the medications used to treat scleroderma, such as prednisone in very high doses, may also lead to irregular cycles and decreased fertility (but unlike cyclophosphamide, this decrease is temporary not permanent).

"If a woman has a lot of GI involvement and has lost a fair amount of weight, that will affect ovulation and menstrual cycles. A certain amount of body fat is needed to convert the hormones for starting menstruation. You see amenorrhea in women with anorexia because of low estrogen. In scleroderma, if you've had a fair amount of weight loss and you've lost a great deal of body fat, you may have the same situation," remarks Dr. Mayes.

Birth control pills do not seem to affect scleroderma. In fact, studies suggest that women taking oral contraceptives may have less skin thickening.

Treatment with cyclophosphamide can cause sterility and trigger an early menopause. The chances of becoming infertile rise with increasing doses given for longer periods of time and with increasing age (even a woman at age 35 is at risk for sterility caused by cyclophosphamide).

Pregnancy

Like Karen, almost half of women with scleroderma have their first symptoms before age 40, and childbearing is an important issue.

Early studies reported a high incidence of miscarriages, premature births, and smaller-than-average babies among women with scleroderma. But research led by Dr. Steen found that most women with scleroderma are no more likely than healthy women to suffer these complications of pregnancy.

"We did see a much higher percentage of preterm births in women with early diffuse disease," remarks Dr. Steen. "Patients who have had diffuse disease for a long time had a significantly greater risk of miscarriage than the other groups." The majority of patients had no change in their symptoms during pregnancy, but 34 percent experienced a worsening of Raynaud's, arthritis, and skin thickening.[10]

"We encourage women to have an early consultation with their rheumatologist to assess the type and activity of their disease. We discourage women with early diffuse disease from becoming pregnant during that period, because of the risk of kidney problems," says Dr. Steen.

Dr. Mayes advises women newly diagnosed with scleroderma to wait two to three years to see how their illness develops; limited scleroderma may be less risky for a pregnancy than diffuse disease (although there's some increase in prematurity). The disease must be stable (with no signs of hypertension or lung problems) because most medications must be stopped before a woman tries to conceive.

While many women with scleroderma have uneventful pregnancies, they should be under the care of an obstetrician who specializes in high-risk pregnancies because of the risk of premature birth. Blood pressure must be carefully monitored. High blood pressure, *preeclampsia* (severe high blood pressure with protein leakage from the kidneys, *proteinuria*), and even more serious kidney damage have been reported more often in women with scleroderma.

Preeclampsia may arise in scleroderma because of thickening and narrowing of blood vessels in the placenta, which hampers delivery of oxygen and nutrients to the fetus and the removal of wastes. If untreated, it can progress to eclampsia (seizures), which can result in maternal death. Preeclampsia develops most often in the third trimester. If blood pressure cannot be managed, the baby may have to be delivered early. If untreated, it can progress to eclampsia, which can cause seizures and death. ACE inhibitors are not given during pregnancy unless other medications fail to control high blood pressure. If a woman develops preeclampsia and her blood pressure doesn't respond to medication, cesarean delivery is required.

The most common symptoms of pregnancy—morning sickness in the early months, and heartburn as the pregnancy progresses—are more pronounced in women with scleroderma.

Menopause

Menopause is still largely uncharted territory in scleroderma, and its effects on the disease itself are unclear.

Menopause in all women is associated with some skin thinning and collagen loss due to low estrogen. Studies find a 1 to 2 percent decline in collagen per year after menopause. One recent study suggests that menopause has a substantial effect on skin thickening in diffuse systemic sclerosis, with postmenopausal women having a lower mean *mRSS* compared to premenopausal women.[11]

Canadian researchers find that estrogen supplementation in postmenopausal women may increase skin scores by increasing collagen content in the skin.[13] "I have no problem prescribing hormones for women who are experiencing hot flashes, because my data does not suggest there's a problem with taking hormones," comments Dr. Steen.

The atrophy of vaginal tissues that occurs as estrogen levels drop in menopause can also occur independently in women with scleroderma and Sjögren's syndrome (see page 148). "Perhaps 10 percent of women with scleroderma have true autoimmune Sjögren's syndrome. Probably 30 to 40 percent of women with scleroderma have overlapping symptoms with Sjögren's, but when their parotid glands are examined, they are fibrotic," says Dr. Steen. Anti-Ro and La antibodies point toward Sjögren's syndrome.

In both cases, vaginal tissues may feel dry; there may be itching, burning, and irritation as well as painful sex. If the problem is due to menopause, oral estrogen therapy or estrogen cream can help relieve vaginal dryness. (If you have an intact uterus you need to take progestin to protect against endometrial hyperplasia.) Vaginal dryness can also be relieved by special moisturizers. (See pages 191 to 192.)

Systemic estrogen does carry the risk of blood clots, is not advisable for women with vascular or clotting problems, and is not recommended for the secondary prevention of heart disease. So a woman needs to discuss the pros and cons with her physician. One study did suggest a slightly increased risk of Raynaud's among women taking estrogen therapy.[12]

"In general, we have not seen an increased risk of osteoporosis in scleroderma patients as there is with rheumatoid arthritis," adds Dr. Steen.

Sexuality

In any chronic illness, there's a higher risk of depression. This can affect sexuality, as can a negative body image from the changes caused by scleroderma. The fatigue of scleroderma can interfere with having an active sex life, and uncomfortable vaginal dryness can cause some women to avoid sex altogether.

However, a 2009 study of 101 women with scleroderma found that 60 percent remained sexually active despite their disease. And the main causes of inactivity could be helped, the researchers say.[13]

The most common symptoms reported by the group that influenced sexual function were fatigue (60 percent), vaginal dryness (42 percent), body pain (40 percent), depression, and vaginal discomfort (38.3 percent). Among those women who reported decreased sexual function, the problems of vaginal dryness, vaginal discomfort, Raynaud's phenomenon, and depression were more common; more than 28 percent of the women reported depression.[14]

If you're suffering depression along with sexual problems, a combination of counseling and medication can help.

Hand Function

The hands can be severely affected early in scleroderma. Skin thickening and contracture can cause loss of flexibility in the fingers, loss of wrist motion, and a decline in fine motor skills, such as writing. Women, particularly those with diffuse scleroderma, need to do range-of-motion exercises to help slow or avoid loss of motion. Such exercises include stretching the tiny joints of the fingers by using the palm of one hand to press down the back of the finger joints of the other hand, flexing and extending the wrist, and doing rotations, two to three times a day. Women are often sent to an occupational therapist to help with exercising.

"There are also some individuals who will have a true arthritis with joint inflammation that contributes to the hand and wrist decreased range of motion in scleroderma," says Dr. Mayes. "It's sometimes difficult to figure whether the pain and swelling in the hand are due to the general puffiness that goes along with scleroderma, or to true arthritis joint inflammation that's making the joint swollen. Ultrasound examination of the joints of the hands and wrists can be very helpful in identifying true joint inflammation from the soft tissue swelling from leaky blood vessels."

The arthritis that can occur in scleroderma is treated with the same anti-inflammatories and arthritis drugs used to treat RA, like methotrexate. There may be a potential for gastric bleeding with some pain medications, so the *COX-2 inhibitor celecoxib (Celebrex)* may prescribed.

Psoriasis

Psoriasis is a chronic, inflammatory skin disease diagnosed in 150,000 people each year. According to the National Institutes of Health, as many as 7.5 million Americans in every racial group are affected (2.6 percent of Caucasians), and it is slightly more common in women than men.

In some patients, a form of arthritis—psoriatic arthritis—can develop over a period of years. Both can also occur with other autoimmune diseases (such as Crohn's disease). For this reason, we've decided to include both diseases in this book.

Psoriasis is frequently diagnosed in a woman's late twenties to midthirties, but it can develop at any time, from childhood to old age. In some cases, skin injury, infections, stress, and certain drugs may trigger psoriasis.

Heredity may also play a role. One out of three women with psoriasis has a family history of the disease, says noted psoriasis researcher Mark Lebwohl, MD, professor and chairman of the department of dermatology at the Mount Sinai School of Medicine in New York City. "If one parent has it, the likelihood a woman may also develop psoriasis is around 10 percent. If both parents have it, there's a 30 to 50 percent risk," he says. "Different genes may cause psoriasis. What we call psoriasis probably can be thought of as a group of very closely related disorders. But the genetic abnormalities lead to the same pathway. That's why there are different patterns, and why some treatments work for some people and not others."

No one knows exactly what causes psoriasis; specific autoantibodies have yet to be identified.

"What we can say is that psoriasis is a disorder of the immune system in which T lymphocytes are activated in response to some yet to be identified antigen, and then cytokines cause skin cells to multiply too quickly and cause inflammation," explains Dr. Lebwohl. A normal skin cell matures around every 28 days and is then shed from the skin's surface. "In psoriasis, skin cells can turn over every two to four days."

Warning Signs of Psoriasis

- Red, scaly patches of skin topped by silvery scales that appear on the elbows, knees, scalp, and elsewhere (patches may be small, then increase in size and number)
- Itching and scaling of the scalp
- Sudden eruptions of inflamed skin, with tiny pustules or weeping lesions
- Dramatic, extensive sloughing and inflammation of the skin

Some studies show stress may play a role in the onset and exacerbation of psoriasis and, for some people, living with a chronic skin condition can lead to depression and anxiety.[14]

As many as 30 percent of women with psoriasis (usually moderate or severe) will develop *psoriatic arthritis*. Like RA, psoriatic arthritis (PsA) causes inflammation and stiffness in the soft tissue around joints, often involving the fingers and toes, as well as the wrists, neck, lower back, knees, and ankles. In severe cases, psoriatic arthritis can cause joint destruction and disability. PsA may develop as long as 10 years after a diagnosis of psoriasis. It can come on slowly or quickly, with more severe symptoms.

Psoriatic arthritis is classified as a *spondyloarthritis* (*spondyloarthritides*), a family of inflammatory arthritic diseases that usually involve the spine, the *sacroiliac* joints in the pelvis, and areas where ligaments and tendons attach to bone (*entheses*).

Psoriatic arthritis is characterized by swelling, tenderness, and inflammation in areas where ligaments attache to bone (*enthesitis*) like your Achilles tendon, often with a gradual onset of pain that improves with activity and gets worse with rest. "Inflammatory arthritis that affects the spine is called *spondylitis*, which occurs in PsA," he explains. "So one of the things we look for is inflammatory back pain, characterized by pain that improves with activity and gets worse with rest, lasting longer than three months," he explains. There can also be *sacroiliitis*, inflammation of the sacroiliac joints (located on either side of your tailbone) seen best on MRI.

Psoriatic Arthritis

Psoriatic arthritis may sometimes be overlooked by a dermatologist, who may not be aware of the connection between psoriasis and PsA and so may miss some key signs of the disease, observes Philip J. Mease, MD, director of rheumatology research at the Swedish Medical Center in Seattle and a clinical professor of medicine at the University of Washington.

"We did a study in which rheumatologists paired with dermatologists evaluated almost 1,000 patients who were diagnosed with psoriasis and found that 30 percent had PsA; of these, 41 percent were not previously aware they had PsA," says Dr. Mease.[15]

Other characteristics of PsA are *dactylitis*, sausage-like swelling of fingers or toes or fingernails or toenails that look infected, are unusually thick, or are separating from the nail bed. You may also have eye redness and pain (*conjunctivitis*) and inflammation (*uveitis*).[16]

To make a diagnosis of psoriatic arthritis, your rheumatologist will examine your joints, skin, and nails, looking for specific patterns of inflammation, psoriatic skin and nail lesions, as well as order x-rays and/or MRIs of your joints and lab tests for markers of inflammation, such as C-reactive protein (CRP).

A major factor that distinguishes psoriatic arthritis from rheumatoid arthritis (RA) is the presence of circulating autoantibodies in blood tests; people with RA have them, those with PsA do not.[17] PsA patients have little or no rheumatoid factor in blood tests (versus high levels in RA). Inflammatory cytokines do play a role in both PsA and RA, but the mechanisms are different, says Dr. Mease.

In contrast to RA, which affects the same joints on both sides of the body, PsA usually has an asymmetrical pattern of joint swelling and pain.

One form of psoriatic arthritis, *symmetric PsA*, does affect the same joints on both side of the body, but these other factors (like enthesitis) must also be also present.

There are four other forms of PsA:

- *Oligoarticular PsA:* affects just a few joints in an asymmetrical pattern and is usually milder.
- *Arthritis mutilans:* a rare and severe form of PsA that causes extreme pain and deformities in the small joints of the hands and feet.
- *Distal interphalangeal predominant (DIP) PsA:* affects primarily the finger and toe joints closest to the nails (the *distal joints*).
- *Spondylitis*, which predominantly affects the spinal column from the neck to the lower back.

Just as with RA, early diagnosis and treatment is the key to slowing and preventing joint damage and loss of function in PsA.

Patients often try nonsteroidal anti-inflammatory drugs (NSAIDs) to ease pain before they even see a rheumatologist. "These may be adequate for mild disease, but are not adequate for more severe symptom," remarks Dr. Mease.

According to the latest treatment guidelines, nonsteroidal anti-inflammatory drugs (NSAIDs) are the first-line therapy for joint symptoms, usually given for the shortest possible duration.[18] "NSAIDs are often tried by patients as a first line of therapy. These may be adequate for mild disease but are not adequate for more severe symptoms," says Dr. Mease.

Many of the same disease-modifying anti-rheumatic drugs (DMARDs), such as methotrexate, used in RA (and psoriasis) are also prescribed for people with PsA. Four *tumor necrosis factor alpha (TNFa)* blockers are used in PsA: *infliximab (Remicade)*, *etanercept (Enbrel)*,[19] *golimumab (Simponi)*,[20] *certolizumab pegol (Cimzia)*.[21]

Around a third of women with PsA can't take TNF blockers, because they either don't work well or cause severe side effects (including, rarely, psoriasis-like lesions). In this case, new drugs that target other inflammatory cytokines may be effective. *Ustekinumab (Stelara)*, which inhibits *IL-12* and *IL-23*, is approved for active PsA and plaque psoriasis.[22] Other drugs that target members of the *IL-17* family, *secukinumab* and *ixekizumab*, and *guselkumab*, an anti-IL-23 agent, are in the pipeline.

The first oral drug for PsA, *apremilast (Otezla)*, is taken twice a day.[23] Apremilast acts as an anti-inflammatory, inhibiting the enzyme *phosphodiesterase 4 (PDE4)*, and regulates the immune network within cells, says Dr. Mease. Side effects include diarrhea, nausea, depression, weight loss, and drug-drug interactions. Because of its GI side effects, your rheumatologist may start you out on a lower dose of apremilast then slowly increase it. There's only limited safety data available for its use during pregnancy. It is also approved for plaque psoriasis (see page 157).

Types of Psoriasis

There are several forms of psoriasis. The most common, *plaque psoriasis*, is characterized by red, inflamed patches of skin topped by a layer of silvery white scales.

Other forms of psoriasis include:

- *Guttate*, characterized by small dot-like lesions
- *Pustular*, characterized by pustules over inflamed skin
- *Inverse*, characterized by intense inflammation and little scaling in body folds
- *Erythrodermic*, characterized by intense sloughing and inflammation of the skin

Plaques can be limited to a few patches on the elbows or knees, or they may involve more extensive areas of the skin, including the scalp, nails, palms, soles, torso, genital area, and, in rare cases, the face. Plaques may be symmetrical, in the same place on the right and left sides of the body.

For many people, the disease tends to be mild, but in some cases it can be disabling and even deadly. "In the more severe forms of psoriasis, the erythrodermic and the pustular forms, some patients will literally be covered by lesions overnight. Generalized erythrodermic and pustular psoriasis can be life threatening because they can affect 90 to 100 percent of the body surface, and people lose the protective functions of the skin," says Dr. Lebwohl.

The skin is actually an organ that serves as the body's first defense against infection and helps regulate body temperature. But when large areas of skin are affected in severe psoriasis, these functions are lost. "People lose protein and nutrients through the skin. They lose fluid, so their blood pressure can fall. They lose heat, so they can have low body temperature or develop fevers. In rare cases, a bacterial infection can cause death," says Dr. Lebwohl. According to the National Psoriasis Foundation (NPF), as many as 400 people die of complications related to psoriasis each year.

Because each form of psoriasis has a characteristic appearance, a physical examination by a dermatologist is needed to make a diagnosis. However, the first signs of psoriasis may not cause concern, allowing plaques to become more extensive. "Some people with mild psoriasis will treat scaly patches with moisturizers and never mention it to their physician," remarks Dr. Lebwohl. "There's no marker of who's likely to get psoriasis. Women with Crohn's disease may be unaware of the increased risk, and psoriasis plaques may not be noticed by a gastroenterologist."

Psoriatic arthritis can develop years before or after psoriasis. If you have joint pain and psoriasis you need to be evaluated by a rheumatologist.

Treating Psoriasis

While you may have a spontaneous remission, in many cases psoriasis requires continuous treatment. There are many options that can control or even eradicate plaques. However, some cause birth defects and cannot be used if you're planning a pregnancy (see pages 158 to 159).

Topical Treatments

For people with mild psoriasis, creams, ointments, and solutions such as *calcipotriene (Dovonex)* and *calcitriol (Vectical)*, both derivatives of vitamin D_3, and *tazarotene (Tazorac)*, a vitamin A derivative, can be used alone or, in more severe cases, combined with topical corticosteroids. These include *halobetasol propionate (Ultravate)*, which comes in cream and ointment form, *diflorasone diacetate (Psorcon)*, *fluticasone propionate (Cutivate)*, and *mometasone (Elocon)*. They can also be used with systemic therapies like methotrexate.

The prescription scalp solution and ointment *Taclonex* contains both *calcipotriene* and the potent steroid *betamethasone dipropionate*, which slow down skin cell growth and reduce inflammation and itch.

Topical steroids cause atrophy and thinning of the skin and are typically used only for limited periods. But if medium- or high-potency steroids are combined or alternated with Dovonex, for example, their use can be extended. Both Tazorac and Dovonex can be irritating, especially on the face and places where skin rubs against skin, like the groin or the armpit. Combining Dovonex and Ultravate can extend a period of remission or improvement up to six months. A common regimen is to use Dovonex and Ultravate twice a day for two weeks, then apply Ultravate only on weekends (but not on the face or areas like the groin).

Dovonex can also be alternated with other "superpotent" topical steroids, such as *clobetasol (Temovate)* or *Psorcon*, which otherwise must be used for limited periods because of their thinning effects on skin. For scalp psoriasis, a two-week cycle of Temovate scalp application solution twice a day is followed by a cycle of Dovonex solution twice a day on weekdays and Temovate twice a day on weekends. Dovonex also increases the effectiveness of systemic therapies, allowing lower doses to be used and reducing the number of treatments with PUVA (ultraviolet light combined with the light-sensitizing drug psoralen—see "Light Therapy" later in this chapter).

Tazorac works best for women with thick, stable plaques rather than inflamed patches or thin skin. It must be used sparingly, however, because it can cause irritation and redness on unaffected skin surrounding treated plaques. Using Tazorac at night and a topical steroid in the morning can minimize this problem. As with other vitamin A derivatives, it cannot be used during pregnancy.

An older topical prescription, *dithranol (anthralin, Dritho-Scalp)*, is used to treat plaque psoriasis. It slows down the growth of skin cells associated with psoriatic plaques.

Tacrolimus (Protopic) and *pimecrolimus (Elidel)* are topical nonsteroidal, anti-inflammatory treatments approved for eczema that can also help improve psoriasis in sensitive areas such as the face, genitals, and skin folds.

Light Therapy

Women with psoriasis may undergo therapy that exposes affected areas to ultraviolet light B (UVB), with or without medications that sensitize the skin to UV.

Ultraviolet light has several wavelengths. Most of the solar radiation that penetrates the earth's atmosphere is ultraviolet A (UVA), which penetrates more deeply into the skin and causes wrinkling and other signs of sun damage. UVB is a shorter wavelength and is the chief culprit in sunburn. Both UVA and UVB have been implicated in skin cancer.

For some people, moderate exposure to natural sunlight can help psoriasis. More intense but controlled exposure to UVB produces more of the reaction in the skin that helps clear plaques. In PUVA, the light-sensitizing drug psoralen produces a greater reaction by the skin when a person is exposed to ultraviolet A. PUVA does carry an increased risk of skin cancer.

"Phototherapy UVB is not the same spectrum of light as sunlight. It's given in graded fashion, starting with low doses and increasing gradually to try to avoid burns, and we often cover the face," explains Dr. Lebwohl. "Study after study shows there's no increase in skin cancers in people treated with UVB for psoriasis. But PUVA is clearly carcinogenic. About one out of six PUVA-treated patients will develop a skin cancer during his or her lifetime—typically squamous cell carcinoma, which usually is easily cured. The more PUVA you get, the more likely you are to get skin cancers."

The *Excimer laser* is a small (less than an inch in diameter) intense beam of ultraviolet B light (UVB) that can be aimed at single lesions. The Excimer laser is recommended for women with lesions in specific areas of the body. It may take several sessions with the laser to completely clear an area.[24]

Systemic Therapies

Women with psoriasis may be put on oral medications, such as the immunosuppressant *cyclosporine (Neoral, Sandimmune)*, *methotrexate*, and derivatives of vitamin A called *retinoids.*

Acitretin (Soriatane) is the only oral retinoid specifically approved for psoriasis. It promotes the normal growth of skin cells and speeds up shedding. It keeps working in the body after it is discontinued, so pregnancy must be avoided for two to three years after stopping the drug (see page 159).[25]

You can't donate blood for transfusion during treatment and for up to three years afterward, and women of childbearing potential shouldn't drink alcohol while on the drug and for two months after discontinuing it. Alcohol can convert the short-acting acitretin to a longer-acting form that can stay in the body 60 times longer, increasing the chances of side effects.

It should also not be taken with vitamin A, either in multivitamins or separate supplements, because the accumulation of vitamin A in the body can cause problems with vision, skin, and bone loss. Like other vitamin A therapies, it can cause birth defects. Soriatane can't be combined with other retinoids, such as oral *isotretinoin (Accutane)* or topical *tretinoin (Retin-A, Renova).*

"Pustular psoriasis responds well to isotretinoin, formerly known as Accutane, which stays in the body for a much shorter period than acitretin; 31 days after you stop using it, it's out of your system. Isotretinoin also works well with ultraviolet light. So as long as we know a woman is not planning on becoming pregnant (and for at least 31 days after finishing the drug), she can go on isotretinoin," says Dr. Lebwohl. "Methotrexate and cyclosporine are very effective for psoriasis. But they do have serious drawbacks. Cyclosporine can damage the kidney; methotrexate can damage the liver and causes fetal death."

Another oral medication, *apremilast (Otezla)*, is approved for people with moderate to severe plaque psoriasis for whom phototherapy or systemic therapy is not appropriate.[21] It works differently than other psoriasis medications by targeting an enzyme called *phosphodiesterase 4 (PDE4)* to regulate the inflammatory network within cells. It is taken twice a day.

Alefacept (Amevive) was the first "biological" therapy approved for psoriasis. It causes a decline in the "memory" T cells, which trigger psoriasis plaques by setting off inflammation and abnormally rapid growth of skin cells.[26]

Treatment involves weekly intravenous or intramuscular injections for 12 or 24 weeks and can produce remissions that last as long as 18 months.

In RA and in psoriasis, the inflammatory molecule *tumor necrosis factor alpha (TNFα)* is produced in elevated levels, leading to bone and tissue damage in the joints. The anti-TNF drugs *infliximab (Remicade)*, *etanercept (Enbrel)*, and *golimumab (Simponi)* block TNFα by binding to it, preventing it from triggering inflammation, and can produce very dramatic improvements in psoriasis and psoriatic arthritis.

Infliximab is given by intravenous (IV) infusion in a doctor's office. Etanercept is given by self-injection just under the skin once or twice per week, and golimumab is also injected subcutaneously, but only once a month.

Ustekinumab (Stelara), a new drug that inhibits two other inflammatory cytokines, *interleukin 12* and *23* (*IL-12, IL-23*), is approved for plaque psoriasis and psoriatic arthritis.[27] The first injection (given by a healthcare provider under the skin, or *subcutaneously*) is followed by a second at four weeks and then every 12 weeks.

How Psoriasis Can Affect You Over Your Lifetime

Psoriasis doesn't usually flare premenstrually and may improve in some women during pregnancy. "A rare form of pustular psoriasis called impetigo herpetiformis occurs during pregnancy," cautions Dr. Lebwohl. "Women can develop pustules all over, starting out small but often growing larger so that they merge and cover larger areas."

Pregnancy and Breast-Feeding

The biggest problem for women involves medications used to treat psoriasis, some of which cause birth defects. Soriatane and Accutane stay in the body for varying periods of time. With Soriatane (which is stored in fatty tissues), women must use two forms of birth control beginning a month before treatment is started and for two to three years after it ends. Accutane stays in the body for 31 days, so women must avoid pregnancy during treatment and for 31 days after stopping the drug.

Breast-feeding is not recommended while taking the drug and for two to three years after treatment is stopped. Methotrexate is also teratogenic (harmful to the fetus) and not recommended during pregnancy or breast-feeding. Information is limited on the safety of Ultravate during pregnancy.

"There's a tremendous amount of data among women who underwent organ transplants and were on cyclosporine during pregnancy. So it does appear to be very safe. The adverse effect appears to be a reduction in birth weight," comments Dr. Lebwohl.

PUVA is not approved for use during pregnancy. While there do not appear to be any PUVA-related birth defects, there is a slight risk of miscarriage. "It certainly merits discussion with the patient. PUVA does involve a drug that you take by mouth; it gets into your skin and requires activation by ultraviolet light. However, the fetus isn't exposed to ultraviolet light, so it should be safe," he adds. Some women develop a facial rash or discoloration called melasma during pregnancy when exposed to ultraviolet light. Called "the mask of pregnancy," melasma can also occur in pregnant women undergoing PUVA therapy, on the arms as well as the face.

Acitretin also may interfere with low-dose, progestin-only oral contraceptives (such as *Micronor*), so women are advised to use birth control pills containing both estrogen and progestin. Oral contraceptives may affect levels of cyclosporine.

The TNF inhibitors Remicade and Enbrel should only be used during pregnancy if necessary; no harmful effects have been seen on a developing fetus, but risk can't be completely ruled out. (See pages 50 to 51.)

You and your doctor need to go over all of your psoriasis medications if you plan on becoming pregnant.

Menopause and Beyond

Psoriasis doesn't seem to be affected by hormonal fluctuations, so it may or may not improve with menopause. There are no known interactions between psoriasis medications and the estrogens or progestins used in hormone replacement (although there has been no research in the area).

Psoriasis medications have not been well studied in older adults. But it is known that older people are more likely to experience side effects, and medications can stay in the body longer than in younger people. "For example, methotrexate is excreted more slowly when you're older because your kidneys don't work as well. Methotrexate also increases the risk of high blood pressure in people over 65. Cyclosporine directly raises blood pressure, as well," says Dr. Lebwohl. Older women should discuss all medications with their physician, including any unusual side effects they may be experiencing.

Alopecia Areata

Alopecia areata is an autoimmune skin disease that affects hair follicles, causing hair loss on the scalp and elsewhere on the body. The National Alopecia Areata Foundation (NAAF) estimates that over 4.5 million people in the United States are affected, many of them women.

What Causes Alopecia Areata?

We actually lose hair all the time; each day you may shed as many as 100 hairs as part of the normal growth cycle. Each hair on your head grows about a half inch per month for an average of four to seven years, then enters a "resting" phase (or telogen) lasting two to three months. About 85 percent of the hair on your scalp is growing at any given moment; 15 percent of your hair is in the resting stage. At the end of the resting stage, the hair falls out and a new hair grows in its place.

In alopecia areata, hair follicles are attacked by cell-killing (cytotoxic, NK) T cells, resulting in the arrest of the hair growth stage, explains Madeleine Duvic, MD, professor of Medicine, Interim Chair, Department of Dermatology, and director of the Alopecia Areata National Registry at the M. D. Anderson Cancer Center at the University of Texas in Houston. "The hair breaks off because of the

---

Warning Signs of Alopecia

- One or more round bald patches on the scalp
- Loss of hair in the eyelashes or eyebrows
- Sudden or progressive loss of hair on the scalp or body

---

inflammatory infiltrate, so you get a little stubble. But the hair follicles are still there—they are just damaged and that is why hair breaks off," explains Dr. Duvic.

Recent research has uncovered multiple immune signaling pathways that promote attacks on hair follicles.[28] It's unclear how those immune signals may influence the severity of the attacks, how long they last, or why they can suddenly stop. But hair regrowth often resumes spontaneously, says Dr. Duvic.

According to the NAAF, the autoimmune attack causes hair follicles to go into a dormant state where they become very small and produce barely visible hairs (or no hair) for months or even years. The scalp is the most commonly affected area, but any hair-bearing site can be affected alone or together with the scalp. Illness and stress may play a role, though most people with alopecia areata are otherwise healthy. "When there's a stressor like an illness, or a fever, or a loss of blood that can synchronize your hair. And after you've been sick, your hair starts falling out, you lose the resting hairs that are synchronized; that's telogen effluvium, which is reversible and different from alopecia areata," says Dr. Duvic.

Alopecia areata occurs in men and women of all ages and races, but it often begins in childhood. Genes play a role; at least one out of five persons with alopecia areata has someone else in the family with the disorder. When the disease occurs before age 30, it's more likely there's a family history. Alopecia areata often occurs in families whose members have asthma, allergies, eczema, or other autoimmune diseases such as thyroiditis, diabetes, rheumatoid arthritis, lupus, vitiligo, pernicious anemia, or Addison's disease.

Recent research indicates that some people may have genetic markers that both increase their susceptibility and influence the severity of the autoimmune attacks on hair follicles.[29]

Alopecia areata may cluster with vitiligo (see page 161), rheumatoid arthritis, lupus, ulcerative colitis, celiac disease, and Hashimoto's thyroiditis, as well as the nonautoimmune skin disorders atopic dermatitis and eczema.

Symptoms of Alopecia Areata

Alopecia usually begins with one or two small, roundish bald spots that appear on the scalp, or with diffuse shedding of hair. Some people may lose eyelashes in one area of the eyelid or eyebrow hair. In some people, the nails develop stippling that looks as if a pin had made rows of tiny dents; in rare cases, the nails become severely distorted. Some people may have coexisting vitiligo, a loss of pigment in patches of the skin (the pigment melanin is present in hair root bulbs) or regrowth of white hair.

Some women develop only a few bare patches that regrow hair within a year. In others, extensive patchy loss occurs. When all scalp hair is lost, the condition is referred to as *alopecia totalis*; when hair is lost from the entire scalp and body, it's called alopecia universalis. (This does not cause scarring, which can occur in lupus.)

Alopecia areata does not appear to be influenced by hormones. "A lot of my patients say they get worse in the spring or the fall; there's a 30 percent incidence of allergy and atopy in alopecia areata patients. So it's possible that they're allergic and the pollens in spring or fall set the reaction," says Dr. Duvic.

Some women may have alopecia areata and not even know it because hair loss occurs in the back of the scalp. In some cases, hairdressers are the ones who spot it.

Diagnosing Alopecia Areata

While the coin-sized patches of baldness characteristic of alopecia areata are the key symptom, a dermatologist will take a medical history, including when the problem began, if there was any associated life stress, what kind of medications are being taken, what the hormonal status is, any unusual diet, and whether there's a family history of baldness.

A dermatologist will also examine the scalp carefully for any scarring caused by trauma, lupus, or a skin disorder, which can be confirmed with a scalp biopsy. In some cases, a few hairs will be examined under a microscope. If there's a root bulb at the end of a strand, it indicates a telogen hair. Hair lost during the growth phase has a club-like shape on its root end and can indicate a reaction to medication, among other things. Blood tests may also be done to see whether a woman has thyroid disease, a hormonal imbalance, lupus, or anemia.

"You have to rule out fungal infection of the scalp, which is often localized like alopecia areata, and there may be broken-off hairs, called 'exclamation point hairs.' If you don't see specific patches and there's a generalized loss, you look for an infection. However, generalized hair loss can also occur during telogen effluvium," says Dr. Duvic. "Low iron, which can cause anemia as well as hair loss, may be a contributing factor in some patients. There's about a 30 percent incidence of thyroid problems in adults with alopecia areata; it can precede it or develop after it."

"A biopsy is the most definite way to make a diagnosis. You will see lymphocytes around the root bulb of the follicle," she stresses.

Treating Alopecia Areata

The choice of treatment depends mainly on a woman's age and the type of alopecia. Alopecia areata occurs in two forms: a mild patchy form where less than 50 percent of scalp hair is lost and an extensive form where greater than 90 percent of scalp hair is lost. These two forms of alopecia areata behave quite differently, and treatment depends on which form you have.

Current approved treatments do not affect the autoimmune process that underlies alopecia but are aimed at stimulating the hair follicle to grow hair again. Treatments need to be continued until the disease process turns itself off. Treatments are most effective in milder cases.

Cortisone Injections

In cases of mild, patchy alopecia areata, multiple injections of cortisone are done in and around bald patches and repeated once a month. If new hair growth occurs, it's usually visible within four weeks. Local cortisone injections do not prevent new patches from developing, but they do kill T cells locally. Other than the needle prick and a slight tingling afterward, there are few side effects. Occasionally, temporary depressions in the skin result from the local injections, but these dells usually fill in by themselves. Topical, over-the-counter steroids don't work with alopecia areata.

Topical Minoxidil

A solution of 5 percent topical *minoxidil* applied twice daily to the scalp and eyebrows may help regrow hair. If scalp hair regrows completely, treatment can be stopped. Over-the-counter, 2 percent topical minoxidil solution is not effective by itself in alopecia areata; response may improve if cortisone cream is applied 30 minutes after the minoxidil. Topical minoxidil does not lower blood pressure in people with normal blood pressure. Neither 2 percent nor 5 percent topical minoxidil solution is effective in treating women with 100 percent scalp hair loss.

"Some people respond beautifully to minoxidil. However, those people may have grown back hair anyway. Alopecia areata is a hard disease to evaluate because a lot of people regrow hair no matter what, and there's no way to predict who will regrow hair," says Dr. Duvic.

Topical minoxidil hasn't been studied among pregnant women, although animal studies suggest it may cause problems during pregnancy. It's also not known whether topical minoxidil passes into breast milk. Limited tests have been conducted among older adults (up to age 65), and it appears to work better in younger patients. People with low blood pressure need to be careful about using too much and over large areas because topical minoxidil is actually a form of a drug used to treat hypertension.

Anthralin Cream or Ointment

Anthralin is a synthetic, tarlike substance that is used for psoriasis. It's applied to bare patches once daily and washed off after 30 to 60 minutes. Anthralin can be combined with minoxidil for an increased effect.

"Anthralin irritates the scalp; it attracts other T cells and they kind of override the hair-specific autoimmune attack. And then probably the immune system tries to shut off that reaction and takes the alopecia away. That's how we think it works," explains Dr. Duvic.

If new hair growth occurs with anthralin, it will be visible in 8 to 12 weeks. Side effects include irritation and temporary brownish discoloration, which can be lessened by shortening treatment times. Care must be taken not to get anthralin in the eyes. Hands must be washed after applying.

Anthralin may be absorbed through the skin, but no studies of its effects on pregnancy, in either humans or animals, have been done, and it's not known whether it can pass into breast milk. No data are available on whether anthralin works differently in older women.

Systemic Corticosteroids

Oral corticosteroids (such as prednisone) are sometimes prescribed when there is extensive scalp hair loss. "If someone is going completely bald really quickly, and it is her first episode of alopecia areata, we try systemic steroids. Because if you can cut it off before it becomes established, then you might make a difference," says Dr. Duvic.

The main problem is that any regrown hair is likely to fall out when the cortisone pills are stopped. In addition, there are health risks, such as bone loss, high blood pressure, diabetes, ulcers, and cataracts (see pages 42 to 43).

Topical Sensitizers

Topical sensitizers are medications that, when applied to the scalp, provoke an allergic reaction that leads to itching, scaling, and eventually hair growth. Two topical sensitizers are used in alopecia areata: *squaric acid dibutyl ester (SADBE)* and *diphenylcyclopropenone (DPCP).* Approximately 40 percent of patients treated with topical immunotherapy regrow scalp hair after about six months.[30] However, the treatment must be continued to maintain hair regrowth.

Photochemotherapy

Photochemotherapy combining the light-sensitive drug *psoralen* and UV light, used most commonly for psoriasis, can be used in alopecia areata. PUVA is usually given two to three times per week at a specialized center. However, when used for long periods, PUVA may increase your risk of developing skin cancer.

What's Next?

A synthetic DMARD approved for RA, *tofacitinib (Xeljanz),* which disrupts the signaling of cytokines called *Janus-associated kinases (JAK)* may hold promise as a treatment for alopecia areata.

Studies in 2010 revealed that signals from JAK-associated cytokines in hair follicles cause NK cells to attack the follicles.[22] "We found that a 'danger signal' in the hair follicles of patients—not previously linked to alopecia areata—attracts the immune cells to the follicle and sparks the attack," explained researcher Angela M. Christiano, PhD, professor in the Departments of Dermatology and of Genetics and Development at Columbia University Medical Center in New York.[31]

Later experiments in mice with alopecia found that interrupting those signals with JAK inhibitors completely restored hair within three months. The research prompted small clinical trials in alopecia patients of tofacitinib and *ruxolitinib (Jakafi)*, another JAK inhibitor approved to treat blood disorders. Preliminary results, reported in 2014 in the journal *Nature Medicine*, show ruxolitinib produced complete hair regrowth within five months in three patients with moderate-to-severe alopecia.[21]

Tofacitinib and ruxolitinib are oral medications taken twice a day. A cream formulation is also under investigation.

A Little Artifice Aids Appearance

Women with extensive hair loss often opt for wigs. Some newer, well-made wigs of synthetic or human hair have special tiny suction caps that keep them firmly in place, even during active sports. Another option is special double-sided tape, which can be purchased in beauty supply outlets. Cosmetic tattooing can be done on the eyebrow area and along the eyelids for an eyeliner effect. Then again, some women are proudly showing off their bald heads, rejecting the notion that the only way a woman can be beautiful is with long, thick hair.

Vitiligo

Vitiligo is caused by an immune attack on melanocytes, the skin cells that produce melanin, the pigment that gives skin its color. The result is white patches of skin, which may enlarge and increase in number. In some cases the condition may stabilize and then start up again.

Vitiligo affects 1 to 2 percent of Americans, and while it's less obvious in light-skinned people, it can be traumatic for African Americans and other women of color. Half of women with vitiligo develop the disorder between the ages of 10 and 30, and it may be genetic in some cases.

Vitiligo is also associated with other autoimmune disorders. As many as 30 percent of women with vitiligo may develop thyroid disease. Women with vitiligo also have an increased risk of *pernicious anemia* or *Addison's disease* (see page 228).

People with vitiligo must protect their skin from the sun; without the protection of melanin the affected patches of skin can become seriously sunburned. Women must use sunscreen with a *sun protection factor (SPF)* of at least 30 on exposed skin year-round (there are special sunscreens, like 60 SPF *Total Block*, designed for people with extreme sun sensitivity and those at high risk of skin cancer). Long sleeves and pants and wide-brimmed hats should be worn during long periods spent outdoors. Sun-protective clothing, made from special fabric that blocks out UV light, should have a hang tag that gives its *ultraviolet protection factor (UPF)* value and detail the testing standards it has met.

Treating Vitiligo

There's no cure for vitiligo, but there are treatments that help restore lost melanin. The mainstay of treatment is PUVA, which can effectively darken white skin patches, especially if vitiligo is extensive. If vitiligo patches are very limited, occasionally psoralen can be applied directly to the skin before ultraviolet A treatment. At least a year of twice-weekly PUVA treatments is needed to restore melanin production.

PUVA is 50 to 70 percent effective in restoring pigment to vitiligo patches on the face, trunk, upper arms, and legs. However, the hands and feet respond poorly to PUVA. PUVA is not approved for use in pregnant or nursing women (see page 156).

If patches are small, corticosteroid creams may help restore pigment. However, chronic use of steroids can result in thinning and atrophy of the skin.

According to the American Academy of Dermatology, topical treatments work best for people with darkly pigmented skin. They work best on the face and are least effective on the hands and feet.

Excimer Laser

The *Excimer laser*, a small, intensely focused UV laser, is now used to treat limited vitiligo (covering less than 30 percent of the body's surface) and stable vitiligo patches.[24] Laser therapy is more effective when used early in the disease. Localized lesions are treated twice weekly for an average of 24 to 48 sessions, so the treatment can be costly. Adding tacrolimus ointment to laser therapy may improve results.

Notes

1. Scleroderma Foundation. What is scleroderma? http://www.scleroderma.org/site/PageNavigator/patients_whatis.html#.VWiX3M9Viko.
2. van den Hoogen F, Khanna D, Fransen J, et al. 2013 classification criteria for systemic sclerosis. *Arthritis Rheum*. 2013. doi:10.1002/art.38098.
3. Kowal-Bielecka O, Landewé R, Avouac J. EULAR recommendations for the treatment of systemic sclerosis: a report from the EULAR Scleroderma Trials and Research group (EUSTAR). *Ann Rheum Dis*. 2009;68:620–628. doi:10.1136/ard.2008.096677.
4. Herrick AL, van den Hoogen F, Gabrielli C, et al. Modified-release sildenafil reduces Raynaud's phenomenon attack frequency in limited cutaneous systemic sclerosis. *Arthritis Rheum*. 2011;63(3):775–782. doi:10.1002/art.30195.
5. van Laar JM, Farge D, Sont JK, et al. Autologous hematopoietic stem cell transplantation vs intravenous pulse cyclophosphamide in diffuse cutaneous systemic sclerosis: a randomized clinical trial. *JAMA*. 2014;311(24):2490–2498. doi:10.1001/jama.2014.6368.
6. Burt RK, Shah SJ, Dill K, et al. Autologous non-myeloablative haemopoietic stem-cell transplantation compared with pulse cyclophosphamide once per month for systemic sclerosis (ASSIST): an open-label, randomized phase 2 trial. *Lancet*. 2011;378(9790):498–506.
7. Skoro-Sajer N, Lang IM. Selexipag for the treatment of pulmonary arterial hypertension. *Expert Opin Pharmacother*. 2014;15(3):429–436. doi:10.1517/14656566.2014.876007. Epub 2014 Jan 7.
8. Hudson M, Russell Steele R, Canadian Scleroderma Research Group (CSRG), and Baron M. Update on indices of disease activity in systemic sclerosis. *Semin Arthritis Rheum*. 2007;37:93–98.
9. Muangchan C, Harding S, Khimda S, et al., Canadian Scleroderma Research Group. Association of C-reactive protein with high disease activity in systemic sclerosis: results from the Canadian Scleroderma Research Group. *Arthritis Care Res*. 2012;64(9):1405–1414. doi:10.1002/acr.21716.
10. Steen V. Pregnancy in scleroderma. *Rheum Dis Clin*. 2007;33(2):345–358. http://dx.doi.org/10.1016/j.rdc.2007.03.001.
11. Vinet E, Bernatsky S, Hudson M, Pineau CA, Baron M. Effect of menopause on the modified Rodnan skin score in systemic sclerosis. *Arthritis Res Ther*. 2014;16:R130. doi:10.1186/ar4587.

12. Fraenkel L, Zhang Y, Chaisson CE, et al. The association of estrogen replacement therapy and the Raynaud phenomenon in postmenopausal women. *Ann Intern Med.* 1998;129(3):208–211. doi:10.7326/0003-4819-129-3-199808010-00009.
13. Impens1 AJ, Rothman J, Schiopu1 E, et al. Sexual activity and functioning in female scleroderma patients. *Clin Exp Rheumatol.* 2009;27(suppl 54):S38–S43.
14. Golpour M, Hamzeh Hosseini SM, Khademloo M, et al. Depression and anxiety disorders among patients with psoriasis: a hospital-based case-control study. *Dermatol Res Pract.* 2012. doi:10.1155/2012/381905.
15. Mease PJ, Gladman DD, Papp KA, et al. Prevalence of rheumatologist-diagnosed psoriatic arthritis in patients with psoriasis in European/North American dermatology clinics. *J Am Acad Dermatol.* 2013;69(5):729–735. doi:10.1016/j.jaad.2013.07.023.
16. Gottlieb A, Korman NJ, Gordon KB, et al. Guidelines of care for the management of psoriasis and psoriatic arthritis. *J Am Acad Dermatol.* 2008;58(5):851–864.
17. Veale DJ, Fearon U. What makes psoriatic and rheumatoid arthritis so different? *Rheum Musculoskeletal Dis, RMD Open.* 2015;1:e000025. doi:10.1136/rmdopen-2014-000025.
18. Gossec L, Smolen JS, Gaujoux-Viala C, et al. European League Against Rheumatism recommendations for the management of psoriatic arthritis with pharmacological therapies. *Ann Rheum Dis.* 2012;71(1):4–12. Epub 2011 Sep 27.
19. Ritchlin CT, Kavanaugh A, Gladman DD, et al. Treatment recommendations for psoriatic arthritis. *Ann Rheum Dis.* 2009;68:1387–1394.
20. Eder L, Thavaneswaran A, Chandran V, Gladman DD. Tumour necrosis factor α blockers are more effective than methotrexate in the inhibition of radiographic joint damage progression among patients with psoriatic arthritis. *Ann Rheum Dis.* 2014; 73:1007.
21. Cimzia (certolizumab pegol) Fact Sheet, 2015. https://www.psoriasis.org/document.doc?id=2755.
22. Stelara (ustekinumab) Fact Sheet. 2013. https://www.psoriasis.org/document.doc?id=661.
23. FDA approves Otezla to treat psoriatic arthritis. FDA Press Release, March 21, 2014. http://www.fda.gov/NewsEvents/Newsroom/PressAnnouncements/ucm390091.htm.
24. Mudigonda T, Dabade TS, Feldman SR. A review of protocols for 308 nm excimer laser phototherapy in psoriasis. *J Drugs Dermatol.* 2012;11(1):92–97.
25. Soriatane Prescribing information. http://www.drugs.com/pro/soriatane.html.
26. FDA, Alefacept package insert. http://www.fda.gov/downloads/Drugs/Development ApprovalProcess/HowDrugsareDevelopedandApproved/ApprovalApplications/TherapeuticBiologicApplications/ucm086009.pdf.
27. Stelara (ustinumab) Fact Sheet. https://www.psoriasis.org/document.doc?id=661.
28. Xing L, Zhenpeng Dai Z, Ali Jabbari A, et al. Alopecia areata is driven by cytotoxic T lymphocytes and is reversed by JAK inhibition *Nat Med.* 2014. Advance online publication. doi:10.1038/nm.3645.

29. Petukhova L, Duvic M, Hordinsky M, et al. Genome-wide association study in alopecia areata implicates both innate and adaptive immunity. *Nature.* 2010;466(7302):113–117. doi:10.1038/nature09114.
30. Singh G, Lavanya MS. Topical immunotherapy in alopecia areata. *Int J Trichology.* 2010;2(1):36–39. doi:10.4103/0974-7753.66911.
31. FDA-approved drug restores hair in patients with alopecia areata. Columbia University Medical Center press release, August 17, 2014.

6

More Than a Dry Spell—Sjögren's Syndrome

I started having dryness symptoms in my middle forties. I kept complaining about dry mouth to my dentist, but he didn't seem concerned about it. I had lots of cavities, and I didn't realize then that lack of saliva can cause your teeth to deteriorate. I had dry mouth for three or four years, but it started to become much worse. I found I couldn't eat anything. I was totally without saliva and could hardly swallow. As it turned out, there was a saliva specialist at the university where I work.

My husband urged me to see him, but I said, "Why should I see a saliva specialist if I don't have any saliva!" But my husband insisted, and I finally went. The specialist told me right away I probably had Sjögren's.

I had never heard of it before. When he asked me about dry eyes and eye pain, until then I hadn't realized that the shooting pains in my eyes were from dry spots. I simply connected my dry mouth to my eyes.

EVELYN, 52

Having *Sjögren's syndrome* is like wandering in a desert, thirsting for a cool drink of water. Sometimes you're so dry that nothing can quench your thirst or make your mouth feel moist. Your eyes feel gritty and painful, and after a while other parts of the body, such as the vagina, can become dry as well.

Sjögren's syndrome is actually the second most common autoimmune rheumatic disease after rheumatoid arthritis. The Sjögren's Syndrome

Foundation (SSF) estimates that two to four million people may be affected, 90 percent of whom are women. Sjögren's often accompanies other autoimmune disorders like rheumatoid arthritis or lupus (in this case, it's called *secondary Sjögren's*), but 50 percent of patients have Sjögren's that occurs on its own (*primary Sjögren's*).

Years ago, you might never have heard of Sjögren's unless you were diagnosed with it. But all that changed in 2011 when tennis champion Venus Williams revealed that she had Sjögren's, putting the disease on the map. She's now the Honorary Chairperson of the Sjögren's Syndrome Foundation Awareness Ambassador Program.

Williams, 35, who has won more than 45 singles titles in her career, including Grand Slams like the U.S. Open and Wimbledon, doesn't comment much publicly on her Sjögren's. It has caused her back pain and fatigue, but she doesn't let it slow her down.

"What else am I going to do, get down?" she told sportswriters in Cincinnati in 2013. "The same amount of time you spend down is the amount of time you can spend up. I don't like being down."[1]

Still, she's made some accommodations. "In the past, I would train until I died. Now, because of Sjögren's syndrome, I have to be careful. If I train too hard, then I won't be able to do anything the next day. There would be times when I'd park my car at home, and I fell asleep behind the wheel because I was so tired! It's a balance between pushing myself as much as I can and being reasonable about what I can achieve and what my body will tolerate," she told *ESPN Magazine* in July 2014.[2]

"You are so tired it hurts," she continues. "At my worst point, I wasn't able to play tennis at all. Just the whole quality of my life was compromised—and uncomfortable. It's very difficult to understand unless you've gone through it. Especially as a professional athlete, there's never any acceptable excuse. You push and you push and you'll die on the court if you have to, but you get it done. The whole experience is just foreign as an athlete. You have to accept that you're never going to be 100 percent. So, how do you get past those roadblocks?"

"There is never not an answer," says Williams. "For me, that's the solution. If I have to work hard or think hard or just copy somebody else that's doing it better—whatever it takes, I'm going to find that solution. That's the drive that keeps me going."[2]

Warning Signs of Sjögren's

- Dry, scratchy eyes
- Chronic dry mouth
- Reduced salivary flow
- Burning oral mucous membranes (burning mouth syndrome)
- Frequent cavities
- Dry vagina and painful intercourse
- Fatigue
- Neuropathy
- Lung inflammation

What Causes Sjögren's Syndrome?

In Sjögren's, the disease process targets the body's moisture-producing glands: the *lacrimal* glands that produce tears (located within the upper and outer margins of the eye socket and in the eyelid) and the three glands that produce saliva—the *sublingual* salivary gland (located under the tongue), the *submandibular* salivary gland (beneath the jaw), and the *parotid* glands (deep within the angle of the jaw in front of the ear). These are called *exocrine* glands because they have ducts and don't secrete hormones and other substances directly into the blood. Sjögren's also targets moisture-producing tissues, including mucous membranes in the nose, vagina, and lungs.

The moisture-producing glands are regulated by the *autonomic nervous system* that governs automatic functions like breathing and blood pressure. As these glands become damaged by activated immune cells, they may be less able to respond to signals from an area of the brain that handles sensory input and triggers production of tears or saliva (for example, your mouth watering at the sight or smell of food). At the same time, inflammatory molecules (*cytokines*) released by immune cells may lead to damage to nerves (as well as diminished production of *neurotransmitters*) that stimulate the salivary or tear glands. In addition, these activated immune cells don't undergo normal programmed cell death, so they accumulate to perpetuate the autoimmune response.

The dry eyes of Sjögren's are caused by low tear production due to destruction of the lacrimal glands and dysfunction of the tiny glands behind the eyelashes that secrete oil that prevents tears from evaporating (*meibomian glands*).

Your tears are actually made up of three layers: the *mucin* layer on the surface of the eye is made up of secretions from the cornea and glands scattered throughout the *conjunctiva* (the mucous membrane covering the lining of the eyelids and outside of the eyeball); the middle, *aqueous*, layer is largely made up of water and proteins from the lacrimal glands; the outer layer, called the *lipid layer*, is made up of fatty secretions from oil glands in the eyelids (*meibomian glands*).

The mucin layer provides lubrication for the cornea; without it, dry spots develop and cause discomfort. The aqueous layer of tears provides key proteins that protect the eye against bacteria. The lipid layer of the tear film prevents excessive evaporation of tears; if the lipid layer is inadequate, the tear film evaporates. Every time you blink, your eyelids distribute the tear film over the surface of the eye and lubricate it; if there's not enough tear film, the eyelid won't move as smoothly over the surface of the eye, causing

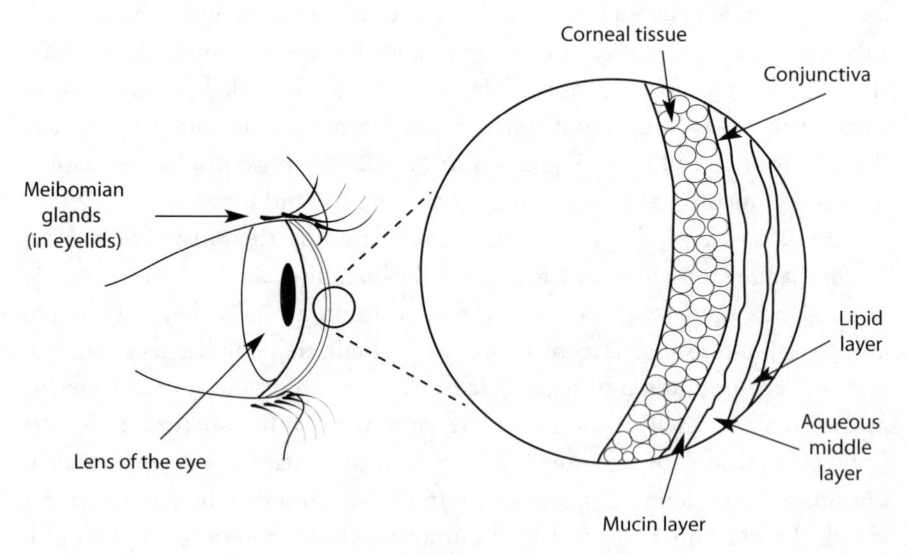

Tear Film Layers

the gritty sensation that also characterizes Sjögren's. In fact, this evaporative problem is thought to contribute to 80 percent of all cases of dry eye, says David A. Sullivan, MS, PhD, senior scientist at the Schepens Eye Research Institute in Boston.

"It used to be thought that inadequate aqueous tears were the main problem in Sjögren's. But women with Sjögren's also have meibomian gland dysfunction and don't have enough oil in the tear film. So the tear film is unstable and evaporates," explains Dr. Sullivan, also an associate professor of ophthalmology at Harvard Medical School.

One underlying risk factor for the development of evaporative dry eye may be androgen deficiency (low levels of male hormones).[3] Androgens play a key role in the function of the meibomian glands and also serve to dampen inflammation in the lacrimal glands, says Dr. Sullivan.

While Sjögren's can emerge at any age, women typically develop the syndrome between ages 45 and 55, when androgens and estrogens decline.

In the case of mucous membranes and other tissues that produce moisture, cytokines may interfere with the normal passage of fluid onto the surface of those tissues, such as those in the vagina. Without moisture, these tissues become uncomfortably dry and ulcerated. Almost 70 percent of women with Sjögren's experience dry vagina, and most of them find sex uncomfortable if not painful.[4] The disorder can also affect organs such as the lungs, kidneys, and liver, as well as blood vessels.

What triggers the autoimmune reaction in Sjögren's is unknown. Several genes are associated with Sjögren's, and the disorder tends to cluster in families. According to the Sjögren's Syndrome Foundation, around 12 percent of patients have one or more relatives (usually female) with Sjögren's.

It's possible that a viral infection or other injury may set off an immune reaction in genetically susceptible people. Some research suggests a role for *Epstein-Barr virus (EBV)*. The virus lies dormant in the salivary glands for years and can be reactivated, perhaps during other viral infections. However, since most people have been exposed to EBV, the virus alone is not thought to be a trigger. EBV has also been implicated in multiple sclerosis and lupus.[5]

Symptoms of Sjögren's

When you have Sjögren's, you'll typically have a gritty or burning sensation in the eyes, eyelids that stick together, mucus accumulation in the inner corners of the eyes usually when you awaken, itching, sensitivity to light, blurred vision, and discomfort and difficulty reading or watching television. You may notice a "filmy" effect that interferes with vision. Symptoms often worsen as the day goes on.

The symptoms of dry eye result from increased friction due to insufficient tears and evaporation of the tear film. In some cases, the eyelid may actually stick to the conjunctiva or corneal surface and can literally pull epithelial cells away from the surface, causing erosions. Dry eye, discomfort, inflammation, and defects in the surface layer of the conjunctiva and cornea are called *keratoconjunctivitis sicca (KCS)*. Ironically, people with dry eyes may notice excessive tearing at first, as the eye compensates by producing more "reflex" tears, tears usually produced when there's a foreign body in the eye or other irritation. But women with Sjögren's are less able to produce reflex tears.

Sjögren's also affects the production of saliva. Saliva is actually a mixture of mucins, water, nutrient proteins, and growth factors that provide lubrication for the tongue for speaking, swallowing, and washing away bacteria and toxins from the surface of the teeth and mucous membranes. Loss of saliva is associated with increased cavities; fillings may also loosen or break down more quickly, you may also get oral yeast infections, and you have mouth discomfort.

Dry mouth symptoms (*xerostomia*) can include a burning sensation on your tongue or mucous membranes in the mouth ("burning mouth syndrome"), and you may have problems with chewing or swallowing food. For example, being unable to swallow dry foods like crackers without fluid is a frequent complaint. Your mouth may feel dry and sticky and you can develop cracks in the tongue or corners of the mouth (often due to yeast), problems with taste or smell, and a constant need to drink liquids. Many women need to keep water at their bedside. The combination of dry eyes and dry mouth is also called *sicca syndrome*.

The *parotid glands*, the largest of the salivary glands (the same glands affected by the mumps) may also be enlarged or hardened. In fact, if you had mumps as a child and seemed to get it again as an adult, it's not mumps but may be a sign of Sjögren's. You may also have yeast infections in the mouth.

There can be drying of the nasal passages with crusting and nosebleeds and throat hoarseness, as well as dry and irritated vaginal tissues.

Around 40 to 50 percent of primary Sjögren's patients have what's called "small fiber neuropathy," with pain, prickling, tingling, or burning in the forearms and legs and, in some cases, problems with bowel motility or difficulty sweating.[6] It's believed to be caused by dysfunction or reduced numbers of tiny nerve fibers beneath the *epidermis* (the tissue just under the skin's surface), and other areas.

Another major problem is fatigue—experienced by 60 to 70 percent of women with Sjögren's syndrome.[7] Again, we're not talking about feeling tired from lack of sleep, but a unique kind of tiredness that you can't predict or control. Rheumatologists are now paying more attention, but it's still something you need to bring up with your doctor.

In a recent report in *Arthritis Care & Research*, a group of Sjögren's patients described how when fatigue hit, their body would stiffen up and become painful and feel as if it had "run out of energy," "given up," or "had flat batteries," forcing them to put their life on hold[7]:

> *"I never felt tired when I was healthy—I was always very involved in things and had lots of energy. So this is a real difference. Of course I was often tired when I had small children and was pregnant and everything, but you know, then you could just go to sleep and afterwards it was better. But this doesn't work now. Now it feels sort of lethargic, my body feels heavy and I never get my energy back. It's like my body's lost all its fervor in a way. I just don't have the energy I used to have. In my head I want to do everything I did before and then it just doesn't work. It's exhausting just peeling potatoes—everything takes so long,"*[7] one woman remarked. *"When I have my usual tiredness I just decide that today I'll do what I have to. But I can't do this when I get these waves of tiredness—I just have to sort of give up. It goes up and down a bit but I have this sort of constant tiredness all the time, and sometimes I feel absolutely empty of energy."*[7]

There may also be joint pain, fever, dry skin, allergic skin reactions, and sleep disturbances, waking up with a dry mouth, drinking water, and then having to urinate more often, as well as gastrointestinal problems like constipation, all of which people may not associate with the disorder.

Sjögren's can also affect many systems in the body, including the nerves, kidneys, and lungs. It can cause peripheral nerve problems (*neuropathy*), lung inflammation (*interstitial pneumonitis*), and kidney dysfunction (*renal tubular acidosis*). Symptoms of lung problems in Sjögren's are shortness of breath and exercise intolerance.

Sjögren's symptoms can also mimic other conditions. The drying of vaginal tissues is often blamed on menopause; eye irritation may be attributed to conjunctivitis. Joint pain and fatigue may be blamed on lupus or rheumatoid arthritis, and nerve-related symptoms can be similar to multiple sclerosis. Not surprisingly, Sjögren's can be tricky to identify. A survey of SSF members found that 25 percent spent over five years trying to get an accurate diagnosis.

Women with Sjögren's also have an increased risk of *lymphoma* (malignancy of the lymph glands). So it's imperative to be carefully followed by an internist. Any lymph node lump in the neck, underarm, or groin should be investigated immediately. However, less than 10 percent of Sjögren's patients develop lymphoma.

Evelyn's story continues:

At the salivary dysfunction clinic, the first test I had was a "resting saliva" test. I sat for five minutes without swallowing and then spit into a little cup, and he looked at what I produced, which was a little blob of what looked like glue. He turned the cup upside down and it didn't move. Then he gave me a stimulated saliva test, where you chew a little piece of wax to stimulate saliva production. As you chew you spit out what's in your mouth, and I didn't produce much of anything. Then he ran a series of blood tests, then sent me to an ophthalmologist, who confirmed the diagnosis. Getting a diagnosis was extremely helpful to me. I now do a fluoride treatment with my teeth every night, and I avoid eating foods with sugar. Without saliva, there's nothing to protect your teeth. That made a real difference. I've had a few cavities, but nothing like the kind of major dental work I had before.

Diagnosing Sjögren's Syndrome

As with Evelyn, it often takes years before a woman is properly diagnosed. Sometimes the symptoms are blamed on aging, says Ann Parke, MD, a noted rheumatologist who specializes in Sjögren's at St. Francis Hospital and Medical

Sjögren's Clusters

While dry eyes are a common symptom in autoimmune diseases, secondary Sjögren's frequently accompanies a number of diseases, including the following:

- Rheumatoid arthritis
- Systemic lupus erythematosus
- Hashimoto's thyroiditis
- Graves' disease
- Primary biliary cirrhosis
- Autoimmune hepatitis
- Multiple sclerosis
- Scleroderma
- Myasthenia gravis

Center in Hartford, Connecticut. "I have patients who come in and say they were perfectly fine until age 40 or 45, and that's when they start to develop their complaints. But frequently they are not diagnosed for another 10 years. To a certain extent we associate dry eyes, dry mouth, and dry vagina with aging, but I think a lot of people don't take these complaints seriously," says Dr. Parke, a member of the Sjögren's Foundation medical and scientific advisory board. "The fatigue associated with Sjögren's also complicates things. Women go in to see their primary care physicians and say, 'I'm tired,' and they are labeled as having 'empty-nest syndrome' or being depressed. They are not asked the important questions: 'Do you have dry eyes? Do you have a dry mouth? Do you sleep OK?' It's a major problem."

According to the 2015 screening guidelines from the Sjögren's Syndrome Foundation, patients answering "yes" to any of the following questions need a full ocular examination:[8]

- How often do your eyes feel dryness, discomfort, or irritation? Often or constantly?
- When you have eye dryness, discomfort, or irritation, does this impact your activities (e.g., stop or reduce your time doing them)?
- Do you think you have dry eye?

Other causes of the symptoms associated with Sjögren's must also be ruled out, such as the drying effects of drugs, eye diseases or infection, the effects of allergies (and allergy medications), and lymphoma (which can sometimes involve the salivary glands).

A workup should begin with a complete history and physical to assess the possibility of autoimmune, connective tissue, or glandular diseases. Your eyes, mouth, skin, and glands in your face and neck should be carefully examined.

Tests You May Need and What They Mean

After an assessment of your symptoms, a number of blood tests can help confirm a diagnosis of Sjögren's, the most important of which are autoantibodies reactive with SSA/Ro and SSB/La. Other tests may include an *erythrocyte sedimentation rate* (*ESR*, a general indication of inflammation, see page 33), as well as measuring levels of blood proteins called *immunoglobulins*. An elevation of the ESR and total IgG levels are often observed in patients with Sjögren's but are not specific.

Specific antibody tests that are performed include:

Antinuclear antibodies (ANAs) are a group of antibodies that react against the components of a cell nucleus. ANAs are present in a variety of autoimmune diseases, including lupus, but about 70 percent of patients with Sjögren's will also have a positive ANA test (see page 72).

Rheumatoid factor (RF), an antibody associated with rheumatoid arthritis, is found in 60 to 70 percent of people with Sjögren's (see page 32).

Sjögren's syndrome-associated A antigen (SSA/Ro) and Sjögren's syndrome-associated B antigen (SSB/La) are separate autoantibodies. Anti-SSA/Ro antibodies react with intracellular proteins that can be found in the cytoplasm (white of a cell as in an egg) or the nucleus (yellow center). Anti-SSB/La reacts with a nuclear protein. These antibodies are often found in pairs, but anti-SSA/Ro is more common. It is seen in the majority of patients with SS and in about 40 percent of patients with SLE. Anti-SSB/La is also seen in the majority of patients with SS but only about 15 percent of patients with SLE.

Recent research indicates that ANAs and other autoantibodies may be present years before obvious symptoms even appear.[9]

Antithyroid antibody and thyroid stimulating hormone (TSH) levels will be checked, since autoimmune thyroid diseases can cluster with Sjögren's and share symptoms like dry skin and fatigue. Therefore tests will be done to measure antithyroid antibodies and assess thyroid function, including the level of TSH.

The 2015 screening guidelines from the Sjögren's Syndrome Foundation include the following tests to evaluate dry eye.[8]

The Schirmer test is the simplest and most common eye test to assess tears and tear production. Small pieces of filter paper are placed between your eyeball and lower lid, and the amount of wetting produced within five minutes indicates the level of tear production. No anesthetic is required. A result of less than 5 mm would be strongly suggestive of Sjögren's.

A slit-lamp examination measures the amount of tears produced by the eye in its normal resting state. A lamp indirectly illuminates your eye to avoid producing reflex tears, and magnifies the surface so the normal layer of tears along the lower eyelid can be seen. The tear film may appear thickened with excessive debris. There may be inflammation of the conjunctiva.

Rose Bengal staining determines the quality of the mucin layer of the tear film and its distribution over the surface of the eye. *Rose Bengal* is a harmless vegetable dye. A single drop is administered after rinsing with a preservative-free tear preparation; reddish stain remains on the cells that have lost their mucin coating, a pattern of staining characteristic of keratoconjunctivitis sicca syndrome. The number of cells is counted, or scored. Another test, using a dye called *lissamine green*, can reveal scratches on the surface of the eye.

The degree of severity is graded, based on the results of ocular staining. Fluctuations in vision, decreased vision, and sensitivity to light also factor into the severity grading.[8] A dentist or oral pathologist may also measure your saliva production. As in Evelyn's case, this is done by stimulating saliva production using an acidic or sour substance, and then measuring the amount of saliva produced.

Salivary gland biopsy may be performed in some cases. The procedure involves making a small incision in the lower lip and removing five to ten tiny salivary glands, which are examined under a microscope for immune cell infiltration. Ultrasound to examine the salivary glands may provide additional information.

In cases of severe neuropathic pain, a small "punch" biopsy to count these fibers may be done *(epidermal nerve fiber density, ENFD)*. A lower nerve fiber count is considered diagnostic.[10]

A combination of symptoms, positive antibody tests, and positive tests for dry eye and/or decreased salivary production substantiate the diagnosis of Sjögren's. However, there's no single standard for diagnosis. American College of Rheumatology (ACR) has proposed simple criteria that your rheumatologist may use:[11]

1. Positive tests for anti-SSA or SSB antibodies, or positive RF plus elevated ANA.
2. A minor salivary gland biopsy to remove tiny salivary glands from the lips, which shows a specific pattern of inflammation (*focus areas of infiltration*).
3. Dry eye (*keratoconjunctivitis sicca*) with an ocular staining score of 3 or more.

Two of these tests should be positive for a diagnosis of Sjögren's syndrome, according to the ACR.[10]

However, many patients do not want to undergo salivary gland biopsies. In some clinical settings physicians will diagnose Sjögren's based on three or more of the following (provided that there is also some objective clinical testing).

- Symptoms of dry eyes
- Symptoms of dry mouth
- Objective evidence of dry eyes
- Objective evidence of dry mouth
- Anti-SSA/Ro or SSB/La antibodies
- Abnormal small salivary gland biopsy

The Female Factor

As many as 60 percent of pre- and postmenopausal women suffer from dry eyes. While estrogen appears to play a role in some autoimmune diseases, androgen deficiency appears to be a more critical factor in dry eye.[3] "Premenopausal women normally make about two-thirds of the amount of androgen than men do, and we have found that women with Sjögren's are androgen deficient. We have also learned that androgens are important for optimal lacrimal and meibomian gland function," says Dr. Sullivan. "Androgens can significantly influence the nature of the lipids produced in the meibomian glands, and they appear to promote the formation of the tear film lipid layer, thereby enhancing tear film stability. Consequently, androgen deficiency may promote the development of dry eye."

Androgen deficiency can occur with aging, during menopause (peak years for Sjögren's), and with certain autoimmune diseases, like lupus and Sjögren's. Androgens seem to dampen inflammation; studies indicate that dry eye improves in people given androgens. Dr. Sullivan adds. "In contrast, estrogen may worsen inflammation of the lacrimal glands, and may suppress meibomian gland function."

In fact, a 2001 study coauthored by Dr. Sullivan found the risk for dry eye was greater among women taking postmenopausal hormones. Researchers from the Schepens Eye Research Institute and Brigham and Women's Hospital in Boston looked at data from the Women's Health Initiative (WHI), which included 25,665 postmenopausal women, and found that almost 7 percent of women taking HT reported dry eye syndrome (keratoconjunctivitis sicca, KCS). More than 9 percent of women using estrogen therapy (ET) alone had KCS. The longer a woman used hormones, the greater the risk; for each three years that women used HT there was a 15 percent increase in the likelihood of being diagnosed with KCS or having severe symptoms.[12] However, the study was limited since diagnostic tests were not done.

Dry eyes can also occur in women with *autoimmune premature ovarian failure (POF)*, now called *primary ovarian insufficiency* (*POI*, see page 231). While women with premature menopause (before age 40) seem to have worse symptoms and more ocular damage, they don't appear to have reduced tear production.[13]

Evelyn's story continues:

The hardest thing for me are the social interactions. I always feel so self-conscious; I feel like everyone can see how dry I am. When I start a conversation with someone, and I don't have water with me, I can't have a conversation. It's impossible; I can't talk long without water. And it certainly affects eating. I have to have lots of liquid. At a cocktail party, I kind of ignore the food because I need to have something to drink and I can't juggle a plate and a glass. But I manage. I have it easier than people who also have arthritis or other painful syndromes. I have found ways to cope with the dryness. I have tried artificial saliva, and the sprays, but I can't stand the taste, and they are very short-acting. I took pilocarpine for two years, but it had a lot of side effects. The biggest way Sjögren's affects me is actually the fatigue. By nine o'clock at night, I just collapse.

Treating Sjögren's Syndrome

While there's no cure, there are a variety of treatment options for symptoms of Sjögren's syndrome.

Dry Eye

For some women, over-the-counter "artificial tears" can temporarily soothe dry eyes. However, these lubricating drops don't have lasting effects and, in severe cases, must be used frequently, increasing the risk of problems from preservatives says Janine Austin Clayton, MD, director of the Office of Research on Women's Health at the National Institutes of Health (NIH). Ocular lubricant ointments can be helpful if used before bedtime but can blur vision, causing problems during the day, so apply only a small amount.

Use preservative-free eyedrops (drops used to relieve redness and allergies often contain preservatives and can cause rashes under the eye). OTC drops include *Refresh Tears, Bion Tears*, and *TheraTears.*[14] TheraTears has also been shown to increase production of mucin in a rabbit model, adds Dr. Clayton, who served as deputy clinical director of the National Eye Institute at NIH. Some products provide the staying power of an ointment without blurring vision.

Several new gels have a consistency somewhere between eyedrops and ointment. *GenTeal* is a water-based gel and is among the lubricants and eyedrops containing "disappearing preservatives," which break down once the product is exposed to air.

"*Lacrisert* is a very tiny pellet, kind of like ointment in a pellet that is placed between the eye and the lower lid, and it dissolves over a 24-hour period. But it's only effective in patients who have some tears, because it needs tears to dissolve," explains Dr. Clayton.

A prescription eyedrop formulation of the anti-inflammatory drug *cyclosporine A (Restasis)* is the first therapy specifically aimed at dampening the underlying inflammation of dry eye.[15] Approved for treating Sjögren's and other forms of dry eye, Restasis appears to prevent T cell activation on the ocular surface and in the lacrimal gland. The drops increase tear production (as measured in a Schirmer test).

Corticosteroid eyedrops (such as *Pred Forte, Pred Mild, Lotemax*) can also reduce inflammation.[12] However, they can cause glaucoma and cataracts and are not safe to use for long periods. They are generally used as a short-term therapy for people who have not responded to other treatments. "If the eye is extremely inflamed, other measures won't work. If you can bring down the inflammation, other treatments may have a better chance of helping," says Dr. Clayton, an ophthalmologist who has researched dry eye and other ocular disorders.

A prescription eye "cleanser" called *Avenova (hypochlorous acid)*, for people with meibomian gland dysfunction and inflammation (*meibomitis*), can relieve symptoms of dry eye such as a gritty sandy feeling, crusted lids on awakening, and meibomian cysts (*chalazions*).[16] It is *not* a treatment for dry eye or for Sjögren's, however.

Tiny silicone plugs (called *punctal plugs*) can be placed in your tear ducts near the corner of the eyes and can help tears stay around longer. "In women with Sjögren's who have very low tear flow, punctal plugs may make things worse. If you have no outflow of tears, as the tears evaporate, inflammatory proteins can concentrate on the surface of the eye and cause discomfort. So you need to use other measures to keep the surface of the eye lubricated and flushed," explains Dr. Clayton. In rare cases, the plugs can become contaminated and cause infections, and ducts may become damaged.

Special goggles for outdoor use decrease tear evaporation or slow it, and some goggles have special inserts or patches that increase humidity around the eye. There are also plastic side shields for glasses and wraparound sunglasses. Humidifiers can make a big difference in the bedroom and elsewhere.

Recent research suggests that supplements containing essential fatty acids including omega-3 fats, found in fish like salmon (see page 45), may help relieve dry eye.[17] Now omega-3s are being tested in a randomized clinical trial, the Dry Eye Assessment and Management (DREAM) Trial. A supplement, *Thera Tears Nutrition*, is marketed specifically for dry eye.[12]

What's Next?

New therapies may include androgen eyedrops. "Animal data suggest that topical androgens may suppress lacrimal gland inflammation and correct the meibomian gland dysfunction in Sjögren's syndrome, aiding tear formation and production of a lasting tear film," explains Dr. Clayton. "It's also thought that androgens have anti-inflammatory properties, and that there's a relative androgen deficiency locally in the eye that may allow inflammation to progress on the surface of the eye."

There are also receptors for androgens and estrogens in the eyelid, the conjunctiva, the cornea, the lacrimal gland, and even in the retinal pigment epithelium. "We're learning more about how complex the ocular surface is, and it's not something that you can just rewet. Really what's needed is something that will produce physiologic tears," comments Dr. Clayton.

The androgen eyedrops developed by Dr. Sullivan and his colleagues at Harvard are in clinical trials.

Tests are also under way of an experimental eyedrop preparation, *diquafosol tetrasodium (INS365)*, that acts on receptors in the eye (*P2Y2, purinergic receptors*) that regulate and stimulate secretion of tears and mucin.[18] "It causes an increase in fluid on the surface of the eye. It's not tear fluid, but transudate, fluid that comes from underneath the conjunctiva that moves onto the surface of the eye. It results in an increase in tear volume on the surface of the eye by that mechanism. It's the only drug that works that way," explains Dr. Clayton. So far, studies show the drops appear to be safe and reduce some dry eye symptoms.[19]

In addition, a clinical trial is also underway to test the ability of *lubricin* to alleviate the signs and symptoms of dry eye. Lubricin is the body's antifriction and anti-adhesion protein that Dr. Sullivan and colleagues recently discovered is produced not only in joints but also by the human cornea and conjunctiva.[20] Lubricin reduces friction 20 times better than Teflon, he remarks.

However, inflammation, which typically occurs in ocular surface tissues in dry eye, is known to shut down lubricin production. This would lead to increased stress, friction, and more inflammation. Consequently, Dr. Sullivan and colleagues have made human recombinant lubricin, which is being used in the clinical trials. So far, clinical tests show that a single drop of lubricin dramatically decreases dry eye symptoms for at least eight hours.[21]

Other potential treatments in development include an *interleukin1 (IL-1)* receptor blocker *EBI005*, and *lifitegrast*, which targets another cytokine involved in ocular surface disease inflammation.[17]

Dry Mouth

Salagen (pilocarpine hydrochloride) and *Evoxac (cevimeline)* are oral medications that stimulate saliva production, helping patients chew, swallow, speak, and even sleep more easily. Evoxac is also being studied for its effect on dry eyes.[22] Salagen may have effects on dry eye, and some people using Salagen are using it in addition to other therapies.

Toothpastes containing detergents can cause mouth irritation. Detergent-free brands include *Biotene* (toothpaste and rinse) and *Oral Balance* (gel).

Artificial saliva, which contains ingredients such as methylcellulose, sorbitol or xylitol (artificial sweeteners), and salts like magnesium, can help moisten and lubricate the mouth. Preparations include lozenges (*SalivaSure*), sprays (*Aquoral, Biotene*), and rinses (*Biotene, Oasis*). *Medactive*, a saliva enhancer, is available in lozenges, gel, and spray formulations. These can also help reduce tooth enamel erosion.

A chewable product for dry mouth, *BasicBites*, acts in similar ways to saliva. The sugar-free chocolate soft chews contain *arginine bicarbonate* and *calcium carbonate*, which help maintain the normal pH of the mouth and protect teeth by coating them with calcium.

A lozenge containing *interferon alpha (IFNα)* that may stimulate saliva production is also in clinical trials. IFNα may treat the secretory dysfunction in the salivary glands. In clinical trials, patients using the lozenge had more than twice the increase in saliva production as a placebo group.[23]

Researchers are even exploring possible gene therapy that would be delivered to the salivary glands and even implantable artificial salivary glands.

If you have dry mouth or dry eyes, avoid medications such as antihistamines, which can dry mucus membranes.

Dry Vagina

A number of vaginal moisturizers (including *Replens*, *Feminease*, *Vagisil Intimate Moisturizer*, and *KY Liquid*) can relieve dryness, itching, and burning, and a number of lubricants that can make sex more comfortable are available (see pages 191 to 192).

Since vaginal dryness in Sjögren's before menopause is not due to the absence of estrogen, local estrogen therapy (such as vaginal creams or suppositories) may not help younger women. A new nonhormonal therapy, *ospemifene (Osphena)*, is a once-a-day pill that can help relieve painful intercourse (*dyspareunia*). It combats vaginal dryness and atrophy, but it can have estrogen-like effects on the lining of the uterus and may increase the risk of blood clots, as estrogen does. (For more, see page 192.)

Systemic Therapies

Systemic therapies used for Sjögren's include corticosteroids, *azathioprine*, *cyclophosphamide*, the antimalarial *hydroxychloroquine*, *mycophenolate mofetil*, and the B cell depleting drug *rituximab (Rituxan)*. However, none have been shown to change the course of Sjögren's, and there are still conflicting reports on their effectiveness.

Rituximab has been shown to produce greater improvements in salivary flow, dry eye, and tear production than more conventional DMARDs.[24] But unfortunately a recent study suggested it had lesser effects in recently diagnosed patients.[25] It has been approved for treating rheumatoid arthritis, but not yet for Sjögren's.

Many primary Sjögren's patients find dryness, muscle and joint pain, and fatigue are improved with the DMARD *hydroxychloroquine (Plaquenil)*. However, a recent randomized 24-week study from France suggests that it may be no better than a placebo.[26] The drug only is approved for treating lupus and rheumatoid arthritis.

While studies have found Sjögren's patients have increased levels of the inflammatory cytokine *tumor necrosis factor alpha (TNFα)* in their salivary and lacrimal glands, TNFα blockers such as *etanercept (Enbrel)* have not been shown to be effective as Sjögren's treatments.

Studies continue of *dehydroepiandrosterone (DHEA)* in primary Sjögren's syndrome. DHEA, a supplement, has been used to treat women with lupus and has shown some effectiveness in Sjögren's patients.

"The thought is that androgens could affect the multiple systems involved in Sjögren's. It could decrease inflammation in the mouth, the eyes, the joints, and perhaps in the blood for some of the inflammatory markers of Sjögren's," adds Dr. Clayton. However, DHEA treatment has not been approved to treat Sjögren's.

For severe cases of small fiber neuropathy, *neuroleptic* medications (drugs originally developed for epilepsy that also relieve nerve and muscle pain) such as *gabapentin (Neurontin)*, *pregabalin (Lyrica)*, or *topiramate (Topamax)* may be recommended.[6]

Evelyn's story continues:

You have to manage dry eyes and dry mouth to prevent other health problems. You should not just accept the fact that your eyes bother you. I make sure to keep my eyes moist, and I avoid certain environments that dry out my eyes—like air-conditioned stores, which are very dry—and I wear special sunglasses that have side panels so the wind doesn't dry my eyes. I'm careful about eating sugar and make sure to rinse my mouth or brush my teeth if I eat something sweet. I avoid eating any acidic foods, because they bother me—my tongue burns like crazy. Eventually this becomes part of you and you do things automatically.

How Sjögren's Can Affect You Over Your Lifetime

Sjögren's doesn't directly affect reproduction, but some of the antibodies associated with it can cause problems.

Pregnancy

Forty percent or more of women with Sjögren's have antibodies to *SSB/La*, also associated with lupus. These antibodies to normal cellular components can be harmful to a growing fetus and can lead to cardiac, skin, or blood-related problems, which are all grouped under the term *neonatal lupus*. If you are pregnant and have Sjögren's, you need to have your serum (the clear part of the blood) tested for the presence and amount of these antibodies with a test called an (ELISA, see pages 73 and 355).

Sjögren's patients who have antibodies to SSA/Ro and/or SSB/La can face the prospect of have a child with a condition called *neonatal lupus* (see page 89). Happily this is a rare problem. The name *neonatal lupus* is misleading since the mother may not have lupus at all and the baby doesn't either. The condition is actually related to the presence of these antibodies. The most common problems associated with these antibodies include injury to the heart, skin, liver, and blood cells. The good news is that except for the heart problem the other features are transient and disappear when the antibodies are cleared from the child's circulation at about six to eight months of age. The most serious problem involves the heart, called *heart block*. This occurs in one of 50 women with these autoantibodies.

If you are found to have antibodies to either *Ro* or *La*, your pregnancy is managed just as in women with lupus who have these antibodies.

Women with Sjögren's may also have *antiphospholipid antibodies*. These antibodies are related to *antiphospholipid syndrome* (see pages 347 to 362). These antibodies may predispose women to form clots in the placenta, hampering blood flow to the fetus, and are associated with recurrent miscarriages (most often during the second trimester). Women found to have these antibodies are prescribed blood thinners, such as aspirin or heparin. Pregnancies in women with Sjögren's found to have these antibodies are managed the same way as in women with antiphospholipid syndrome.

Gynecological Issues and Menopause

The major gynecological issue facing you with Sjögren's syndrome is vaginal dryness and painful intercourse. However, not all vaginal dryness that occurs in women with autoimmune diseases is related to Sjögren's.

Vaginal lubrication does not come from moisture-producing glands but mostly from fluid that's passed from the bloodstream through the vaginal walls. "So dryness that occurs in Sjögren's may be due to autoimmune effects on the blood vessels and the circulation in the vaginal area," explains

Lila E. Nachtigall, MD, professor of obstetrics and gynecology at the New York University School of Medicine. Other autoimmune diseases, such as lupus and diabetes, can affect circulation and vaginal secretions; the stress of any chronic illness may also reduce vaginal moisture.

Before menopause, estrogen helps stimulate the normal growth and development of vaginal cells, as well as vaginal secretions. As estrogen levels drop in the years before and after menopause, vaginal tissues gradually begin to thin and atrophy, producing fewer secretions (surgical menopause, removal of the ovaries, causes a more rapid onset of vaginal dryness).

"Since Sjögren's is most often diagnosed in women age 40 and over, some cases of vaginal dryness may be blamed on aging," remarks Dr. Nachtigall. Low estrogen levels occur during other times of life, such as during breastfeeding, and lead to vaginal dryness. Primary ovarian insufficiency (premature ovarian failure) also causes dry eye and dry vagina (see page 231). Other causes must be ruled out before attributing the problem to Sjögren's.

You and your partner should be reassured that this is a physical problem and not related to any failure of sexual arousal, stresses Dr. Nachtigall. Lubricants can make sex more comfortable. These are different from "personal moisturizers." Lubricants are designed for use during sexual activity. "The ideal lubricant is odorless, tasteless, colorless, water soluble, and of a consistency that allows it to remain in the vagina. Never use oil-based products like petroleum jelly. They will interfere with the vagina's natural self-cleansing mechanism," she explains. Lubricants include *KY Jelly* and *Astroglide*.

Vaginal moisturizers are designed for regular use to relieve dryness and irritation and to attract liquid to the dry vaginal tissues. Moisturizers include *Replens* (containing *pilocarpine*, which adheres to vaginal tissues), *Feminease* (containing *Yerba santa*, made from an aloe-like plant), and *Vagisil Intimate Moisturizer*. Both lubricants and moisturizers have an acidic pH that helps prevent vaginal infections and are nonhormonal. Replens is applied three times a week.

Although menopausal vaginal atrophy is somewhat worse in the Sjögren's patient, it does respond to local estrogen therapy, either as a cream or a slow-release ring (*Estring, estradiol* made from yams) or a suppository, *Vagifem* (*estradiol*, also synthesized from yams), which release a small continuous dose of estrogen to vaginal tissues.

You may also want to ask your gynecologist about prescription *ospemifene (Osphena)*, a *selective estrogen receptor modulator (SERM)* approved to combat postmenopausal vaginal dryness and painful sex. SERMs are estrogen *agonists*, compounds that act on estrogen receptors to produce estrogen-like actions in various tissues in this case, preventing atrophy of vaginal tissues. However, like estrogen, they can also affect the lining of the uterus and increase the risk of blood clots. So you need to discuss the risks and benefits with your doctor. Osphena is taken as a pill once a day.[27]

Dry eye can be a component of menopause, so you need to mention it to your gynecologist, as well. "I think it's very critical for women to recognize that Sjögren's can affect nearly every system in their body. Lung problems can cause shortness of breath; there may be nerve problems, which a woman may not connect to her Sjögren's," stresses Dr. Smith. "Women need to communicate to their physicians when they have problems or changes, because if they don't there's no hope of those problems being addressed."

But the problems of Sjögren's are not unsurmountable.

"I wouldn't say I 'enjoyed' the challenge. But I'm up for the challenge. Sjögren's syndrome has been a life-changing experience, that's for sure," says Venus Williams of living with Sjögren's—on and off the tennis court.[2] "I don't like being defeated by anything. It makes me creative, that's for sure. You have to figure out ways to win when you don't feel well. You have to find different avenues in order to get your top health level, and you have to be tough. You can't make any excuses, even though you have one of the biggest excuses available. It's a roller coaster, but thankfully I've enjoyed roller coasters since I was a child."

Notes

1. Rhoden WC. Venus Williams pushes back hard, at the twilight. *New York Times*, August 24, 2013, F5.
2. Ain M, Venus Williams bares all. *ESPN, the Magazine*. July 2014. http://espn.go.com/tennis/story/_/id/11072501/how-tennis-star-venus-williams-got-body-back-game-espn-magazine-body-issue. Retrieved July 10, 2014.
3. Sullivan DA, Sullivan BD, Evans JE, et al. Androgen deficiency, meibomian gland dysfunction, and evaporative dry eye. See comment in PubMed Commons below. *Ann N Y Acad Sci.* 2002;966:211–222. doi:10.1111/j.1749-6632.2002.tb04217.x.
4. Maddali Bongi S, Del Rosso A, Orlandi M, et al. Gynaecological symptoms and sexual disability in women with primary Sjögren's syndrome and sicca syndrome. *Clin Exp Rheumatol.* 2013;31(5):683–690.

5. Hanlon P, Avnell A, Aucott L, Vickers MA. Systematic review and meta-analysis of the sero-epidemiological association between Epstein-Barr virus and systemic lupus erythematosus. *Arthritis Res Ther.* 2014;16:R3. doi:10.1186/ar4429.
6. Birnbaum J. Peripheral nervous system manifestations of Sjögren's Syndrome: clinical patterns, diagnostic paradigms, etiopathogenesis, and therapeutic strategies. *Neurologist.* 2010;16:287–297.
7. Mengshoel AM, Norheim KB, Omdal R. Primary Sjögren's syndrome: fatigue is an ever-present, fluctuating, and uncontrollable lack of energy. *Arthritis Care Res.* 2014;66(8):1227–1232. doi:10.1002/acr.22263.
8. Foulks GN, Forstot SL, Donish PC, et al., Guidelines for the management of dry eye associated with Sjögren disease. *Occular Surf.* 2015;13(2):118–132.
9. Jonsson R, Theander E, Sjöström B, Brokstad K, Henriksson G. Autoantibodies present before symptom onset in primary Sjögren syndrome. *JAMA.* 2013;310(17):1854–1855.
10. Carteron N. Small fiber neuropathy and Sjögren's. *Sjögren's Syndrome Q.* 2014 Summer;9(3):1–2.
11. Shiboski SC, Shiboski CH, Criswell LA, et al. American College of Rheumatology classification criteria for Sjögren's syndrome: a data-driven, expert consensus approach in the Sjögren's International Collaborative Clinical Alliance Cohort. *Arthritis Care Res.* 2012;64:475–487.
12. Schaumberg D, Buring JE, Sullivan DA, Dana MR. Hormone replacement therapy and dry eye syndrome. *JAMA.* 2001;286(17):2114–2119. doi:10.1001/jama.286.17.2114.
13. Smith JA, Vitale S, Reed GF, et al. Dry eye signs and symptoms in women with premature ovarian failure. *Arch Ophthalmol.* 2004;122(2):151–156. doi:10.1001/archopht.122.2.151.
14. Phadatare SP, Momin M, Nighojkar P, et al. A comprehensive review on dry eye disease: diagnosis, medical management, recent developments, and future challenges. *Adv Pharmaceutics.* 2015, Article ID 704946. http://dx.doi.org/10.1155/2015.
15. Information on Restasis (cyclosporine ophthalmic emulsion) 0.5%. http://www.restasis.com/.
16. http://avenova.com/.
17. Rand AL, Asbell PA. Nutritional supplements for dry eye syndrome. *Curr Opin Ophthalmol.* Jul 2011;22(4):279–282. doi:10.1097/ICU.0b013e3283477d23.
18. Kamiya K, Nakanishi M, Ishii R, et al. Clinical evaluation of the additive effect of diquafosol tetrasodium on sodium hyaluronate monotherapy in patients with dry eye syndrome: a prospective, randomized, multicenter study. *Eye (Lond).* 2012;26(10):1363–1368. doi:10.1038/eye.2012.166.
19. Lau OCF, Samarawickrama C, Skalicky SE. $P2Y_2$ receptor agonists for the treatment of dry eye disease: a review. *Clin Ophthalmol.* 2014;(8):327–334. doi:http://dx.doi.org/10.2147/OPTH.S39699.
20. Schmidt TA, Sullivan DA, Knop E, et al. Transcription, translation, and function of lubricin, a boundary lubricant, at the ocular surface. *JAMA Ophthalmol.* 2013;131(6):766–776. doi:10.1001/jamaophthalmol.2013.2385.
21. Murphy R. OSD: help is on the way. *Ophthalmol Manage.* 2015;19(5):2628, 2630.

22. Ono M, Takamura E, Shinozaki K, et al. Therapeutic effect of cevimeline on dry eye in patients with Sjögren's syndrome: a randomized, double blind clinical study. *Am J Ophthalmol.* 2004;138(1):617.
23. Cummins MJ, Papas A, Kammer GM, Fox PC. Treatment of primary Sjögren's syndrome with low-dose human interferon alfa administered by the oromucosal route: combined phase III results. *Arthritis Rheum (Arthritis Care Res).* 2003;49(4):585–593. doi:10.1002/art.11199.
24. Carubbi F, Cipriani P, Marrelli A, et al. Efficacy and safety of rituximab treatment in early primary Sjögren's syndrome: a prospective, multi-center, follow-up study. *Arthritis Res Ther.* 2013;15:R172. doi:10.1186/ar4359.
25. Devauchelle-Pensec V, Xavier M, Jousse-Joulin S, et al. Treatment of primary Sjögren's syndrome with rituximab. *Ann Intern Med.* 2014;160(4):233–242.
26. Gottenberg JE, Ravaud P, Puéchal X, et al. Effects of hydroxychloroquine on symptomatic improvement in primary Sjögren syndrome. The JOQUER randomized clinical trial. *JAMA*. 2014;312(3):249–258. doi:10.1001/jama.2014.7682.
27. Osphena. http://www.osphena.com/.

7

Vanishing Hormones—Type 1 Diabetes, Addison's Disease, Primary Ovarian Insufficiency, and Other Endocrine Problems

I had all the symptoms: the blurry vision, the enormous thirst, the ravenous appetite, and I would feel the deep, deep fatigue. But I didn't recognize them as diabetes. I was going through a divorce at the time and single motherhood, so not feeling "well" felt normal. So I missed the warning signs. Fortunately, I didn't have any damage. I had been diagnosed with another autoimmune disease, sarcoidosis, in 1973 and I was seeing a doctor every month to monitor my lungs for nodules. So the diabetes was found with a routine blood test. I didn't think about the symptoms or report them to the doctor until after he noticed the high glucose level and started asking me questions. It seemed so obvious after we got the blood test results, but it was so easy for me to overlook.

Mary Kay, 67

Type 1 Diabetes

Our bodies need fuel in order to run smoothly. We get that fuel from the carbohydrates and proteins we eat, which are converted to glucose and transported into cells by the hormone insulin. Normally the body keeps levels of blood glucose tightly regulated. But in diabetes that delicate balance is upset.

According to the American Diabetes Association (ADA), there are four categories of diabetes:

Type 1 diabetes, or insulin-dependent diabetes mellitus (once called *juvenile-onset diabetes*), is strongly genetic and usually results from an autoimmune attack on the insulin-producing *beta* (or *islet*) cells in the pancreas that leads to insulin deficiency. Lack of insulin causes blood glucose to soar, wreaking havoc on the body.

Type 2, or non-insulin-dependent diabetes mellitus, is a metabolic disorder frequently brought about by obesity, causing the body to gradually lose its ability to use insulin properly. Once termed *adult-onset diabetes*, an epidemic rise in obesity has increased its occurrence among children. **Gestational diabetes** is an often transient form of diabetes that arises during pregnancy, in which the body temporarily loses responsiveness to insulin. It usually resolves shortly after delivery, but the risk to develop type 2 diabetes in the future remains elevated. Other types of diabetes result from genetic defects in insulin action, pancreatic disease, or are drug- or chemical-induced.[1]

Over 29 million American have diabetes,[2] and more than 347 million people are affected worldwide.[3] Ten percent have type 1 diabetes, which usually arises in early childhood or before age 30. Most people with diabetes have type 2, which typically occurs after age 40 and is related to obesity. However, later in life the two forms of diabetes often merge.

There has been a virtual epidemic of type 2 diabetes, fueled by soaring rates of obesity. However, the incidence of type 1 diabetes has also been increasing around the world, rising by as much as 4 percent a year, mostly among children, and it's unclear why.[4] The most striking rise has been in Finland, which has the highest incidence of childhood type 1 diabetes in the world,[5] but all over Europe rates are expected to increase 60 percent by 2020.[4] In the United States, the incidence rose by 30 percent from 2001 to 2009 and is projected to keep increasing. Potential causes could be environmental, experts say, but most of the cases have been among genetically susceptible children.[6]

While type 1 diabetes affects women and men about equally, it often clusters with other autoimmune diseases common in women, including *thyroid disease*, *celiac disease*, *pernicious anemia*, *Addison's disease*, *myasthenia gravis*, and *vitiligo*.

The pancreas is part of the network of *endocrine* glands (including the thyroid, ovaries, and adrenal glands; see pages 222 to 223) that secrete hormones directly into the bloodstream.

As insulin-producing pancreatic *beta* cells are progressively destroyed by an autoimmune attack, the body produces less and less insulin and becomes less able to convert food into glucose and bring it into cells. As a result, glucose accumulates in the bloodstream. The blood vessel damage caused by high glucose leads to heart attacks, stroke, kidney disease, and blindness. Women with diabetes are at greater risk than nondiabetic women for cardiovascular disease (CVD). High glucose can also cause nerve damage, poor circulation, and tissue death in the legs, sometimes leading to amputations.

But high glucose may produce few or no symptoms in its early stage. The blurry vision and extreme thirst Mary Kay experienced only occur after blood glucose is greatly elevated. While type 1 diabetes can come on abruptly during childhood or adolescence, researchers now believe many middle-aged people thought to have type 2 diabetes actually have type 1 diabetes, but are misdiagnosed because they may not have a rapid progression to full-blown disease since the autoimmune destruction of beta cells often occurs more slowly. Type 1 diabetes is more common in Caucasians, while type 2 is more prevalent in African American, Latina, Native American, and Asian American women.

Warning Signs of Type 1 Diabetes

- Unusual or excessive thirst
- Frequent desire to urinate
- Weight loss
- Fatigue, excessive tiredness
- Blurred vision
- Severe itching in the lower legs
- Chronic vaginal yeast infections

What Causes Type l Diabetes?

In type 1 diabetes, autoantibodies target not only the insulin-producing beta cells in the pancreas, but also proteins made by beta cells that sit on the cell surface, and even insulin itself. Other types of islet cells in the pancreas escape unharmed. Autoantibodies may be present years before symptoms of type 1 diabetes appear. In fact, 70 percent of people with type 1 diabetes screened for the national Diabetes Prevention Trial had one or more of the diabetes autoantibodies but no symptoms. As many as 70 to 80 percent of people newly diagnosed with type 1 diabetes have antibodies to islet cells; 80 to 95 percent have antibodies to a protein made by beta cells called *glutamic acid decarboxylase (GAD)*; two-thirds have antibodies to insulinoma antigen-2 (1A-2); and up to half have antibodies to insulin. Type 1 diabetes can come on gradually, but people with more antibodies may develop it more quickly.

There are a number of autoantibodies involved, but insulin and GAD appear to be the early targets of the attack in type 1 diabetes. The beta cells are destroyed, but they may actually be innocent bystanders of an immune attack on a virus that invades those cells.

You'll recall that some viruses and bacteria may have the same shape as cells in the body, a phenomenon called molecular mimicry. A small area of the GAD protein on beta cells looks almost identical to a protein called *P2-C* on the *Coxsackie virus B* (one of a family of viruses that causes polio).

During an infection, T cells target an invading virus and destroy it. But once the infection is over, T cells on the prowl may see the GAD protein sitting on beta cells, think it's a virus, and attack. Because viruses must first invade cells, some scientists believe they may change something about the islet cells that provokes a T-cell attack. The Coxsackie virus, as well as other enteroviruses (Coxsackie virus A and B, echovirus)[7] cytomegalovirus, adenoviruses, and viruses that cause mumps have all been implicated in type 1 diabetes.[7]

Other immune system problems also contribute to type 1 diabetes—among them, not having enough *natural killer T cells (NK cells)* or the *T-regulator (T-reg)* cells that tell the NK cells which cells to target and which to ignore. In type 1 diabetes (and other autoimmune diseases), another step in giving instructions to NK cells also goes awry. T-cell receptors, which function kind of like TV antennae, need to pick up a signal from *antigen presenting cells (APCs)* to tell them which cells are foreign invaders and which aren't. The APCs display bits of antigens on their surface within special molecules, kind of like hot dogs in a bun, explains Denise Faustman, MD, PhD, who heads the immunobiology laboratory at Massachusetts General Hospital. If the antigens are not properly displayed, or if the presentation process is somehow incomplete, the T cells never get the message to bypass the beta cells, she says.

No matter what triggers the attack, as beta cells are progressively killed off the pancreas produces less and less insulin. Insulin is critical to keeping the body's cellular machinery running smoothly, fueling our cells. Think of insulin as a gas pump, and your cells as tiny cars. The "gas" is blood glucose, processed by the body from sugar in carbohydrates (all carbohydrates—whether doughnuts or fruits—are technically sugar). If the gas pump isn't working properly, cells don't get enough fuel and start to stall. The excess fuel in the pump backs up and spills over into the blood, and over time that high glucose can damage your blood vessels, your eyes, your kidneys, and your nerves. Insulin also helps the body store extra fuel as fat; to get badly needed fuel, the body taps into this reserve, and that's why people with type 1 diabetes lose weight.

In young children, the destruction of beta cells and the loss of insulin can be dramatic, but in adults (especially older adults), it can occur more gradually. By the time type 1 diabetes is diagnosed in adults, the majority of the insulin-producing cells have been destroyed. While there's no way at present to reverse that loss, researchers say it may one day be possible to regrow beta cells or trigger their regeneration (see pages 212 to 213).

Although the disease can run in families, 85 percent of people who develop it have no family history of type 1 diabetes (although family members may have other autoimmune diseases). The risk for people with a parent or sibling with type 1 diabetes is about 6 percent; the risk is 30 percent among identical twins. Even nonidentical twins or siblings have a greater risk of getting type 1 diabetes than people without a family history. More than a half-dozen genes are associated with the disease; some are more common among specific ethnic groups (such as Scandinavians), making them more vulnerable to environmental triggers, like viruses.

Mary Kay's story continues:

I went into a diabetic coma a few months after I was diagnosed with diabetes in 1984. I think it was the result of a collision of medical events, including surgery that preceded it by six months, and an infection I developed afterward. The night before I went into the coma I had gotten the flu, and being newly diagnosed I wasn't aware that dehydration and the flu are very dangerous for people with diabetes; it shoots your glucose level way, way up. So even though I had taken my insulin that day, because I was so sick

I got dehydrated. I developed ketoacidosis and went into a coma in my sleep. Fortunately, I was staying with a friend at the time, who noticed that my breathing was irregular the next morning and that I wouldn't awaken. I was in a coma for nine days. If I had been home it might not have been noticed right away. I was a single mother with two small children; they were seven and nine at the time, and I don't think they would have known to call 911. They know now. In fact, in the months following that, they did become quite frightened, and if I tried to sleep in on a Saturday morning, they would shake me and say "Mom, are you all right?"

Symptoms and Complications of Type 1 Diabetes

In healthy people, the body carefully regulates the amount of glucose and insulin in the blood. When blood glucose becomes elevated (such as after eating), more insulin is produced to help remove it; when glucose falls, insulin secretion also drops. In people with diabetes, the body isn't producing insulin, so glucose builds up in the blood instead of being transported into cells.

High blood sugar, *hyperglycemia*, causes intense thirst, dry mouth, and frequent urination. Some of the excess glucose leaks into the urine, and the excess glucose causes the kidneys to produce more urine, which can result in dehydration. Your doctor can detect glucose levels by dipping a specially treated paper into a urine sample. When cells don't get enough glucose, the body starts breaking down fat to use for energy, which also produces weight loss.

As fats are broken down for energy by the liver, waste products called *ketones* are produced. If ketones build up faster than they can be excreted in urine, they begin to accumulate in the bloodstream, causing the blood to become acidic. This is called *diabetic ketoacidosis*, and it can come on suddenly with life-threatening consequences. In addition to the classic signs of hyperglycemia, ketoacidosis produces a fruity-smelling breath, shortness of breath, dry mouth, loss of appetite, nausea and vomiting, muscle weakness, dry flushed skin, blurry vision, and sleepiness. In severe cases, ketoacidosis can cause coma. (Symptoms are similar to *Addison's disease*—see pages 223 to 230.)

Ketoacidosis is usually triggered by a sharp drop in insulin (if you forget to take a dose of insulin), but it can also be brought on by illness or a major life stress (like a car accident), says Carol J. Levy, MD, CDE, an associate professor of medicine, endocrinology, diabetes and bone disease and director of the Diabetes Center at Mount Sinai Hospital in New York City. "When you're under stress, stress hormones tell the liver to release stored glucose (glycogen). But these hormones also block the effects of insulin," she explains. If your insulin is low to begin with, a bout with the flu or extreme stress could bring on ketoacidosis, which requires immediate treatment with insulin and fluids. The risk of ketoacidosis is 50 percent higher in women, according to the ADA.

Sometimes diabetes can cause (or be associated with) menstrual irregularities, infertility, and pregnancy complications, and it is associated with primary ovarian insufficiency (previously referred to as premature ovarian failure) and an earlier menopause.

As high blood glucose damages blood vessels in the eye, fluid leaks from the tiny blood vessels behind the retina. *Diabetic retinopathy* is the most common cause of blindness in people aged 20 to 75. Often the first sign of a problem is a blurring of vision. This damage may be visible during a routine eye exam.

Diabetes also injures blood vessels in the legs, impeding circulation and causing pain (*intermittent claudication*) while walking. Women are 76 times more likely than men to suffer damage to small blood vessels in their extremities (*peripheral vascular disease, PVD*).

When blood supply to nerves is diminished, the nerves become damaged and don't send out pain signals when there's an injury. So a small cut you may not feel can become ulcerated. If diabetic ulcers go untreated, the tissue can die and become gangrenous, and the limb may need to be amputated.

As glucose accumulates in the bloodstream, it can damage large blood vessels, making it easier for fatty plaques to accumulate inside artery walls, narrowing key arteries and impeding blood supply to the heart. If those plaques rupture and form blood clots, it can completely block an artery, leading to heart attack and stroke. If you have diabetes, you're three to four times more likely to suffer a heart attack and stroke than people without diabetes because the high glucose levels reduce the protective effects of estrogen on cholesterol and blood vessel flexibility before menopause.

You're also at increased risk of bone loss and hip fracture, which studies suggest is partly due to a hormonal disruption and to lower levels of vitamin D and magnesium. You can also have an overactive *parathyroid gland* (see pages 229 to 230), which causes the body to leach calcium from the bones. So you may need regular bone density scans and possibly bone-building drugs.

Between 10 and 21 percent of women with diabetes develop kidney disease. Damage to kidney cells, *diabetic nephropathy*, is the most common reason for kidney dialysis (needed to help rid the body of waste products) or a kidney transplant.

Diabetes also causes skin problems, including fungal infections in the corners of the mouth and under the breasts and armpits. One of the common symptoms of diabetes is itching brought on by dry skin and poor circulation, especially in the lower legs. Women can develop a skin condition called *diabetic dermopathy*, which produces brown spots, especially on the legs. Atherosclerosis can also affect the skin when it narrows blood vessels in the legs, causing it to thin and feel cool; your toenails may thicken and become discolored, and your toes may feel cold. You can also suffer chronic vaginal yeast infections, gum disease, and infections of the tiny glands in the eyelid (*styes*).

Unexplained weight loss is also a symptom of exocrine pancreatic insufficiency (EPI), stemming from inadequate digestion of food and malabsorption of nutrients.[8] Other symptoms of EPI that can occur in diabetes include nausea, appetite loss, gas, bloating, abdominal pain, diarrhea, and *steatorrhea* (unabsorbed fat in the stools), oily, foul-smelling stools that float, which also occurs in celiac disease (see page 270). You can also have bone loss and vitamin deficiency (notably vitamin B_{12}, calcium, and vitamin D), as well as muscle cramps, bone pain, and easy bruising. If you start to have these symptoms or GI problems along with your diabetes, it's wise to see a pancreatic specialist, since EPI can arise in diabetes.[8]

Diagnosing Type 1 Diabetes

Unlike other autoimmune diseases, it's not always necessary to test for autoantibodies to diagnose type 1diabetes. A complete medical history, the presence of classic symptoms (especially extreme thirst, frequent urination, and weight loss), and high blood glucose are often all that's needed to confirm a diagnosis.

However, since some people can develop a late-onset disease that initially can look like type 2 diabetes, autoantibody testing may help diagnosis in those cases. Almost everyone who develops type 1 diabetes has one or more autoantibodies to insulin, islet cells, and/or GAD at the onset of the disease.

The FDA recently approved the first autoantibody test that can distinguish type 1 diabetes from other types of the disease, the *Zinc Transporter 8 Autoantibody (ZnT8Ab) assay.*[9] ZnT8Ab is only produced by people with type 1 diabetes.

Such testing may help find the disease in its earliest stages. In fact, genetic testing of newborns at risk for type 1 diabetes is now being done around the country, along with monitoring for autoantibodies. Such autoantibodies may begin to appear in early childhood.

Endocrinologists also recommend that close family members be tested for autoimmune diseases, including type 1 diabetes. "If someone has the classic symptoms of diabetes and they're not overweight, chances are it's type 1. If someone is very overweight, has a strong family history of type 2 diabetes, and no other symptoms other than elevated glucose, chances are it's type 2. But autoantibody screening can help separate less clear-cut cases," adds Dr. Levy. "I routinely test women for autoimmune thyroid disease. If a woman has fatigue, irregular bowel habits, and trouble with certain types of foods, and if she has another autoimmune endocrine disease, I will test for celiac disease and send her to a gastroenterologist for diagnosis. If she has classic symptoms of Addison's—a change or darkening in skin color, fatigue, increasing hypoglycemia—I immediately screen for adrenal insufficiency."

Tests You May Need and What They Mean

Hemoglobin A1C is a test now used to diagnose diabetes as well as to monitor blood sugar control. *Hemoglobin*, a protein inside red blood cells that carries oxygen to the body, also links up (*glycates*) with glucose in the bloodstream. The higher your blood glucose, the more hemoglobin is glycated, says the ADA. Measuring the percentage of A1C provides an average of blood glucose over two to three months. An A1C level of 6.5 percent or greater is among the revised diagnostic ADA criteria for diabetes.[1] For treatment monitoring purposes; A1C testing is typically done two to four times a year.

Fasting plasma glucose (FPG) is a second blood test for diagnosing type 1 diabetes. The day before the test, your doctor will ask you not to eat for 8 to 10 hours. The next morning, a sample of your blood will be taken and the glucose level measured. Normally, your glucose would be 100 milligrams per deciliter (mg/dL) of blood after not eating for that many hours.

But if you have diabetes, your glucose will be 126 mg/dl or over, according to the ADA criteria. Levels in between are considered *impaired fasting glucose* and indicate a high risk of developing diabetes.

Postprandial glucose (PPG) may be an earlier indication of impending diabetes than an FPG for some patients. Postprandial glucose is the level seen two hours after eating. In this test you're given oral glucose after an overnight fast. If postprandial glucose is over 200, then you have diabetes. If it's between 140 and 200, you have *impaired glucose tolerance*, or *prediabetes*.

Urinalysis (for *ketones*, *protein*, and *sediment* from red or white blood cells) is also done. The presence of ketones in the urine can indicate the beginnings of ketoacidosis. (It can also just mean that you haven't eaten for a long time.) Protein in the urine and sediment are signs of kidney dysfunction.

eGFR (estimated glomerular filtration rate) tells how well your kidneys are working. It's a number based on results of a blood test for *creatinine*, a waste product of muscles. Healthy kidneys filter creatinine out of your blood. An eGFR is calculated from a blood creatinine level, your age, race, gender, and other factors. A normal eGFR is 60 or above; if the rate is lower, your kidneys aren't functioning properly. An eGFR is also used to diagnose *chronic kidney disease (CKD)*.

Since one out of every 100 with type 1 diabetes will develop Graves' disease, and one in 20 will develop *Hashimoto's thyroiditis*, your doctor will likely order a test to measure *thyroid stimulating hormone (TSH)*.

You and your immediate family also run a high risk (approximately one in 20) of developing *celiac disease*. Many people with celiac are asymptomatic, and if the condition goes untreated it can lead to anemia, bone loss, and even cancer. Diagnosing it early can help prevent those problems (see page 270).

Measuring the level of vitamin B_{12} and folic acid in your blood helps to diagnose *pernicious anemia*. One in 50 adults with type 1 diabetes also develops this autoimmune disease, in which the stomach is unable to absorb vitamin B_{12}; telltale symptoms include anemia and weakness. Testing for autoantibodies against the *parietal cells* in the stomach lining indicates autoimmune disease; low plasma B_{12} indicates malabsorption.

There are a number of tests for EPI, among them stool tests to measure the pancreatic enzymes *trypsin* and *elastase*, and a blood test for *trypsinogen (immunoreactive trypsin)* another enzyme reduced in pancreatic sufficiency. (For more details on testing for EPI, see page 202.)[10]

The ADA recommends repeating all diagnostic tests to rule out lab errors and confirm a diagnosis, unless classic symptoms of diabetes are present.[1]

Mary Kay's story continues:

When I was first diagnosed with diabetes, I had to mix two kinds of insulin in my morning injection, one was long-acting and the other was fast-acting. I also needed to eat breakfast. I was never a breakfast eater, and you need to eat approximately four hours after your first injection. My appetite has always been zero first thing in the morning, and it sort of grows during the day. Now on a different insulin regimen things are a bit easier with eating. Everyone thinks it must be hard or painful to give yourself shots, because we all remember those painful immunizations we got as kids. But it's really not like that at all. In fact, I don't really feel the injections; they have these itty-bitty fine needles now. The most difficult part for me is the constant paying attention to eating and what you are consuming. I mean, diabetes makes you eat a healthy diet. And you can certainly lead a normal life with it. . . . But it means never going anywhere without candy bars or fruit in your purse, in case your blood sugar gets too low, and never skipping meals. And always making sure if you've taken your insulin. It's been many years, and I can often tell when my glucose is low. I can feel the symptoms of hypoglycemia before it really gets bad. For me, it feels very much like a hot flash. And I have such a rapid metabolism I never seem to get enough calories.

Treating Type 1 Diabetes

The goal of treatment in type 1 diabetes is to keep blood sugar levels normal, or as close to normal as possible. Replacement insulin is needed to achieve that tight control, along with a well-managed diet, regular exercise, and avoidance of obesity.

The landmark Diabetes Control and Complications Trial (DCCT), a major clinical trial conducted from 1983 to 1993 among 1,441 men and women, showed that tight control can help slow the development and progression of complications of type 1 diabetes, especially diabetic eye, kidney, and nerve disease. A follow-up study found a significantly reduced risk of heart disease, heart attacks, and stroke with tight control. After 27 years, tight control reduced deaths from *all* causes among participants in the DCCT.[11] So the long-term outlook is good.

Replacing Insulin

How much insulin you need depends on your glucose level, and that requires testing blood glucose throughout the day (see page 208).

After you eat, the body normally releases just enough insulin to process glucose; with a schedule of insulin injections timed before meals, you can mimic the normal release of insulin. If you're eating three meals a day (and one or two snacks), you might use a short-acting insulin just before each meal, and intermediate- or long-acting insulin once or twice a day to maintain a basic-level (*basal*) insulin.

Your body may respond better to a particular type of insulin, or a combination of insulin preparations, depending on how quickly they work, when they peak, and how long they last. The most commonly used preparations are human insulins produced by genetic engineering, which act just like natural insulin. Some are faster-acting than others.

There are four basic types of insulin[12]:

- **Rapid-acting insulin** begins to work about 15 minutes after injection, peaks in about 1 hour, and continues to work for 2 to 4 hours. These include: *Insulin glulisine (Apidra)*, *insulin lispro (Humalog)*, and *insulin aspart (NovoLog)*.
- **Regular or short-acting insulin** usually reaches the bloodstream within 30 minutes after injection, peaks anywhere from 2 to 3 hours after injection, and is effective for approximately 3 to 6 hours. These include: *Humulin R, Novolin R.*
- **Intermediate-acting insulin** generally reaches the bloodstream about 2 to 4 hours after injection, peaks 4 to 12 hours later, and is effective for about 12 to 18 hours. There are currently two: *Humulin N* and *Novolin N.*
- **Long-acting insulin** reaches the bloodstream several hours after injection and tends to lower glucose levels fairly evenly over a 24-hour period. The two long-acting insulins are *insulin detemir (Levemir)* and *insulin glargine (Lantus, Toujeo).*

Instead of a syringe that must be filled from a separate vial, insulin these days often comes in a "pen," either a prefilled injector or a pen that uses an insulin cartridge. You dial the insulin dose on the pen and inject your insulin through a small needle. Cartridges and prefilled insulin pens contain a single type of insulin, so if you use two forms of insulin you'll need an injection from each device.

Insulin works fastest when injected in the abdomen, the ADA says, and gets into the blood a little more slowly from the upper arms and slower still from the thighs and buttocks. For best results, especially with mealtime insulin, inject it in the same general *area* each time—but not in the same exact *spot*, which may cause fatty deposits or hard lumps to develop. For example, injecting your before-breakfast insulin in the abdomen and your before-supper insulin in the leg each day gives more similar blood glucose results.

There's now a rapid-acting inhaled human insulin powder, *Afrezza*.[13] Afrezza is used in combination with long-acting insulin. It's not recommended for treating diabetic ketoacidosis. Afrezza is inhaled at the beginning of each meal.

"If a woman is eating a low-fat diet, which many women do, she'll do much better with short-acting insulins or insulin analogues in combination with a long-acting insulin like Lantus. However, if you go out to dinner and eat higher-fat items, like pizza, then these insulins don't work as well," says Dr. Levy. Taking several injections of fast-acting insulin can give you more flexibility in planning meals (you can take a little extra to cover a second helping of pasta, for example).

Some women prefer to wear insulin pumps that can be programmed to release different doses of insulin at different times of the day. "The only issue for some women is body image; you have to wear a pump 24 hours a day, seven days a week, and some women don't feel comfortable with that," says Dr. Levy. Insulin pumps can be useful in pregnancy, when blood sugars can be erratic, she adds.

Pumps can be programmed to deliver insulin as steady, continuous "basal" dose or as a surge or "bolus" dose around mealtime to control the rise in glucose after you eat. The pump is attached to a flexible plastic catheter with a small needle at the end. As with an insulin injection, the needle is inserted into the fatty tissue under the skin, then you tape it in place. A recent study from Sweden suggests that patients using insulin pumps may have better long-term outcomes compared with people taking insulin injections.[14]

However, insulin therapy is a highly individualized process that should be worked out with a specially trained healthcare provider, such as a certified diabetes educator. They can also help you learn when and how and where to give yourself injections or how to use an insulin pump. (An indispensable reference to help you manage insulin treatment is the *American Diabetes Association Complete Guide to Diabetes*, see Appendix B for more information.)

Pregnancy and oral estrogens can also affect blood glucose and the amount of insulin you need, so you may need more frequent glucose testing if you've just begun taking oral contraceptives or hormone replacement. Illness and stress can also affect glucose, requiring adjustments in insulin.

You need to match the amount of insulin you take with the amount of food you eat (which raises glucose) and the amount of exercise you get (which lowers glucose). But even if you ate the same amount of food each day and exercised the same amount daily, your need for insulin could still fluctuate, so self-monitoring of glucose is vital.

Studies show that three or four injections of insulin a day give the best blood glucose control and can prevent or delay the eye, kidney, and nerve damage caused by diabetes, according to the ADA.

Glucose Self-Monitoring

If your goal is keeping glucose levels as close to normal as possible, you may need to test up to five times a day. The standard times to self-test are before breakfast, lunch, and dinner (and before eating a larger snack), one to two hours after eating, and before bedtime. According to new guidelines set by the ADA,[1] acceptable blood glucose ranges are 80 to 120 milligrams per deciliter of blood (mg/dl) before meals and 100 to 140 mg/dl before bedtime. People without diabetes generally have a glucose level of less than 110 mg/dl before meals, and under 120 mg/dl before going to bed, but you may not be able to achieve those levels.

Glucose home monitoring is usually done with a disposable *lancet* device; you prick a finger to produce a drop of blood and apply it to a specially treated piece of paper or to a handheld glucose meter.

You can also keep track of blood sugar with a monitor (*MiniMed Continuous Glucose Monitoring System*), which your doctor can order for you.

However you test, you should keep track of the results in a small notebook. The patterns you see (for example, a rise in glucose after eating certain foods, or during the premenstrual period) can help you make adjustments in your insulin intake.

Monitoring your glucose and preventing problems like ketoacidosis may get easier in the future with new technology now being tested.

New Diabetes Diet Guidelines

In the past, women with diabetes were told to avoid sugary foods because they would send blood glucose soaring. But updated dietary guidelines from the American Diabetes Association (ADA) say it's OK to have sweets occasionally—as long as your blood sugar levels are well controlled.

According to the revised guidelines, issued in 2014, it's not so important what kind of carbohydrates you eat, but that you keep an eye on your total carbohydrate intake. However, you are advised to eat more nutritious carbohydrates, like fruits, vegetables, and complex carbohydrates like whole grains, which are digested more slowly and don't cause spikes in glucose. Cut sodium to less than 2,300 milligrams a day, limit artery-clogging saturated fat, and eat more fiber (25 to 20 grams a day).[15]

"I let my patients eat what they want as long as they can appropriately cover it with insulin and exercise," remarks Dr. Levy. "As long as you eat a healthful diet, there are no limitations if you don't have problems with weight or cholesterol. But you really need to be careful to balance your carbohydrate intake."

People with type 1 diabetes may process protein faster, but because most of us eat 50 percent more protein than we need (15 to 20 percent of our daily calories), you won't suffer protein deficiency. If you follow a vegetarian diet, be sure to include plant proteins (like beans, nuts, sweet potatoes, and avocado) to avoid deficiency.

Calorie-free sweeteners approved by the FDA—including *saccharine* (*Sweet'N Low*, *Sugar Twin*), *aspartame* (*NutraSweet*, *Equal*), sucralose (*Splenda*), and *stevia/rebaudioside* (*Truvia*, *Pure Via*)—can safely be used by people with diabetes. Apart from the natural sugar (*free fructose*) in fruits, which may aid glycemic control, the ADA advises avoiding foods and beverages with *fructose* added as a sweetener.[10]

Alcohol can trigger both high and low blood sugar, depending on the amount that's consumed and whether it's taken with food. It can also raise blood pressure. But moderate alcohol consumption is not harmful, so follow the standard recommendation for women of one or fewer drinks per day (one drink is considered to be 12 ounces of beer, 5 ounces of wine, or 1.5 ounces of spirits).

The ADA guidelines stress that regular exercise is as important as diet to maintain normal blood sugar. In fact, moderate exercise can lower blood sugar to the extent that you may even need less insulin. Exercise can also help raise "good" high density lipoprotein (HDL) cholesterol and lower blood pressure, which can lessen the risk of cardiovascular complications, notes Dr. Levy.

Intensive diabetes care means a solid education in controlling glucose; balancing diet, exercise, and insulin; and the support of an active healthcare team (including a diabetes nurse specialist, a dietitian, and a physician) to provide regular follow-up.

Your care team can also help reduce your risk of heart attack and stroke. Your goals are to keep blood pressure below 130 mm Hg systolic and less than 80 mm Hg (diastolic, the resting rate) and maintain a *low density lipoprotein (LDL)* cholesterol under 100 mg/dl, an HDL above 50 mg/dl, and triglycerides below 150 mg/dL. Your A1C should be below 7 percent, according to the ADA.[1]

Women who develop high blood pressure or kidney disease will need medications to control those conditions, such as *angiotensin-converting enzyme (ACE) inhibitors*. If retinopathy develops, there are treatments to coagulate leaky blood vessels and prevent vision loss with laser therapy.

Avoiding Hypoglycemia

The one time sugar *does* come in handy is during an episode of hypoglycemia, or low blood glucose. This can occur if you don't take enough insulin, skip a meal or a snack, eat a meal unusually late, or drink alcohol on an empty stomach. You can also suffer low blood sugar if you exercise too vigorously (it can even occur during sex). Even if you're doing everything right, you can still have an episode of hypoglycemia, since the body may not always use insulin consistently; hypoglycemia is also more common during pregnancy. Warning signs can occur at any time—even waking you up from a sound sleep (sometimes you may have a nightmare due to the effects of low blood sugar on the brain).

Warning Signs of Hypoglycemia

- Shakiness
- Dizziness
- Sweating
- Feeling faint
- Rapid heartbeat
- Headache
- Hunger
- Chills
- Clammy, pale skin
- Confusion, difficulty concentrating
- Sleepiness
- Clumsy or jerky movements
- Sudden mood changes, like sadness or anxiety

The first thing to do when those symptoms hit is to test your glucose—hypoglycemia is generally considered to be a glucose level of 50 mg/dl or under, but some women can have symptoms with slightly higher levels. If glucose is low, eat something containing sugar. It's a good idea to carry things like hard candy to help raise your glucose quickly if needed; you can also carry glucose tablets, available in most drugstores. Something as simple as a half cup of orange juice or a handful of raisins (both of which contain 10 to 15 grams of carbohydrates) can raise your blood sugar and head off a more serious reaction, such as seizures or loss of consciousness. After you've eaten, wait 15 to 20 minutes and then retest. Sometimes, you may need a second snack to get your blood glucose back to where it should be. Even if you don't have your test kit with you, treat hypoglycemia immediately.

After you've had diabetes for a number of years, it's not unusual to lose the ability to feel the early warning signs, and you may suffer from more severe episodes. Hypoglycemia unawareness can also occur during pregnancy. This is another reason why testing is crucial.

Type 1 Diabetes Clusters

There's a high risk of thyroid disease in type 1 diabetes, and it can also occur in the autoimmune polyglandular syndrome type 2 (see page 227). Other diseases that cluster with type 1 diabetes include:

- Thyroid disease
- Celiac disease
- Alopecia areata
- Primary ovarian insufficiency
- Addison's disease
- Myasthenia gravis
- Pernicious anemia
- Vitiligo

Mary Kay's story continues:

I was diagnosed with thyroid disease many years ago during a routine wellness exam, and I have been taking a very low dose of Synthroid ever since. My doctor said it was "borderline" hypothyroidism. There was no history of diabetes in my family or other autoimmune diseases; no arthritis, no thyroid disease. When they were searching for the cause of my lung nodules in 1984, I was tested for lupus and for rheumatoid arthritis, and all those tests were negative. But here I am with thyroid disease and diabetes. And my brother has had the same lung nodules I had . . . but he hasn't had a diagnosis of sarcoid. They only found the lung nodules by accident with a routine x-ray. He was also diagnosed with gout, and that's a form of arthritis. So it's possible that there is some genetic component.

What's Next?

Research into reversing or preventing type 1 diabetes has greatly accelerated in recent years. Tests are being conducted of gene therapy, immune-based drug therapies, vaccines, transplants of insulin-producing islet cells, and several artificial pancreas device systems (APDS).

This wearable technology, using already-approved insulin pumps and glucose monitors, is designed to maintain blood sugar within a target range or at a target level, using an algorithm managed by a smartphone.[16] Using continuous glucose monitoring, the system would automatically increase or decrease insulin delivery when it senses blood sugar is above or below the range or target level. Another type of system, designed to be a backup, would suspend glucose delivery when blood glucose drops below a certain threshold.[17]

However, people would still need to manually tell the pump to dispense insulin at mealtimes, and adjust levels based on factors such as physical activity. Systems being tested use insulin alone (single pump) or a combination of insulin and glucagon (with dual pumps).

The Artificial Pancreas Consortium, supported by the Juvenile Diabetes Research Foundation (JDRF), is funding clinical trials of the devices in the United States, and similar systems are being tested in Europe.[18]

Researchers at Boston University and Harvard report the system improves glucose levels and reduces episodes of hypoglycemia in type 1 diabetes more effectively than a conventional insulin pump.[19]

Transplants of islet cells have also met with some success. Back in 2002, a small study from Edmonton, Canada, using a new protocol for islet cell transplantation, found that half of the patients who'd had a transplant didn't need insulin injections for two years afterward. Since then, a consortium of scientists has been working to perfect new transplant techniques and looking for ways for patients to avoid a lifetime of immunosuppressant drugs. Researchers from Harvard Medical School say they may be able to help *regrow* islet cells—and even get rid of the wayward immune cells that attack the pancreas.

One potential gene therapy would infuse into the pancreas islet cells lacking the genetic defects that lead to type 1 diabetes. Another promising strategy, being tested at the University of California, San Francisco, involves coaxing embryonic stem cells (which can grow into almost any cell type), into becoming insulin-producing beta cells.[20]

Dr. Denise Faustman at Massachusetts General Hospital and Harvard Medical School is researching a possible treatment to reverse type 1 diabetes, using a bacterium called *Bacillus Calmette-Guérin (BCG)* that stops the immune system attack on beta cells, allowing the pancreas to regenerate and produce insulin again.

"These trials are already in Phase II and are the first trials in the world to use a safe immune intervention in people with the disease, not just immune therapy in new onset disease," says Dr. Faustman. "This therapy targets and kills the disease-causing white blood cells and boosts the beneficial T cells called Tregs. The 100-year-old generic BCG drug originally developed as a vaccine for tuberculosis prevention now has appeal as a simple cost-effective approach with global human clinical trials in multiple sclerosis, Sjögren's syndrome, and type 1 diabetes."

Early clinical trials sponsored by the National Institute of Allergy and Infectious Diseases (NIAID) show that two courses of the immune suppressant drug *alefacept (Amevive)* given to people soon after a diagnosis of type 1 diabetes preserved beta cell function for as long as one year, compared to those who received a placebo. The NIAID reports that patients who received alefacept needed less insulin and experienced fewer episodes of hypoglycemia, possibly because their insulin production was sufficient to maintain levels of blood sugar within a target range.[21]

Other immune therapies use cocktails of drugs. One combination uses *thymoglobulin*, a drug initially developed for kidney transplants, to kill immune cells that attack beta cells in the pancreas, while *pegfilgrastim (Neulasta)*, a drug used to treat neutropenia associated with chemotherapy, triggers production of healthy new immune cells. Studies show patients given the dual-drug therapy regained the ability to produce insulin while those given a placebo did not.[22] An experimental drug called *DiaPep277* appears to "reeducate" the immune system rather than suppress it, stops destruction of beta cells, and reduces the need for insulin.[23]

A "reverse" vaccine (called *BHT-3021*) is also being tested. In contrast to conventional vaccines, which stimulate an immune response, BHT-3021 dampens the immune response against insulin. In a recent clinical trial, the plasmid vaccine not only shut down the attack on beta cells, but also seemed to preserve pancreatic function.[24]

How Type 1 Diabetes Can Affect You Over Your Lifetime

Many women with type 1 diabetes were diagnosed during their teenage years, and there's an interaction between the disease and hormonal factors during the reproductive years.

Menstruation and Fertility

Women diagnosed with type 1 diabetes in adolescence often get their periods late (at ages 13 to 15, versus the average age of 12.1), and more than a third have menstrual irregularities.[25] These problems can include the absence of periods (*amenorrhea*) due to anovulation, scanty periods (*oligomenorrhea*), and more frequent menstrual cycles (*polymenorrhea*) with less time in between periods.

The fluctuating levels of hormones that underlie these problems can make it harder to control blood glucose. Some studies suggest that high progesterone may affect the action of insulin within cells, causing a slight insulin resistance and raising blood glucose. At the same time, elevated estrogen levels may improve the action of insulin, so blood glucose may be lower than normal when estrogen is high or "unopposed" by progesterone.

The high levels of both estrogen and progesterone during the premenstrual period can wreak havoc with blood glucose. "Women with diabetes who have this problem typically report that their blood glucose is elevated during the week before they get their period, then after they get their period, their sugars come crashing down," says Dr. Levy, who's also an associate professor of obstetrics, gynecology and reproductive science at New York's Mount Sinai and director of the type 1 diabetes/diabetes in pregnancy program there. "Or, some women will tell me their sugars are crazy at certain times of the month and they can't figure out why. So I will have them chart their glucose in relation to their cycles, which is very helpful. It enables us to tailor the insulin regimen to different times in the menstrual cycle."

For example, if you have regular menstrual cycles, your insulin dose may be increased the week before your period. Once you get your period, the dose may be cut back. "Some women don't have predictable cycles, so they don't know when they are going to get those glucose highs and lows. And other women have pretty severe fluctuations in spite of everything. Those women, we will sometimes put on birth control pills to stabilize their cycle, to try to make things more predictable," says Dr. Levy.

Monophasic birth control pills (which do not change the hormone levels during the 21 days you take the active pill) may help minimize changes in blood glucose. Women who have high blood pressure or peripheral vascular disease or who smoke should not take the pill. Progesterone can cause elevations in glucose, and pills containing newer forms, such as *desogestrel, norgestrel, norgestimate,* and *drospirenone* can make a huge difference, says Dr. Levy. "The risks with birth control pills are in the amount of estrogen, which can increase the risk of blood clots in some women, and the newer pills have a much lower estrogen dose." Low-dose pills contain 20 micrograms of estrogen. Some newer progestins may also have less clotting risk.

If you seem to have lower than usual blood sugar right before your period, discuss with your doctor the advisability of gradually reducing the dose premenstrually. And you may want to up your carbohydrate intake (but go for the healthier carbs, like fresh vegetables). Cut back on alcohol, chocolate, and caffeine; they can affect blood glucose as well as mood. Stick with your meal plans and eat at regular intervals, since large blood glucose swings can affect mood, exacerbating PMS.

If you have type 1 diabetes, you may also have menstrual irregularities, which may make it harder to predict when you'll get your period, possibly interfering with your ability to become pregnant. In women who don't ovulate or menstruate, estrogen is produced but not progesterone (which triggers shedding of the menstrual lining each month). A study from the University of Pittsburgh comparing 143 women with type 1 diabetes to 186 nondiabetic women without diabetes found that, on average, women with type 1 diabetes had a 17 percent decrease in the number of reproductive years.

There's also an increased incidence of polycystic ovary syndrome (PCOS) due to elevated androgens; 30 to 40 percent of women with type 1 diabetes may have PCOS.[26]

"Women with type 1 diabetes have more anovulatory cycles, but the reasons for this are not well understood," comments Mary Loeken, PhD, an investigator in the Section on Islet Cell and Regenerative Biology at the Joslin Diabetes Center in Boston Joslin and an associate professor of medicine at Harvard Medical School. "One of the things we do know is that you need to have a certain amount of fat mass in order to cycle appropriately. Just as athletes who overtrain and lose too much body fat stop cycling, women with type 1 diabetes may lack sufficient fat, especially if the disease is not well controlled. One of the hormones secreted by fat is leptin. It's associated with weight gain, but it's also required for menstruation. There are leptin receptors in the brain, and leptin receptor signaling triggers the release of neurotransmitters that control the hypothalamus and the pituitary and, in turn, the ovaries."

You also need a certain amount of body fat to maintain a pregnancy, adds Dr. Loeken. "So leptin production is nature's way of ensuring that the mother will be nutritionally able to support the pregnancy. In addition, ovarian hormones are also needed to build up the lining of the uterus. If a woman's glucose is out of control, she may have enough body fat to ovulate and conceive, but not enough for normal hormone production, so the embryo will not implant in the uterus. It may die before it's implanted. Women with type 1 diabetes may have unrecognized early miscarriages."

If you have menstrual irregularities, a home ovulation test kit can be helpful to tell when you are ovulating, as can taking your basal (morning) body temperature, which is normally 98.6 degrees and may rise as much as 0.5 to 1 degree at ovulation.

Pregnancy and Lactation

Diabetes can lead to a number of complications during pregnancy, including a higher risk of preeclampsia, a pregnancy-induced disorder characterized by high blood pressure, protein in the urine, headaches, and fluid retention (edema).

Pregnancy may increase (or decrease) the need for insulin at different stages of pregnancy and may requiremore frequent glucose testing.

"Once you become pregnant, there are a lot of changes in the energy requirements, not just for the mother but for the developing embryo, which, because it's growing so rapidly, consumes a lot of glucose. So the mother needs to be able to provide enough fuel," explains Dr. Loeken. "The body also reacts to hormones produced during pregnancy by very rapidly increasing the production of adrenal steroid hormones, mostly cortisol. Those hormones interfere with the action of insulin. They increase glucose output by the liver, change fat composition of the body, and mobilize fat for energy."

However, you need to get your glucose under tight control if you're even thinking about becoming pregnant, says Dr. Loeken. "The formation of major organ structures takes place about the time a woman misses her period and first suspects she's pregnant. If a woman's glucose levels go too high, those organ systems may be formed in an abnormal way and the baby develops a congenital malformation. A woman doesn't usually have her first obstetrics appointment until around 11 weeks, and by then a malformation may have already occurred. So it's important to discuss with your doctor your plans to become pregnant so you can maintain tight glucose control from the start."

While problems with fetal development can arise in the second or third trimester, birth defects do not occur after the first trimester because the organ systems are already laid down. Congenital abnormalities can occur in as many as 6 to 12 percent of babies born to women with diabetes. Potential problems can include abnormalities of the heart, kidney, and central nervous system.

Keeping tight control of blood glucose and carefully monitoring the baby's growth can prevent these problems and others, including having a large baby (*macrosomia*, which can cause injury to the mother and baby during delivery or lead to a Cesarean section) and lung problems. "If the mother is hyperglycemic, glucose is delivered to the fetus at a high concentration, and the baby's pancreas responds by producing insulin. Insulin acts like a growth factor in a fetus. So you get a lot of glycogen storage in the liver and fat deposition, you get a big baby," explains Dr. Loeken. "Insulin also interferes with fetal adrenal steroids that stimulate lung maturation. So high insulin can hamper maturation of the baby's lungs, and the baby can suffer from respiratory distress syndrome."

Because of the genetic component of type 1 diabetes, a child has a greater risk of developing diabetes sometime in his or her life time if either parent is affected. However, for reasons we don't understand, the risk is six times less if the mother has diabetes than if the father does.

If you breast-feed, you will need to consume more calories than if you do not breast-feed, and a lot of the nutrients that you consume will be delivered to the baby in your milk. You should make sure that you stay properly hydrated and monitor your blood sugar frequently to adjust your insulin dose.

Women with diabetes have an increased risk of gum inflammation (*periodontitis*), and the damage can be more severe. So get regular dental care, especially during pregnancy.

An important note here about *gestational diabetes (GD)*: This form of diabetes, which develops during pregnancy, is not an autoimmune disease and about 60 percent of the time resolves itself after delivery or goes into remission. However, in a small percentage of cases, what appears to be GD may actually be the onset of type 1 or type 2 diabetes. "Because we screen every woman for gestational diabetes, sometimes it may actually unmask diabetes, and we can treat a woman before she gets into trouble," remarks Dr. Levy. "If your diabetes doesn't go away after you deliver, you're not overweight, and you don't have a strong family history of diabetes, we have to consider whether this is actually early type 1 diabetes." For women with GD, adopting a low glycemic index (GI) diet may result in lower insulin use and lower birth-weights for their babies.[27]

Mary Kay's story continues:

I started taking estrogen replacement therapy in my mid-forties. I was having very, very strong premenopausal symptoms. I am Irish, and thin, and my mom was on estrogen for a long time to prevent osteoporosis. So when I started having menopausal symptoms, I didn't feel it was dangerous for me to take estrogen—actually, the opposite. For the first month I was on estrogen, I doubled my daily blood testing to see if taking estrogen would affect my glucose level or increase my need for insulin. It didn't, in my case. But I was also switching from one kind of insulin to a more human insulin, so that may have made a difference. My gynecologist never told me to increase my daily testing, even though she knew I had diabetes. I knew about gestational diabetes, how high estrogen affects glucose, and it just made sense to me that taking estrogen could affect my need for insulin. I had no idea that diabetes could bring on menopause early. My gynecologist never mentioned it. But my mother went through menopause in her fifties, and I was in my forties, so I guess I was about six years earlier than my mother.

Menopause and Beyond

Just when you thought you'd gotten the hang of controlling those monthly blood glucose swings, you start to approach menopause and things are thrown out of kilter again. Perimenopause can occur any time after age 35, and, far from being a long decline in estrogen, this transition period can be a hormonal roller-coaster ride, with irregular periods and months where you don't ovulate at all. Increases in hormones can boost blood sugar; decreases can send it plummeting. Low-dose birth control pills can help regulate your cycle.

Recent studies suggest that women with diabetes undergo an earlier menopause, sometimes by six to seven years. One study found that women with diabetes went through menopause at an average age of 41.6, compared to those who didn't have diabetes, whose average age at menopause was closer to 50.[28]

"There's just something about type 1 diabetes that totally disrupts the regulatory cycle for menses, and some women develop a condition called hypothalamic amenorrhea. No one knows for sure why type 1 women develop it, but the pituitary gland just shuts off. We're unsure of the reasons for this, but it might be dependent on blood sugar control, low body weight, or stress levels," remarks Dr. Levy.

"We will measure estrogen and follicle stimulating hormone (FSH) in women who have trouble getting pregnant or whose periods stop. If estrogen levels are low and FSH is high, you've gone through menopause."

During this period, episodes of hypoglycemia may become more frequent and more severe. Low blood sugar can disrupt your sleep, along with hot flashes. In fact, menopausal symptoms can be confused with low (or high) blood sugar, especially moodiness and inability to concentrate or short-term memory loss.

You'll need to test glucose more frequently during the menopausal transition. Loss of estrogen after menopause can decrease the body's sensitivity to insulin, requiring adjustments in your insulin dose.

Lack of insulin affects bone formation and, together with estrogen loss, can increase your risk of osteoporosis.[29] One recent study found that women with type 1 diabetes were more than 12 times more likely to report hip fractures compared to those without the disease. (Falls and fracture risk can be increased by vision problems, nerve damage, and the effects of hypoglycemia.)

For women with osteoporosis, once-a-week formulations of *alendronate (Fosamax)* or *risedronate (Actonel)* can make these drugs easier to take. You're also at increased risk of high blood pressure and high cholesterol—both risk factors for heart disease—and those problems may need to be treated separately with appropriate medications.

There are conflicting data about the effects of postmenopausal estrogen for women with type 1 diabetes. Some studies suggest that combination hormone therapy (HT) with estrogen and progestin can help combat the effects of hormone loss on glucose levels and make them easier to regulate.[30]

"It is true that women with diabetes have a higher risk of cardiovascular disease, but in studies that suggest estrogen can worsen coronary disease, the risk in women who don't have the disease appears to be due to blood clotting, and it may well be the type of estrogen," she comments. "In my clinical experience, on occasion I have seen type 1 diabetes improve in women with HT," remarks Dr. Levy.

Studies are mixed. A 2003 study of 20,000 female nurses age 45 and over in Denmark found that current estrogen users with diabetes had over four times the risk of heart disease, and nine times the risk of heart attack compared with those who never used estrogen.[31] Other recent studies, including the Women's Health Initiative (WHI, see page 53) indicate that HT can not only increase the risk of heart disease and stroke in older women, but that progestin may also increase breast cancer risk. One clinical trial suggests low-dose HT may have less impact on heart risk.[32] However, a recent review says there are still not enough definitive data on the impact of HT on glycemic control and cardiovascular risk in women with type 1 diabetes.[33] So it's important to discuss the risks and benefits with your healthcare team.

The combination of diabetes and menopause can also affect your sex life. Reduced circulation to the genital area may make it harder to lubricate during arousal and more difficult to achieve orgasms. The normal decline in testosterone can also lower your sex drive.[34] Again, some form of hormone therapy may help (see pages 52 to 54).

Autoimmune diseases that affect other components of the endocrine system in women include *Addison's disease (adrenal insufficiency)*, *hypoparathyroidism*, and *autoimmune ovarian failure (or premature menopause)*. Ovarian failure can also occur as part of an *autoimmune polyglandular syndrome* and in connective tissue diseases such as lupus. Ovarian autoimmune disease itself has only recently been recognized as a single entity.

The ductless glands of the endocrine system—the thyroid, pancreas, pituitary, and adrenal glands—secrete hormones that affect almost every body function, including reproduction. You may not think of the ovaries as endocrine glands, but sex hormones (estrogen and androgens) are actually steroid hormones that regulate not only reproduction but many other functions in the body. For example, estrogen is needed to maintain bone density.

The endocrine glands also aid our responses to internal or external stimuli. The adrenal glands secrete "stress" hormones (like *adrenaline*, also known as *epinephrine*) to assist us in the primitive fight-or-flight syndrome by increasing heart rate and breathing, and pushing more blood into the muscles. Endocrine cells can also be found in other organs (e.g., gastric cells in the stomach).

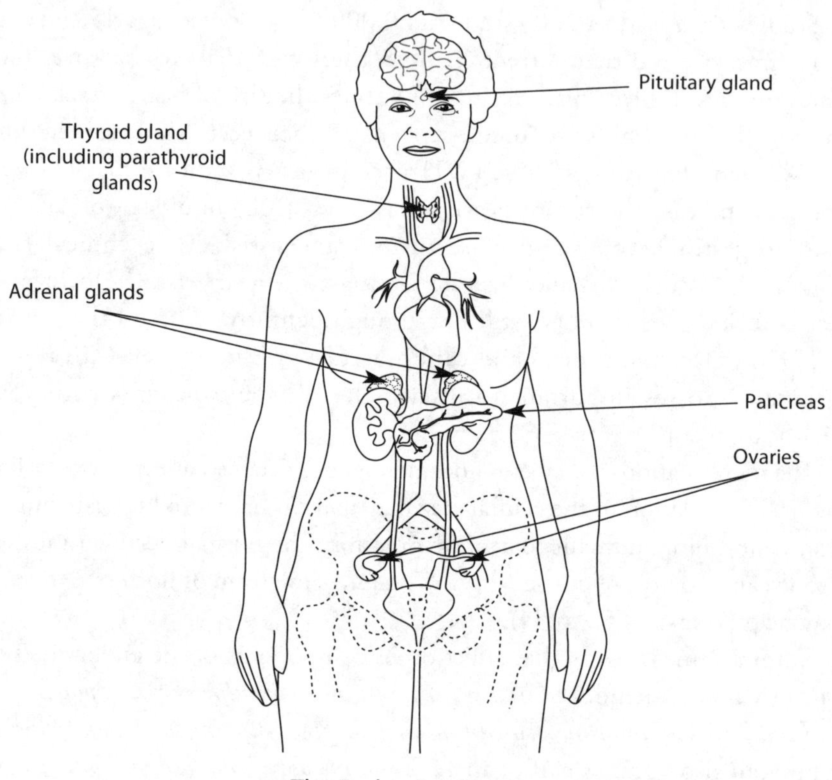

The Endocrine System

Warning Signs of Autoimmune Endocrine Disorders

- Weight loss, fatigue, muscle weakness, brown patches on the skin, low blood pressure (Addison's disease)
- Hot flashes, irregular or stopped periods, infertility (premature ovarian failure)
- Numbness or tingling in the extremities, muscle cramps, anxiety, depression (hypoparathyroidism)

Like the thyroid, other endocrine organs are regulated in a feedback loop by the hypothalamus, an area in the brain that controls the pituitary, in a sense the master of the "master gland." It produces "releasing" hormones, to send a signal to the pituitary, which in turn sends out a chemical messenger to stimulate other endocrine glands. In the case of the ovaries, one chemical messenger is *follicle stimulating hormone (FSH)*, which stimulates the follicles to secrete estrogen and to produce an egg each month. Not surprisingly, when one of the endocrine glands isn't working right, it can throw off the entire system.

But endocrine disorders don't usually come on dramatically; they develop gradually over a period of years, and you may not even pay much attention. The diagnosis usually involves blood tests for hormone deficiency, and the treatment is replacing the lost hormone (or hormones).

Addison's Disease

Among the nonthyroid autoimmune endocrine disorders, *Addison's disease*—autoimmune destruction of the adrenal glands—is the most common among women, typically occurring during the twenties and thirties. In half of those women, Addison's occurs as an isolated disorder, and in the other half it occurs as part of a polyglandular endocrine disorder (see pages 227 to 228) or along with other autoimmune diseases.

The two triangular-shaped adrenal glands, which sit atop the kidneys, are actually two organs in one. The outer region, called the *adrenal cortex*, secretes steroid hormones like *cortisol* (also called *hydrocortisone*), which affects metabolism (how we use food and tap into stored energy) and suppresses inflammation in the body; *aldosterone*, which regulates the amount of salt excreted by the kidneys (helping to maintain blood pressure and blood volume); and small amounts of male hormones, or *androgens*. (The hydrocortisone produced by the adrenal glands is a naturally occurring form of the corticosteroid drugs used to dampen inflammation in autoimmune disease.)

The amount of steroid hormones secreted by the adrenal cortex is regulated by a "negative" feedback loop with the hypothalamus and the pituitary gland. In a negative feedback loop, a drop in one body chemical or hormone triggers a reaction to return levels to normal, restoring balance *(homeostasis)*.

On a chemical signal from the hypothalamus, the pituitary sends out *adrenocorticotropic hormone (ACTH)*, which directly stimulates the adrenal cortex. ACTH is actually produced in a 24-hour cycle, peaking around six o'clock in the morning and falling slowly during the day to hit its lowest level around midnight. If levels of hydrocortisone get too high, it inhibits ACTH production and slows secretion of hydrocortisone. Emotional stress or injury can stimulate the release of ACTH and hydrocortisone, which the body needs to bounce back from stress.

The inner region of the adrenal gland, called the *medulla*, is linked to the sympathetic nervous system and reacts to emotional and physical stresses by secreting hormones like *epinephrine (adrenaline)* and *norepinephrine* (also called *noradrenaline*).

What Causes Addison's?

In Addison's disease, autoantibodies attack the steroid-producing cells of the adrenal cortex, causing inflammation and fibrosis that prevent hormone secretion, and eventually completely destroy the cortex. *Adrenocortical autoantibodies* can target cells that produce specific hormones (autoantibodies can also block ACTH).

There's a genetic component to Addison's (most often in women with adrenal disease associated with autoimmune polyglandular syndrome), but less than a third of women with Addison's have a family history of the disease. Genes associated with Addison's (like DR3) are also linked to Graves' disease and other autoimmune diseases.

It's mainly a disease of reproductive-age women, but "we don't know what precisely predisposes women to Addison's disease," remarks Paul W. Ladenson, MD, the John Eager Howard Professor of Endocrinology and Metabolism and director of the division of endocrinology at Johns Hopkins. "It appears that a variety of genes may be involved, some of which may be gender related, but that does not explain why adrenal insufficiency is more common in women."

Symptoms of Addison's Disease

When the adrenal glands are not working properly, it can cause low blood pressure, often in the form of *postural hypotension* (or *orthostatic hypotension*), where you feel faint as blood pressure suddenly drops when you go from lying down to sitting up, or from sitting to standing. "Addison's disease can present with very nonspecific complaints, such as fatigue or loss of appetite, which makes it hard to recognize," comments Dr. Ladenson. "But almost everyone with this disease has lost weight, whereas most people who have similar symptoms for other reasons have not."

Very often a woman may have a minor illness (like stomach flu) or a physical stress, become extremely dehydrated, and have an episode of low blood pressure that lands them in an emergency room, says Dr. Ladenson. "It's not unusual for a woman to have a history of emergency room visits before an alert physician notices a pattern and picks up on the possibility of Addison's. Laboratory abnormalities, such as low urinary sodium, high potassium, and high calcium are clues that would prompt a good physician to look for adrenal insufficiency."

In an acute adrenal crisis there can be fever, low blood pressure, abdominal pain, and even delirium. Chronic symptoms include loss of appetite, weight loss, fatigue, nausea, diarrhea, abdominal pain, anemia, and orthostatic hypotension. A darkening of the skin and mucous membranes may also occur. "The hardest part of making the diagnosis is to think of the possibility of Addison's disease, because the laboratory testing for it is very straightforward," comments Dr. Ladenson.

Diagnosing Addison's

A number of laboratory tests will be performed to determine whether your symptoms are due to *adrenal insufficiency*. The adrenal glands produce salt-retaining hormones (*aldosterone*), *glucocorticoids (cortisol)*, and weak androgens. Your cortisol level will be measured before and after administration of synthetic ACTH, and imaging of the adrenal glands may also be done to rule out tumors.[35]

However, an intravenous infusion of 100 milligrams of hydrocortisone is usually given immediately when an adrenal crisis is suspected, and followed with 100 milligrams every eight hours until the crisis has passed or the diagnosis of Addison's is confirmed.

Tests You May Need and What They Mean

Adrenocorticotropic hormone (ACTH) is elevated in Addison's. Normally, the ACTH level at midnight should be half of that in the morning (20 to 100 picograms per milliliter of blood, pg/mL).

Cortisol is measured before an injection or intravenous infusion of synthetic ACTH, *cosyntropin (Cortrosyn)*. Then cortisol is measured 30 minutes and an hour later, explains Dr. Ladenson. Cortisol levels that fail to rise to more than 20 micrograms per deciliter of blood (mcg/dl) with administration of ACTH confirm the diagnosis of adrenal insufficiency.

Blood urea nitrogen (BUN), the amount of nitrogen in the blood in the form of urea, a normal waste product (a measure of kidney function), is elevated in people with low blood pressure. The normal BUN level is 7 to 18 mg/dl.

Urine testing to measure sodium, potassium, and calcium, is often done. Sodium is decreased during episodes of low blood pressure (*hyponatremia*). High potassium or *hyperkalemia* compromises the kidneys' ability to excrete potassium. Calcium can also be elevated (*hypercalcemia*) in Addison's disease.

Other blood tests may also reveal high levels of *eosinophils*, a type of white blood cell associated with inflammation and allergies. Low red blood cell counts (anemia) are common in women with Addison's. *Thyroid stimulating hormone (TSH)* may also be measured.

Adrenocortical autoantibodies in the blood can indicate adrenal gland autoimmunity, but hormone deficiency is needed to diagnose adrenal insufficiency.

Treating Addison's Disease

The treatment of Addison's involves replacing the glucocorticoid adrenal hormone with *prednisone*, *hydrocortisone (Hydrocortone, Cortef)*, or *cortisone acetate*, and mineral corticoid with *fludrocortisone (Florinef)*.

"We try to administer synthetic adrenal hormones in a way that approximates the natural pattern of adrenal steroid secretion. Since cortisol is highest in the early morning and lowest late at night, patients will take a larger dose of hydrocortisone or cortisone acetate in the morning and a smaller dose in the afternoon," explains Dr. Ladenson. For example, many patients take 20 milligrams of hydrocortisone in the morning and 10 milligrams in the afternoon. Mineral corticoid therapy is given as a single dose of fludrocortisone.

"Our ability to assess adrenal replacement in the laboratory is limited, so we generally monitor patients' clinical responses. Have symptoms like weight loss, nausea, or loss of appetite gone away? And are there symptoms of excessive replacement, such as weight gain, easy bruising, depressed mood, or muscle weakness?" says Dr. Ladenson. Fludrocortisone therapy is monitored by assessing blood pressure standing and lying down, and measuring serum potassium and plasma renin.

Women need to adjust their doses of hydrocortisone during the third trimester of pregnancy. And if they have an illness accompanied by fever, fludrocortisone may need to be decreased during the premenstrual period, since it can exacerbate fluid retention. Corticosteroids may also increase blood glucose levels. You'll be advised to take in more salt (especially if you work out regularly and perspire) to guard against low sodium, since adequate sodium levels are needed to maintain normal blood pressure. It's a good idea to wear a *MedicAlert* bracelet or necklace so that proper care can be given in an emergency.

How Addison's Disease Can Affect You Over Your Lifetime

Like other autoimmune diseases, Addison's affects women during various stages of their lives.

Endocrine Clusters (Autoimmune Polyglandular Syndromes)

Autoimmune endocrine disorders tend to cluster together, affecting several glands, sometimes with years separating the onset of each disease. There are three types of *autoimmune polyglandular syndromes (APS)*. *Type 1 APS* is more common in childhood and affects both sexes equally. *Type 2 APS* is more common in women and occurs between ages 20 and 40, says Dr. Ladenson, usually with Addison's presenting first and type 1 diabetes (or thyroid disease) occurring later. In *type 3 APS*, autoimmune thyroid disease is accompanied by two other autoimmune diseases, but a woman does not develop Addison's disease.

Type 1 APS

- Hypoparathyroidism
- Adrenal insufficiency (Addison's disease)
- Chronic yeast infections of the skin or nails
- Malabsorption problems
- Alopecia totalis (or universalis)
- Vitiligo
- Sjögren's syndrome
- Chronic autoimmune hepatitis
- Pituitary insufficiency (hypophysitis)
- Gonadal autoimmunity
- Type 1 diabetes (less commonly)

Type 2 APS

- Adrenal insufficiency
- Thyroiditis
- Type 1 diabetes
- Alopecia
- Pernicious anemia
- Myasthenia gravis

Type 3 APS

- Thyroiditis
- Myasthenia gravis (or another nonendocrine autoimmune disease)

Menstruation and Pregnancy

Women with Addison's disease often have menstrual irregularities or primary ovarian insufficiency (see pages 231 to 233). Low-dose oral contraceptives can be used to regulate the menstrual cycle, and hormone therapy (HT) can be used for menopausal symptoms, as there are no cross reactions with estrogen, says Dr. Ladenson. Fluid retention during the premenstrual period may worsen with fludrocortisone, so the dose may be decreased for a few days before menstruation.

In general, women don't need to increase glucocorticoid medication during the first two trimesters. "However, labor and delivery are a physical stress, and glucocorticoid coverage may need to be increased at the time of delivery," says Dr. Ladenson. "We also switch women from oral medication to injectable corticosteroids."

While drugs like prednisone are generally considered safe during pregnancy, fludrocortisone should be used cautiously; too much may cause a baby to be born with an underactive adrenal gland. Fludrocortisone and drugs like prednisone can pass into breast milk and may cause growth problems, so women with Addison's are usually advised not to breast-feed. (Again, check the latest advice about drug use during pregnancy and breast-feeding with your doctor.)

Hypoparathyroidism

The tiny *parathyroid* glands, nestled behind the thyroid gland, produce *parathyroid hormone*, which, along with vitamin D and calcitonin (a hormone secreted by cells in the thyroid gland), regulate the amount of calcium in the body.

In *autoimmune hypoparathyroidism*, autoantibodies attack the four pea-sized glands, destroying hormone-producing tissue. Researchers at Weill Cornell Medical Center reported in 1996 that autoantibodies against the calcium-sensing receptor of the parathyroid glands (which sense how much calcium is available to the body) are frequently observed in this disease.[36] Calcium is not only needed to maintain bone mass, but is also required for muscle contractions. Having too little parathyroid hormone (PTH) leads to tingling and numbness in the hands and feet, muscle cramps, fatigue, irregular heartbeat, depression, and anxiety. It also causes a condition known as *tetany*, a heightened excitability of nerves that causes uncontrollable, painful spasms in the face, hands, and feet; spasms of the larynx; and sometimes seizures.

Hypoparathyroidism can occur in women with autoimmune hypothyroidism, or as part of type 1 autoimmune polyglandular syndrome. It's diagnosed by measuring parathyroid hormone in the blood. (In hyperparathyroidism, too much calcium is removed from the bones and accumulates in the blood, causing excessive thirst and urine output, kidney stones, confusion, seizures, and even coma. It's more common in women, and it is often caused by a benign parathyroid tumor.)

An underactive parathyroid is treated with oral calcium and vitamin D, sometimes in a form called *1,25-dihydroxyvitamin D (Calcitriol)*, to help absorb the calcium. "Because of the lack of parathyroid hormone, the kidney cant convert native vitamin D to its more active form as readily, and very large doses are needed, as high as 50,000 International Units, while the U.S. daily requirement is 600 units for healthy people and 800 IU in those older than 70," comments Dr. Ladenson. "Calcitriol is very potent and easily absorbed by the body. Dosing has to be done carefully, because the toxic range is narrow. However, if you overtreat, you need only withhold a dose or two of Calcitriol, whereas toxicity caused by large doses of native vitamin D can take weeks to go away." Calcitriol is usually taken in capsule form (it's also available by injection).

You need a certain blood level of vitamin D to become pregnant. But the dose must be carefully regulated in pregnancy; taking too much vitamin D can cause the baby to be more sensitive to vitamin D and lead to problems with the parathyroid gland and a heart defect. Only small amounts of Calcitriol pass into breast milk; it has not been reported to cause problems in nursing babies.

An injectable version of parathyroid hormone *teriparatide (Forteo)* is approved for rebuilding bone in osteoporosis, and might have some utility in hypoparathyroidism in a more easily used form, says Dr. Ladenson.

I was absolutely shocked to find out that I was in menopause at age 32. Really shocked. We had been trying to have a baby for a couple of years, and finally went to see an infertility specialist. After he did some tests, he told me the reason I couldn't get pregnant was premature ovarian failure. For some reason, he said, my body had destroyed the eggs in my ovaries. It was really hard to believe—I mean, I didn't have any hot flashes, or anything like that. I thought you went through menopause because your ovaries started to shut down and that only happened when you got older. I cried for days. I know a lot of women have infertility problems. But this was like my body stole something from me . . . it really hurt to think I couldn't have a child. But there wasn't anything we could do about it, so right away we decided to adopt. Now I have a wonderful two-year-old daughter from China. I'm taking hormones and I feel OK otherwise. But I admit I feel different from the other mothers I know, since they're mostly my age and none of them is quote "menopausal" yet.

CELIA, 35

Autoimmune Ovarian Insufficiency

Early menopause, or *primary ovarian insufficiency (POI)* (formerly termed *premature ovarian failure, POF*), is the onset of menopause before age 40. It occurs in 1 to 1.2 percent of women, affecting between 2 and 5 million women.[37] While some cases of this type of ovarian failure have a genetic cause (such as *Turner's syndrome*), or are due to chemotherapy or trauma, studies suggest that many cases may actually be due to autoimmunity.

Approximately 15 percent of women with the problem have other autoimmune endocrine diseases, most commonly thyroid disease, Addison's disease, type 1 diabetes, and autoimmune polyglandular syndromes (as many as 15 percent of women with type 1 APS have ovarian failure). Autoantibodies[38] associated with those disorders (*gonadotropin antibodies*) may also have an effect against the hormone-producing tissue of the ovaries and also react against specific steroid hormone–producing enzymes that are common to the ovary and adrenal gland.

One percent of women with rheumatoid arthritis experience autoimmune ovarian failure, and it's also associated with vitiligo, lupus, myasthenia gravis, and Crohn's disease.

Research conducted by Judith Luborsky, PhD, at Rush University in Chicago suggests that the cause of autoimmune ovarian failure may be immune destruction of ovarian follicles and oocytes.[39] Inflammation from autoantibodies may also compromise ovarian function.[40]

In women with menstrual cycles, an inability to become pregnant may be an early sign. "We believe there is a group of women with autoimmune disease, who have autoantibodies and go through a period of infertility as they progress to a total ovarian failure," says Dr. Luborsky. Women labeled as having "unexplained infertility" (no tubal blockages or other physical problems that prevent pregnancy) may actually have autoimmune infertility. "A significant proportion of these women have anti-ovarian autoantibodies, and this is independent of the hormones typically used to determine ovarian function," she explains.

Blood levels of estrogen and other ovarian hormones, such as progesterone (produced by ovarian follicles after the release of a mature egg) reflect the activity of a group of follicles in the ovary. The total number of active follicles decreases with age or as a result of autoimmune disease or other trauma,[41] observes Dr. Luborsky, now an investigator in the department of biology at the Woods Hole Oceanographic Institute in Woods Hole, Massachusetts.

Autoimmune ovarian failure is not identified by the traditional tests for ovarian function, which include blood levels of *follicle stimulating hormone (FSH)* made by the pituitary gland and estrogen (made by the ovaries). As ovarian function declines with normal aging, estrogen decreases and FSH increases. To be diagnosed with premature menopause (or menopause), FSH must be above 40 International Units per liter of blood (IU/L). For a diagnosis of autoimmune ovarian failure, you need to measure autoantibodies.

"If you measure hormones in individual ovarian follicles during the declining phase, before menstruation ceases completely, you get a different picture than from measuring hormones in the blood. The follicles produce normal amounts of hormones, but because there are less of them in older women, the amount of hormones we see in the bloodstream is less," Dr. Luborsky explains. "However, in patients with anti-ovarian autoantibodies there is more variability in the levels of hormone in the follicles. For instance, in some women with ovarian autoantibodies the follicular cells make huge amounts of progesterone, others may make very little. A lot of these women have functional follicles, but they don't look as normal as in women who are just getting older," she observes.

"Not all women with premature menopause will have an underlying autoimmune disease. If you are having symptoms of an early menopause, you should consider getting tested so you know what's going on," advises Dr. Luborsky.

A workup for autoimmune ovarian failure may include tests for anti-ovarian antibodies and other nonspecific autoimmune markers, such as an elevated *SED rate, antinuclear antibodies,* and *rheumatoid factor (RF),* as well as levels of *thyroid stimulating hormone (TSH),* elevated blood glucose, and the diagnostic tests for Addison's disease (see pages 225 to 226). Accurate diagnosis can help rule out other causes of ovarian failure, such as stress (which may be reversible).

While the causes may be different, the symptoms of autoimmune and nonautoimmune ovarian failure are the same as in a normal menopause, with hot flashes, thinned and dry vaginal tissues (*atrophic vaginitis*), painful sex, infertility, bone loss, and an increased risk of cardiovascular disease caused by estrogen deprivation. As with other endocrine disorders, the treatment is replacing the lost hormones, in this case hormone therapy (HT) with estrogen and progesterone to protect the heart, bones, genital and urinary tract tissues, and the nervous system.

Many cases are diagnosed at infertility clinics. In some women with autoimmune ovarian failure, follicular function may spontaneously resume, and a pregnancy can occur. However, if a woman with this condition wants to become pregnant, aggressive treatment can be tried with hormones to stimulate ovarian follicles to produce multiple eggs, followed by *in vitro fertilization (IVF)*, but the success rate so far is low.

Testing for anti-ovarian autoantibodies may help identify women more likely to succeed with IVF. "Our studies found that women who became pregnant with IVF had a lower frequency of anti-ovarian antibodies compared to the women who did not succeed with IVF," comments Dr. Luborsky. "Women found to have anti-ovarian antibodies may be candidates for future immune-based therapy. A few studies indicate immune suppression may result in a return of normal periods and pregnancy, although this is somewhat controversial," she notes.

The consequences may go beyond infertility. Recent research by Dr. Luborsky has found that autoantibodies found in this type of ovarian failure also appear to be associated with ovarian cancer.[42] However this research is very preliminary and does *not* indicate a cause and effect.

Symptoms associated with menopause should be cause for concern for younger women. Without estrogen therapy, atrophy of vaginal tissue can make sex uncomfortable and lead to frequent urinary tract and yeast infections. Make sure you talk to your gynecologist if you are not comfortable discussing menopausal symptoms with a rheumatologist or other specialist.

Notes

1. Standards of medical care in diabetes—2014. *Diabetes Care*. 2014;37(suppl 1):s14–s80. doi:10.2337/dc14-S014. American Diabetes Association.

2. Centers for Disease Control and Prevention. National diabetes statistics report, 2014 (released June 10, 2014). http://www.cdc.gov/diabetes/pubs/statsreport14/national-diabetes-report-web.pdf.
3. Danaei G, Finucane MM, Lu Y, et al. National, regional, and global trends in fasting plasma glucose and diabetes prevalence since 1980: systematic analysis of health examination surveys and epidemiological studies with 370 country-years and 2.7 million participants. *Lancet*. 2011;378(9785):31–40.
4. Patterson CC, Dahlquist GG, Gyürüs, E, et al. Incidence trends for childhood type 1 diabetes in Europe during 1989–2003 and predicted new cases 2005–2020: a multicentre prospective registration study. *Lancet* 2009;373(9680):2027–2033. doi:http://dx.doi.org/10.1016/S0140-6736(09)60568-7.
5. Harjutsalo V, Sjöberg L, Tuomilehto J. et al. Time trends in the incidence of type 1 diabetes in Finnish children: a cohort study. *Lancet.* 2008;24;371(9626):1777–1782. doi:10.1016/S01406736(08)607655.
6. Gale, EAM. Rising incidence [Internet]. 2014 Aug 13, *Diapedia (The Living Textbook of Diabetes, EASD)*. 21042821128 rev. no. 42. http://dx.doi.org/10.14496/dia.21042821128.42.
7. Lin HC, Wang CH, Tsai FJ, et al. Enterovirus infection is associated with an increased risk of childhood type 1 diabetes in Taiwan: a nationwide population cohort study. *Diabetologia*. 2014. doi:10.1007/s00125-014-3400-z.
8. Hardt PD, Hauenschild A, Nalop J, et al and the S2453112/S2453113 Study Group. High prevalence of exocrine pancreatic insufficiency in diabetes mellitus. A multicenter study screening fecal elastase 1 concentrations in 1,021 diabetic patients. *Pancreatology*. 2003;3(5):395-402. doi:10.1159/000073655.
9. FDA allows marketing of first ZnT8Ab autoantibody test to help diagnose type 1 diabetes. FDA Press Release, August 20, 2014. http://www.fda.gov/NewsEvents/Newsroom/PressAnnouncements/ucm410830.htm.
10. National Library of Medicine, MedLine Plus/LabTestsOnline. What is pancreatic insufficiency? http://vsearch.nlm.nih.gov/vivisimo/cgi-bin/query-meta?v%3Aproject=medlineplus&query=exocrine+pancreatic+insufficiency+&x=22&y=22.
11. Writing Group for the DCCT/EDIC Research Group. Association between 7 years of intensive treatment of type 1 diabetes and long-term mortality. *JAMA*. 2015;313(1):45–53. doi:10.1001/jama.2014.16107.
12. American Diabetes Association: Insulin basics. http://www.diabetes.org/living-with-diabetes/treatment-and-care/medication/insulin/insulin-basics.html.
13. Now available, Alfrezza® inhaled insulin. Sanofi Diabetes. https://www.afrezza.com/.
14. European Association for the Study of Diabetes (EASD) 2014 Annual Meeting, September 15–19, 2014, Vienna, Austria. Abstract #196: Gudbjornsdottir S, Eliasson B, Svensson AM, et al. Observational study of insulin pump treatment: Swedish National Diabetes Register. http://www.easdvirtualmeeting.org/resources/16958.
15. Nutrition therapy recommendations for the management of adults with diabetes. *Diabetes Care*. 2014;37(suppl 1):s120–s143. doi:10.2337/dc14-S120. American Diabetes Association.

16. Kovatchev BP, Renard E, Combelli C, et al. Feasibility of outpatient fully integrated closed-loop control. First studies of wearable artificial pancreas. *Diabetes Care.* 2013;36:1851. doi:10.2337/dc12-1965.
17. Types of artificial pancreas device systems. U.S. Food & Drug Administration, December 10, 2014. http://www.fda.gov/MedicalDevices/ProductsandMedicalProcedures/HomeHealthandConsumer/ConsumerProducts/ArtificialPancreas/ucm259555.htm#TSDS.
18. First U.S. outpatient artificial pancreas trial receives FDA approval. May 2015. http://jdrf.org/key-research-advances/first-u-s-outpatient-artificial-pancreas-trial-receives-fda-approval/.
19. Russell SJ, El-Khatib FH, Sinha M, et al. Outpatient glycemic control with a bionic pancreas in type 1 diabetes. *N Engl J Med.* 2014;371:313–325. doi:10.1056/NEJMoa1314474.
20. Norris J. For type 1 diabetes, islet transplantation gains momentum. UCSF experts improve treatments to prevent rejection. University of California San Francisco Press Release, November 14, 2013. http://www.ucsf.edu/news/2013/11/110271/type-1-diabetes-islet-transplantation-gains-momentum 1/.
21. Rigby MR, Harris KM, Pinckney A, et al. Alefacept provides sustained clinical and immunological effects in new-onset type 1 diabetes patients. *J Clin Invest.* 2015;125(8):3285–3296. doi:0.1172/JCI81722.
22. Curry C. UF sees progress in potential new treatment for Type 1 diabetes. *Gainesville Sun,* June 19, 2014. http://www.gainesville.com/article/20140619/ARTICLES/140619588?p=1&tc=pg.
23. Raz I, Ziegler A, Linn T, et al. Treatment of recent-onset type 1 diabetic patients with DiaPep277: results of a double-blind, placebo-controlled, randomized phase 3 trial. *Diabetes Care.* 2014;37(5):1392–1400. doi:10.2337/dc13-1391.
24. Roep BO, Solvason N, Gottlieb PA, et al. Plasmid-encoded proinsulin preserves C-peptide while specifically reducing proinsulin-specific CD8+ T-cells in type 1 diabetes. *Science Trans Med.* 2013;5(191):191ra82. doi:10.1126/scitransmed.3006103.
25. Schweiger BM, Snell-Bergeon JK, Roman R, et al. Menarche delay and menstrual irregularities persist in adolescents with type 1 diabetes. *Reprod Biol Endocrinol.* 2011;9:61. doi:10.1186/1477-7827-9-61.
26. Codner E, Escobar-Morreale HF. Clinical review: hyperandrogenism and polycystic ovary syndrome in women with type 1 diabetes mellitus. *J Clin Endocrinol Metab.* 2007;92:1209–1216.
27. Viana LV, Gross JL, Azevedo MJ. Dietary intervention in patients with gestational diabetes mellitus: a systematic review and meta-analysis of randomized clinical trials on maternal and newborn outcomes. *Diabetes Care.* 2014;37(12):3345–3355. doi:10.2337/dc14-1530.
28. Dorman JS, Steenkiste AR, Foley TP, et al. Menopause in type 1 diabetic women—is it premature? *Diabetes.* 2001;50:1857–1862.
29. Leidig-Bruckner G, Grobholz S, Bruckner T, et al. Prevalence and determinants of osteoporosis in patients with type 1 and type 2 diabetes mellitus. *BMC Endocr Disord.* 2014;14:33. doi:10.1186/1472-6823-14-33.

30. Ferrara A, Karter AJ, Liu J, Selby JV. Hormone replacement therapy is associated with better glycemic control in women with type 2 diabetes. The Northern California Kaiser Permanente Diabetes Registry. *Diabetes Care.* 2001;24(7):1144–1150. doi:10.2337/diacare.24.7.1144.
31. Økkegaard E, Pedersen AT, Heitmann BL, et al. Relation between hormone replacement therapy and ischaemic heart disease in women: prospective observational study. *BMJ.* 2003;326:1–5.
32. McKenzie J, Jaap AJ, Gallacher S, et al. *Clin Endocrinol.* 2003;59(6):682–689. doi:10.1046/j.1365-2265.2003.01906.x.
33. Mackay L, Kilbride L, Adamson KA, Chisholm J. Hormone replacement therapy for women with type 1 diabetes mellitus. *Cochrane Database Systematic Rev.* 2013;6. doi:10.1002/14651858.CD008613.pub2.
34. Enzlin P, Rosen R, Wiegel M, et al. Sexual dysfunction in women with type 1 diabetes: long-term findings from the DCCT/EDIC study cohort. *Diabetes Care.* 2009;32(5):780–785. doi:10.2337/dc08-1164.
35. Chaker AJ, Vaidya B. Addison disease in adults: diagnosis and management. *Am J Med.* 2010;123:409–413.
36. Li Y, Song YH, Rais N, et al. Autoantibodies to the extracellular domain of the calcium sensing receptor in patients with acquired hypoparathyroidism. *J Clin Invest.* 1996;97(4):910–914.
37. Nelson LM. Primary ovarian insufficiency. *N Engl J Med.* 2009;360:606.
38. Luborsky J. Ovarian autoimmune disease and ovarian autoantibodies. *J Womens Health Gend Based Med.* 2002;11(7):585–599.
39. Edassery SL, Shatavi SV, Kunkel JP, et al. Autoantigens in ovarian autoimmunity associated with unexplained infertility and premature ovarian failure. *Fertil Steril.* 2010;94(7):2636–2641. doi:10.1016/j.fertnstert.2010.04.012.
40. Bakalov VK, Anasti JN, Calis KA, et al. Autoimmune oophoritis as a mechanism of follicular dysfunction in women with spontaneous premature ovarian failure. *Fertil Steril.* 2005;84(4):958.
41. Luborsky JL, Thiruppathi P, Rivnay B, et al. Evidence for different aetiologies of low estradiol response to FSH: age-related accelerated luteinization of follicles or presence of ovarian autoantibodies. *Hum Reprod.* 2002;17(10):2641–2649.
42. Luborsky JL, Yu Y, Edassery SL, et al. Autoantibodies to mesothelin in infertility. *Cancer Epidemiol Biomarkers Prev.* 2011;(9):1970–1978. doi:10.1158/1055-9965.EPI-11-0139. Epub 2011 Aug 16.

8

Tough to Digest—Inflammatory Bowel Disease (Crohn's Disease and Ulcerative Colitis), Celiac Disease, and Pernicious Anemia

I was diagnosed with Crohn's when I was 20. But, looking back, I'd had symptoms ever since I was a child. I would have these strange periods of a week or two where I would have fevers, abdominal pain, and such fatigue and exhaustion that I couldn't move. But my pediatrician used to tell my parents, "She's just trying to get out of going to school. Don't take it seriously." And then during stressful times, I would get really sick. Like during exams or the week of my high school graduation. It took a long time to figure out what was wrong with me. I was going to lots of doctors. I was going to a gynecologist, I was seeing my family doctor, and they were all saying different things. One said I was developing an ulcer and I should reduce the stress in my life, and I needed to take acid reducers. My gynecologist said I had ovarian cysts and that's what was causing the pain. I was told I had irritable bowel syndrome . . . I was put on antibiotics . . . but no matter what they did, nothing helped. When I was at my sickest, I dropped around 20 pounds. I was also having fevers and night sweats, which are all classic symptoms of Crohn's during a flare. But it still took a long time to be diagnosed. And that only happened because I was so sick my gynecologist decided to admit me to the hospital to find out what was wrong. Once I was put in the hospital, they ran some CAT scans and barium tests and they found the Crohn's. But that was only after the pain and inflammation were so bad, and my small intestine became so inflamed that it burst through my bladder. So I had to have a whole section of my intestines removed. If they had caught it early, maybe I could have just had medication and been fine.

Janine, 26

As Janine found out, diagnosing *inflammatory bowel disease (IBD)* is rarely quick or simple. The two types of IBD—*Crohn's disease* and *ulcerative colitis*—are often mistaken for each other, and their early symptoms of diarrhea and cramping are frequently confused with a nonautoimmune problem called *irritable bowel syndrome (IBS)*. Sometimes they even occur together.

However, IBS and IBD are not the same, even though the abbreviations are similar. In Crohn's disease and ulcerative colitis, it's as if something is eating at you, destroying the parts of your body needed to extract vital nutrition from food and protect you from bacteria in the gut. Both are technically "foreign" antigens, and for our intestines to be tolerant of food and protect against invasion by bacteria, the thin mucosal lining must have a tightly regulated immune system. In IBD and *celiac disease* (another autoimmune disease that affects the intestines), this system fails, disrupting normal digestion.

The process of digestion can be likened to an assembly line, with the various parts of the gastrointestinal system moving food along on a conveyor belt powered by smooth muscle tissue. Food is first chopped up into manageable pieces as we chew, moistened by saliva (which also contains enzymes that begin to break down carbohydrates), and, after a minute or two, is loaded onto the conveyor belt with each swallow. The muscles in the esophagus contract (this is called *peristalsis*) to push food down into the stomach, where it's mixed with acid and digestive juices produced by the stomach lining (which help break down proteins). Your stomach continuously churns as it breaks down and mixes food into a semiliquid consistency, and after two to four hours sends it into the many loops of the small intestine.

This part of the GI conveyor belt has three sections: the *duodenum* (the part that connects directly to the stomach), the *jejunum* (the section just below it), and the *ileum* (which connects to the *colon*, or large intestine). In the duodenum, liver enzymes and *bile salts* (produced by the gallbladder)

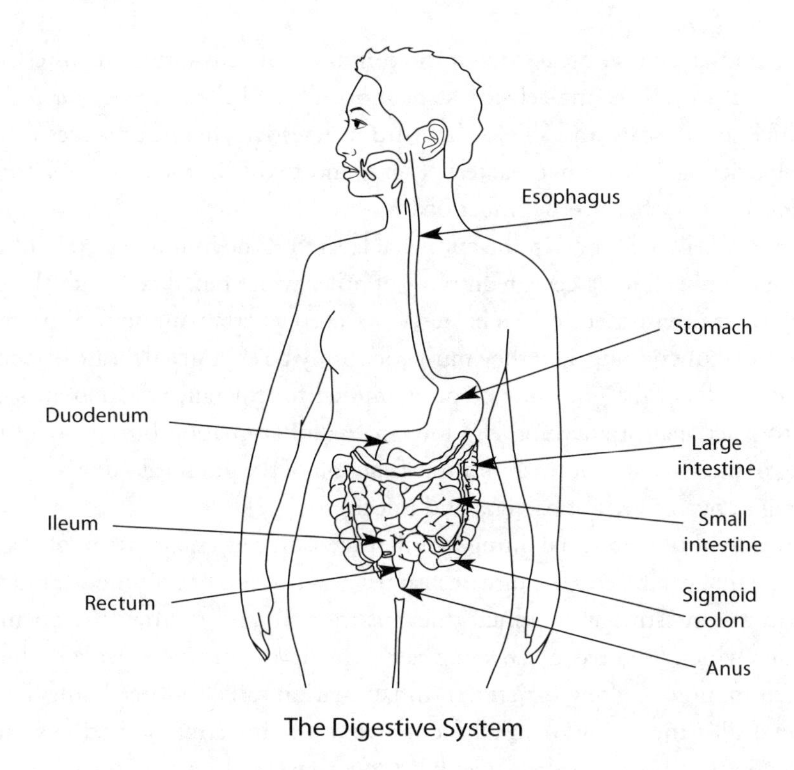

The Digestive System

break down fats, and digestive enzymes from the pancreas continue the breakdown of carbohydrates and proteins. The final breakdown of food is carried out by glands in the lining of the small intestine, and nutrients are extracted by tiny fingerlike projections from the inner lining called *villi*; the layer of cells just beneath the lining helps nutrients pass into the bloodstream.

This process takes anywhere from one to four hours. Finally, the conveyor moves food into the colon. Here, the lining has indentations called *crypts*, which extract most of the water. The solid waste that's left over is moved out of the body as feces. This is actually the longest part of the process, taking anywhere from 10 hours to a couple of days.

The inflammation of IBD speeds up the passage of food, so the intestines empty more frequently, causing diarrhea. Because your body doesn't get enough time to absorb food properly, calories pass out of the system before you can use them, so you start to lose weight.

Inflammation also breaks down the thin layer of cells lining the intestines (*epithelial cells*). This one-cell-thick sheet of cells and the layer of *mucin* they produce to lubricate and shield them from digestive chemicals serves as the only barrier against normal bacteria (*flora*) and toxins in the bowel. Without it, we'd be overwhelmed by infections.

Some T cells are found in the epithelial layer, but the immune system of the intestines only allows a certain amount of other white blood cells into the gut to take care of viruses or excess bacteria (we need a certain amount of bacteria for normal functioning, and they must constantly be kept in a delicate balance). Immune cells in the gut must be programmed for tolerance of food antigens and to react against anything else foreign. As inflammation breaks down the lining of the intestine, normal immune function of the gut breaks down as well, leading to overgrowth of bacteria and infections.

Erosion of the intestinal lining by inflammation causes *ulcerations* or cracks (*fissures*) that can bleed. The disease also triggers overgrowth of smooth muscle cells in the intestine wall, which thickens the wall and narrows the opening through which food passes. In some cases, the narrowing is so severe it blocks food from moving along (*strictures*). Inflammation can also spread outside the bowel wall, penetrating to an adjacent area of the intestine, sometimes causing sections of bowel to stick together (*adhesions*).

Crohn's disease typically affects the lower part of your small intestine (the *terminal ileum*), but it can produce inflammation and ulcerations along any part of the digestive conveyor belt, from the mouth to the anus (as well as nearby tissues) and can cause symptoms in other parts of the body (see pages 245 to 246). The terms *ileitis* and *proctitis* refer to inflammation in the ileum and rectal areas. In *ulcerative colitis (UC)*, inflammation usually occurs only in the lower colon and in the rectum, but may spread to the entire colon.

IBD is actually the second most common chronic inflammatory disorder after rheumatoid arthritis. Crohn's and ulcerative colitis commonly occur between ages 12 and 28, and spikes again after age 50. Opinions are divided as to whether women are more prone to Crohn's disease; some studies show women are two to three times more likely to develop it. Crohn's is a lifelong, chronic disease, but new treatments have made lengthy remissions possible; UC can be cured with surgery to remove the affected area of bowel.

According to the Crohn's & Colitis Foundation of America (CCFA), Crohn's disease and ulcerative colitis affect as many as 1.4 million Americans.[1]

Warning Signs of Inflammatory Bowel Disease

- Chronic diarrhea (more than six weeks)
- Abdominal pain
- Nausea and vomiting
- Fever
- Fatigue
- Night sweats
- Weight loss
- Mouth ulcers, ulcerations in the perianal area (Crohn's disease)
- Joint pain
- Clubbed fingernails

Crohn's Disease

Crohn's disease seems to stem from a combination of genetic and environmental causes, especially bacterial infections. Around 5 to 20 percent of people with Crohn's have a close family member with inflammatory bowel disease. If you have a parent or sibling with IBD, your chances of developing it are increased. "With one affected parent the risk is 3 to 7 percent; with two affected parents it goes up to 33 percent for the child," remarks Sunanda V. Kane, MD, professor of medicine, gastroenterology, and hepatology at the Mayo Clinic in Rochester, Minnesota. Crohn's is also more common in Caucasians and among people of Jewish descent.

What Causes Crohn's Disease?

Back in 2001, scientists at three U.S. universities and in Europe identified the first genetic abnormality that increases susceptibility to Crohn's disease. Today upwards of 70 genes have been found.

Discovery of that first Crohn's gene proved pivotal. The gene involves a protein called *NOD2/CARD15*, which helps immune cells called *macrophages* target bacterial invaders by recognizing a key component of their cell membrane. Macrophages, the Pac-Man-like cells of the immune system, engulf and break down bacteria they encounter, then display crumbs of their meal on their surface as a signal to other immune cells to join in the fight. This signal also helps the other immune cells "remember" their prey. In flawed forms of the *NOD2/CARD15* gene, a small portion of the protein is missing, making it less effective in recognizing the bacteria.[2]

How this triggers the inflammation of Crohn's disease isn't yet clear. Researchers speculate that if macrophages are less efficient in sensing bacteria initially, then the other immune cells that are eventually activated and react to the bacteria may produce an exaggerated, prolonged inflammatory response.

As many as 20 percent of people with Crohn's disease in North America and Europe may have a damaged form of the *NOD2/CARD15*. Having just one copy of a defective *NOD2/CARD15* gene may double the risk of developing Crohn's; having two copies could increase risk 15 to 20 times, according to the CCFA.

While *NOD2/CARD15* is only one of many genes that increase risk, the finding gives an important clue as to how bacteria, even those that normally live in the gut (the *microbiome*) could contribute to Crohn's disease.

For example, *Escherichia coli (E. coli)* bacteria are normally present in the intestines, but if you eat or drink food or water contaminated by fecal matter, certain strains of *E. coli* can cause a diarrheal infection. People with Crohn's are often infected with the bacteria. French researchers reported in 2002 that *E. coli* infection causes cells lining the intestine to produce molecules called *MICA*, which activate natural killer T cells. The T cells then release a chemical signal that causes inflammation. One theory of how inflammatory bowel disease develops is that bacteria may constantly stimulate the mucosal lining of the intestines, and the resulting activation of immune cells and production of inflammatory cytokines (like *tumor necrosis factor alpha, TNFα*) lead to chronic inflammation that eventually breaks down these tissues.[3]

So a big surge in MICA molecules in the intestines due to an *E. coli* infection could set off an immune response that causes Crohn's disease. Or, people with a defective *NOD2/CARD15* gene may be genetically "programmed" to mount a prolonged immune response to the infection, causing chronic inflammation of the intestines that leads to Crohn's. It may also be that toxins produced by *E. coli* (or other bacteria) could also damage the intestinal lining.

One bacterium linked to Crohn's is *Mycobacterium paratuberculosis*, which has been found in biopsies of intestinal tissue from Crohn's patients. Crohn's has been confused with intestinal tuberculosis, and one of the drugs used to treat TB is *para-aminosalicylic acid*, an aspirin-like drug closely related to *5-aminosalicylic acid*, a component of *sulfasalazine (Azulfidine)*, which is used to treat Crohn's disease.

The persistent idea that the measles virus (*Rubeola*) may play a role in Crohn's disease has been largely disproven.

Disruption of the normal balance of gut bacteria (*dysbiosis*), caused by toxins, bacteria, and even stress may lead to Crohn's. As previously mentioned, more than 500 species of bacteria, along with yeast and other organisms, live in the gut. When dysbiosis occurs, the normally "tight junctions" between the epithelial cells lining the intestines may become "leaky," so inflammatory cells and harmful bacteria can get through and cause an abnormal immune reaction.[4] The theory is that inflammation triggers changes in the lining of the gut that eventually lead to Crohn's and other autoimmune diseases such as rheumatoid arthritis.[5]

Smoking is a major risk factor for Crohn's and for developing symptoms outside the gut.[6] But ironically, smoking seems to be protective in ulcerative colitis. One of the theories is that in ulcerative colitis, nicotine may stimulate mucin production, and mucin acts as a barrier to help prevent bacteria in the gut from invading the intestinal wall and stimulating the immune system. In Crohn's disease it seems to be the opposite—mucin production is reduced. However, it's not clear whether it's the nicotine or something else in cigarette smoke that's causing this effect.

I think I must have had this disease my whole life . . . I remember when I was in second grade, I was in a gifted class, and when we would have tests I would have severe stomach pains. I would be doubled over; I was in the bathroom all the time. But when my parents took me to a doctor, they were told I had a "spastic colon," a "nervous stomach." That's what I was told all my life.

I've been living on diarrhea medicines since I was a kid. At times the pain would be so bad I thought I had appendicitis. It was only after I had my second child in 1990 that my doctor said, "I think it's time you got this checked out." I went to a gastroenterologist, who did a colonoscopy—and that's how I found out I had Crohn's. But there had been other signs. In 1985 I suddenly started bleeding vaginally. I went to my gynecologist and found that

I had an ulcer in the vagina that was bleeding. He tried cauterizing it, but no matter what he did nothing worked. Then one night I started to hemorrhage. The ulcer had exposed an artery, and they had to tie it off. That was in 1985. It kept happening. I must have had around 10 to 12 different surgeries for vaginal ulcers. They would seem to heal, then a month or two later another one would open. They lasered them . . . twice they used placental tissue for a graft . . . but it wasn't really that successful. They thought maybe it was Behçet's disease, but I didn't meet all the criteria for that. Then, as suddenly as it started it just seemed to go away . . . years later, after I developed another one and it was biopsied, we confirmed that they were Crohn's ulcers.

Laura, 46

Symptoms of Crohn's Disease

Crohn's can develop gradually over a period of years before you have obvious symptoms. Even when there are some symptoms, you may have thought you were simply prone to diarrhea. In some cases, however, Crohn's can come on suddenly.

The most common symptoms are frequent bowel movements, diarrhea, and abdominal pain, often in the lower right side of the abdomen. In contrast to ulcerative colitis, in which the pain may be intermittent and relieved by a bowel movement (see page 262), if you have Crohn's disease, pain will be more constant and will worsen after you eat. The diarrhea is accompanied by a sense of urgency, and it may come on at night. Abdominal pain after eating is also a symptom of *diverticulitis*, the formation of tiny inflamed sacs in the lining of the intestine (usually the lower part of the colon). Diarrhea and abdominal pain are also symptoms of *celiac disease*, an autoimmune attack on the bowel triggered by a reaction to gluten in wheat (see pages 270 to 284).

It's not uncommon for women with Crohn's to be initially diagnosed with irritable bowel syndrome (IBS) because of the shared symptoms of chronic diarrhea and abdominal pain after meals, remarks Christine L. Frissora, MD, an associate professor of medicine at the Weill Medical College of Cornell University. Adding to the confusion, there's an increased incidence of irritable bowel syndrome (IBS) among women with Crohn's.

"IBS has been called a 'spastic colon,' but we think it may be caused by a loss of synchronization between the small and large intestines. Instead of working in concert with each other, one of the intestines may have a stronger reaction to a food or stressful event, and that can cause altered emptying of the bowel," explains Dr. Frissora. "To be diagnosed with IBS, you must have had abdominal discomfort that's relieved by defecation, associated with a change in stool consistency and frequency, or mucus in the stool and bloating. About a third of women have a diarrhea-predominant form of IBS, a third have more constipation with their IBS, and the remaining third alternate between the two. However, in Crohn's disease, in addition to such bowel dysfunction, you have associated symptoms of inflammation."

Those symptoms include fever, fatigue, and weight loss due to malabsorption, she adds. If your fever is low-grade (up to 100.4 degrees), you may not even be aware you're running a temperature. You may feel lethargic and irritable, but not feverish. If your Crohn's is flaring or severe, you can run a high fever (up to 104 degrees), with night sweats. Diverticulitis also causes fever, abdominal tenderness, and strictures.

Crohn's can cause sores or ulcerations anywhere in the digestive tract or where there are mucous membranes, including the mouth. These include *aphthous ulcers*, tiny shallow sores that often occur between the gum and the lower lip, or along the base of the tongue. While canker sores last a week or two, Crohn's ulcers can last for months.

Some women, like Laura, may develop ulcers in the area between the vagina and rectum, or around the vagina itself. Bleeding may be serious and persistent, leading to anemia. In some cases, a *fistula* (an abnormal, tunnellike opening) can occur between the rectal and vaginal areas or between the bowel and the skin near the anus. (Fistulas can also occur internally between adjacent areas of the bowel.)

"Recurrent oral and genital ulcers also occur in a rare inflammatory condition called *Behçet's disease*, which is also thought to be autoimmune," notes Dr. Frissora. (*Behçet's* is more common in Mediterranean countries, the Middle East, and in Japan, where the disease is a major cause of blindness.) Other symptoms it shares with Crohn's are eye inflammation and raised, red bumps called *erythema nodosum*, often on the shins and ankles (which can also be a sign of increased disease activity in IBD).

Because the intestinal tract isn't absorbing nutrients properly, you may have deficiencies of vitamin B_{12}, calcium, vitamin D, and protein. Malabsorption causes you to lose weight, and unexplained weight loss is another key symptom of Crohn's (and *ulcerative colitis*).

Sores, cracks (fissures) in the anal area, and rectal bleeding can occur in Crohn's, as well as hemorrhoids, skin tags in the anal area, or cauliflower-shaped mounds of thickened tissue; the skin tags and areas of thickened skin can both resemble hemorrhoids. There may be pain in the *perianal* area, abnormal discharge of mucus and pus (if there's an internal rectal abscess), or discharge of pus and fecal material due to false openings in the rectum called *sinus tracts.*

In up to 30 percent of women, Crohn's can also cause symptoms in other areas of the body, most commonly joint pain. Between 10 to 20 percent of people with IBD have inflammatory joint disease in their extremities, with the joint pain accompanying (or following) bowel inflammation. In fact, IBD may be causing your arthritis *without* producing bowel symptoms, possibly by the migration of immune cells related to inflammation to the joint lining (*synovium*). Unlike rheumatoid arthritis (which can cluster with Crohn's), the joint pain associated with IBD is not usually symmetrical and doesn't usually produce changes seen on x-rays. Treating Crohn's usually improves joint problems. Some of the same medications used to treat RA are also used to treat Crohn's.

Women with Crohn's can also develop kidney stones, gallstones, or liver disease. An autoimmune liver disorder, *primary sclerosing cholangitis (PSC)*, the blockage of bile ducts by scar tissue, occurs in a small percentage of women with Crohn's (though it's more common in ulcerative colitis). Fifteen percent of women may have skin rashes, including erythema nodosum, usually on the legs. You may also experience eye inflammation (*uveitis*) or pain, light sensitivity, blurred vision, and dry eye.

Women with Crohn's may already have bone loss when they first present to a physician, remarks the Mayo Clinic's Dr. Kane. "Crohn's disease in itself can cause osteoporosis, due to inflammatory cytokines and malabsorption of calcium and vitamin D. Many Crohn's patients have also avoided dairy products because it makes their diarrhea worse, so they don't get enough calcium to begin with," she says. "Bone mass studies in IBD patients have found that anywhere from a third to 60 percent will have low bone mass, without any other kinds of risk factors." (Steroids and other medications used to treat Crohn's can cause or worsen bone loss, as well.)

A child or adolescent with Crohn's may have growth problems or delayed puberty. Menstrual periods and fertility may be normal, but you may find yourself avoiding sex because of pain in the anal or genital area.

Diagnosing Crohn's Disease

The diagnosis of Crohn's disease is made on the basis of symptoms and findings of diagnostic tests. Blood tests can pick up systemic inflammation, anemia, vitamin deficiencies, and other problems related to Crohn's, but sigmoidoscopy and a barium x-ray of the colon (and sometimes an intestinal biopsy) will reveal the classic inflammation and ulcerations.

The *Crohn's Disease Endoscopic Activity Index of Severity (CDEAIS)* measures the percentage of affected areas of mucosal surface in six segments of the intestines (the ileum, right and left colon, *transverse* and *sigmoid* colon, and the rectum), but the index doesn't really correlate to the severity of disease activity. A series of diagnostic tests, including stool analysis (to detect bleeding and other causes of inflammation, such as parasites or bacteria), may be needed to confirm the diagnosis and assess the extent of Crohn's.

Crohn's disease involves all of the layers of the bowel, and a lot of times the inflammation never hits the surface. So if you do a sigmoidoscopy or a barium study you may not see any changes in the mucosa. If you just do a CT scan, all you might see instead is a thickening of the bowel. But if it's just in a short segment, a single CT may not be able to pick it up. So a combination of tests is often needed.

Tests You May Need and What They Mean

Flexible sigmoidoscopy uses a lighted, flexible fiber-optic scope inserted through the rectum to examine the lower areas of the sigmoid colon. The inner lining of the colon can be seen clearly through the scope. If you have Crohn's disease, your doctor may see patches of red, inflamed tissue, ulcerations, and fistulas (making the diagnosis more likely, especially if it's a rectal-vaginal fistula). Most cases of Crohn's involve both the small and large intestine; 15 percent of cases may involve only the colon (and can be mistaken for ulcerative colitis). However, in Crohn's there may be "skip areas" where patches of diseased bowel occur next to areas of normal tissue and the rectum is usually not affected.

Sigmoidoscopy can be done in a physician's office without much discomfort (some people may need a mild tranquilizer). The only preparation you'll need is a mild enema with tap water to cleanse the colon one or two hours before the test. A more thorough examination of the entire colon can be done with colonoscopy, a similar fiber-optic procedure (see below).

A **barium x-ray (barium enema, barium swallow)** is an x-ray of the colon using barium, a contrast agent that shows up as white on the x-ray. It's usually done if you have symptoms but a sigmoidoscopy is negative or inconclusive. You'll be asked to drink a solution to clean out the colon and take a mild enema an hour or two before the test. Just before the x-ray, a small amount of barium is infused into the colon through the rectum. The contrast agent will coat the inside of the colon (which will look like a white tube on the x-ray). In Crohn's, the normally rounded hills and valleys in the surface of the colon are flattened, and there may be tiny ulcerations or fissures. Diverticula show up as protrusions on the outer surface. The test is performed in a radiology facility.

An **upper GI series** uses barium and X-rays to examine the small intestine, the terminal ileum, and the beginning of the colon. There's no prep involved; you simply don't eat anything after midnight the night before so food is less likely to be present in the ileum. On the morning of the test, you drink a small amount of liquid barium (it's chalky, but comes in several flavors). It takes about two hours for the barium to pass through the loops of the small intestine and reach the colon. In Crohn's, the normal pattern of the intestinal lining (including the villi) is often distorted or lost, and there may be narrowing of the opening inside the intestines (the lumen). Additional x-rays may be taken using a compression paddle on the abdomen to separate adjoining loops of bowel, so the end portions of the ileum can be seen clearly (this is similar to the way compression is used when you get a mammogram, so that the tissues of the breast are more visible on x-ray).

Colonoscopy involves a more detailed examination of the entire colon using a very flexible fiber-optic *endoscope* (*endo* means "inside"). Because the scope must pass through all the pretzel-like loops and curves of the colon, sedation is used to make the procedure more comfortable. The fiber-optic scope used for the procedure magnifies the image of the colon's inner lining up to ten times its normal size so it can be thoroughly examined. Photographs and videotapes can even be made during the procedure by mounting a small camera on the viewing end of the scope. The scope is hollow, so a biopsy device can be passed through it.

You'll be asked to eat a liquid diet for the 48 hours before the test (with only clear liquids during the preceding 24 hours) to minimize the chances of any fecal residue in the colon. In Crohn's disease, colonoscopy may reveal patterns of inflammation (the characteristic "skip" pattern), ulcerations or other lesions, and loss of the normal folds in the inner surface (those folds are needed to thoroughly extract moisture and nutrients). The scope can reveal polyps, and biopsies can be taken. The biopsy may reveal granulomas, a microscopic granular-like lesion caused by an influx of inflammatory cells, seen in up to 10 percent of people with Crohn's. Ulcerations may bleed (and blood may be present in a stool sample). The lining of the colon can also take on a cobblestone-like texture in Crohn's.

Colonoscopy is an extremely valuable test, but it needs to be done by a qualified gastroenterologist. It's only performed in Crohn's when adequate information can't be obtained from other diagnostic tests, or if cancer or polyps are suspected, because inflammation can make the colon more prone to injury during the procedure.

Capsule endoscopy is a fairly new imaging technique used in Crohn's that involves swallowing a small video capsule (larger than a standard medicine capsule) that takes thousands of photographs of the inside of the esophagus, stomach, and the small intestine as it works its way down. You'll need to do the same bowel prep as for a colonoscopy so the photos will be clear. The capsule actually contains video chips that function as cameras, a miniscule battery, a radio transmitter, and even a teeny light bulb. The photos are taken quickly and transmitted to a small receiver, downloaded into a computer and then reviewed by your physician. After the capsule has done its job, it's simply flushed down the toilet with fecal matter. Just as with sigmoidoscopy, this technique only images part of the GI tract, the images can be blurry because the capsule is moving and, like any battery-powered device, the battery can die (average battery life is only about eight hours). You'll need to swallow a dummy capsule first to make sure there are no blockages to trap the capsule. If it does get stuck, it can be retrieved surgically.[7] The technique is also used in Celiac disease and in other conditions.

Gastroscopy involves the examination of the lining of the esophagus, stomach, and the uppermost portion of the small intestine (*duodenum*) with a thinner fiber-optic scope. Crohn's disease can cause inflammation and ulceration of these areas, and the test can help distinguish between Crohn's and ulcerative colitis. Sedation is usually given to reduce discomfort and quiet your gag reflex as the scope is passed down the throat.

Computed tomography (CT) scans can help detect abnormalities in the intestinal mucosa and other areas in Crohn's. Radioactive dyes may also be used to assess the extent of inflammation. Other imaging techniques, like transabdominal ultrasound or magnetic resonance imaging (MRI), may also provide useful information.

Complete blood count (CBC) can reveal iron-deficiency anemia due to bleeding, vitamin B_{12} deficiency due to malabsorption, or depletion of red blood cells. You may also have a low platelet count (thrombocytopenia), a high platelet count (thrombocytosis), or a high white blood cell count, a sign of inflammation.

C-Reactive protein (CRP) is a marker of inflammation found in the blood that will be elevated in Crohn's. CRP is also measured to determine whether a patient is in remission.

Erythrocyte sedimentation rate (SED rate) will be elevated because of inflammation (see pages 32 to 33) in Crohn's, but CRP is more helpful in determining disease activity.

Tests to measure antibodies associated with Crohn's disease can be useful for separating Crohn's from ulcerative colitis and other disorders. They include antibodies against baker's yeast (*anti-Saccharomyces cerevisiae*), present in 50 to 70 percent of Crohn's patients (but only 6 to 14 percent of people with UC). Antibodies to *pancreatic antigens (PABs)*, a protein in pancreatic secretions, are seen in 31 percent of Crohn's patients (and only 4 percent of people with UC). Testing for these antibodies is not yet routine, but may be useful in some cases.

Janine's story continues:

Two years after my surgery I was put on sulfasalazine. First they got me into remission with steroids, then they tapered me off the prednisone and put me on Pentasa, and I've been doing really well with it. I have not let my disease interfere with my life, apart from watching what I eat. I have been active in support groups and on the Internet. I think that getting to know other people with inflammatory bowel disease helps tremendously. You need that emotional support.

Treating Crohn's Disease

The treatment for your Crohn's depends on how much of the bowel is involved and how severe the disease is (for example, if you have fistulas) and any other complications you may have. The goal is to control inflammation; relieve symptoms like abdominal pain, diarrhea, and rectal bleeding; and correct any nutritional deficiencies. Treatment may include medications, surgery, nutritional supplements, or a combination.

You can experience long periods of remission—sometimes years without any symptoms—with proper treatment. But there's no cure for Crohn's, and it can recur periodically. Unfortunately, there's no way to predict when this may happen. Although it can be controlled, Crohn's is a chronic disease, and you'll need regular medical visits, periodic diagnostic tests in the event of a recurrence, and sometimes a change in your medication.

Sulfasalazine (Azulfidine) has been the most common drug for treating Crohn's. It contains a sulfa preparation (*sulfapyridine*) that has antibiotic properties. Sulfasalazine also contains *mesalamine*, an aspirin-like substance that helps control inflammation and is used to treat mild to moderate Crohn's. Sulfasalazine is also helpful in treating flares of Crohn's colitis and ileitis. Side effects include nausea, vomiting, heartburn, diarrhea, appetite loss, and headache. If you've had allergic reactions to other sulfa drugs, you may have a rash in reaction to sulfasalazine; in this case, the drug may be stopped. It can also interfere with the absorption of digoxin and folic acid. Your doctor will continue the medication until symptoms go away. Once you're in remission, you'll be put on a maintenance dose. Sulfasalazine can safely be used during pregnancy (see page 259).

Aminosalicylic acid (5-ASA) agents are aspirin-like drugs that also contain mesalamine, and have largely replaced sulfasalazine. The 5-ASA agents include *balsalazide* (*Colazal* and a generic), *olsalazine sodium (Dipentum)*, and *mesalamine (Pentasa, Asacol, Delzicol, Apriso)*.

These are coated capsules with pure 5-ASA that are delivered either to the small bowel or to the terminal ileum into the early part of the colon; or, if it's the distal colon, Asacol is delivered to that area. Pentasa is delivered to the small bowel. They can also be given orally.

Immunosuppressants are used to treat moderate to severe Crohn's disease. The most commonly prescribed are *6-mercaptopurine (6-MP, Purinethol), methotrexate*, and *azathioprine (Imuran)*, a chemical cousin to 6-MP. Immunosuppressive agents work by blocking the immune reaction that contributes to inflammation. It may take three to four months for 6-MP to show benefits.

These drugs can cause fever, bone marrow suppression, and, in some cases, pancreatitis. While taking these drugs you'll need careful monitoring of your blood counts and liver function tests. Immunosuppressant drugs may also cause side effects like nausea, vomiting, and diarrhea, and may lower your resistance to infection.

Corticosteroids (glucocorticoids) are also used to treat moderate to severe disease, as well as severe or fulminant Crohn's. Among the most commonly prescribed are *prednisone (Deltasone, Orasone)* and *prednisolone (Prelone).*

Budesonide (Entocort EC) is a steroid that's released in the intestine, where it works locally and topically to decrease inflammation, avoiding many of the side effects of systemic corticosteroids. Budesonide capsules are approved for mild to moderate Crohn's disease involving certain sections of the small and large intestines. It is also used along with anti-diarrheal agents (see page 254).

Clinical trials among people with active Crohn's have found that the drug significantly improves symptoms. The most common side effects include headache, respiratory infection, and nausea. In comparison with prednisolone, fewer patients on budesonide experienced facial swelling and acne. Although your doctor may try to avoid the use of corticosteroids because of side effects (like a fatty liver) and the risk of osteoporosis, these drugs may enhance the effects of immunosuppressive drugs. When used in combination with immunosuppressants, the dose of steroids can be lowered. While steroids are very effective in bringing about a remission, nearly half of women may become dependent on them and need to be tapered off the drug. (For more details on corticosteroids, see pages 42 to 43.)

Biologic therapies for IBD and Crohn's target specific enzymes and proteins that are elevated, very low, or defective.

Infliximab (Remicade) blocks the inflammatory cytokine *tumor necrosis factor alpha (TNFα)*, which damages tissue in Crohn's, rheumatoid arthritis, and other autoimmune diseases. It's a monoclonal antibody that targets the

TNF molecule, binds to it, and removes it from the bloodstream before it reaches the intestines, preventing further inflammation. It's also approved for ulcerative colitis.[8]

Remicade is given as an intravenous drip (it takes about two hours) every eight weeks. It's used to treat moderate to severe Crohn's and for people who don't respond to sulfasalazine, 5-ASA agents, or immunosuppressive agents. It is also approved to treat people with fistulas and to induce and maintain remissions of Crohn's. Side effects include an increased risk of serious infection, and a lupus-like syndrome. It is used in combination with 6-MP, azathioprine, or a 5-ASA compound. Remicade should be avoided during pregnancy (see page 259).

Two other TNFα blockers are also approved for treating moderate to severe Crohn's disease—*Adalimumab (Humira)* and *certolizumab pegol (Cimzia)*. Adalimumab is given by self-injection every other week. The first three injected doses of certolizumab are given every two weeks and after that once a month. Infliximab and adalimumab appear to be similarly effective at maintaining remission in Crohn's.[9]

According to the CCFA, approximately 60% of people with IBD respond to anti-TNFα therapies and, among these patients, about 35% will be in remission at the end of one year.

TNFα drugs produce mucosal healing, do away with inflammation, and change the natural history of the disease. One of the big problems of Crohn's is that patients get scarring, stenosis, obstructions, and fistulas, and these drugs shut all that down.

A number of new treatments have been approved by the FDA. These include the intravenous drug *vedolizumab (Entyvio)*,[10] approved for adults with moderate to severe Crohn's and ulcerative colitis who haven't responded well to corticosteroids, immunomodulators, or TNF blockers. Vedolizumab is among a new class of drugs called *integrin receptor antagonists*. These drugs block a protein that sits on circulating inflammatory cells from interacting with a protein on the inner surface of blood vessels, preventing them from migrating into the GI tract.

The first dose of vedolizumab is followed by infusions at two, four, and six weeks, then every two months after that. The infusion takes around a half hour. The most common side effects include headaches, joint pain, nausea, and fever, as well as serious infections and liver toxicity. It's uncertain whether the drug, like another type of integrin receptor antagonist, causes a rare and often infection of the nervous system called progressive multifocal leukoencephalopathy (PML), a disease that affects the myelin sheathe around nerve cells, so patients must be monitored.[11]

Natalizumab (Tysabri) is an *alpha 4 integrin inhibitor.* It interferes with a cell adhesion molecule (which acts as kind of molecular glue) so white blood cells can't stick to receptors in inflamed tissues. The drug, also used to treat multiple sclerosis, is approved for adults with active moderate Crohn's disease who haven't responded to TNF blockers or other drugs.[12]

Natalizumab is given as an intravenous infusion (it takes around an hour to receive a full dose) and is usually administered every four weeks. It has some of the same side effects as vedolizumab and can also lead to PML, and patients being treated for Crohn's or MS with the drug must be monitored for neurological symptoms, such as vision loss, impaired speech, weakness or paralysis, and cognitive deterioration. PML is diagnosed by testing for a virus called the JC virus.

Antidiarrheal agents can be used to relieve the cramps and diarrhea of Crohn's. These include *diphenoxylate (Lomotil)* and *loperamide (Imodium).* In severe cases you may become dehydrated, so you'll need plenty of fluids (such as Gatorade) to replenish electrolytes. Budesonide is also used to relieve symptoms of diarrhea.

A prescription "medical food," *EnteraGam,* is designed for people whose diarrhea prevents them from digesting, absorbing, and metabolizing food.[13] The special proteins in this product (*serum derived bovine immunoglobulin/protein isolate*) remain in the intestine and are not absorbed whole, as are proteins from regular food. It can also help manage diarrhea.

Cholestyramine (Questran) is a cholesterol-lowering agent that can be helpful in controlling diarrhea. Patients with IBD affecting the end portion of the ileum (or who have had surgery) may not be absorbing bile salts in the area, which causes the colon to secrete fluid and electrolytes, leading to watery diarrhea.

Antibiotics are used to treat bacterial overgrowth (and resulting inflammation) in the small intestine caused by fistulas, strictures, or prior surgery. Commonly prescribed antibiotics include *ampicillin, sulfonamide, cephalosporin, tetracycline, ciprofloxacin (Cipro),* and *metronidazole (Flagyl).* These are also used to treat abscesses and perianal fistulous disease.

Nutritional supplements, either oral supplements or injections, may be recommended in people who have deficiencies of vitamin B_{12} or vitamins D, A, or K. The anemia caused by malabsorption of vitamin B_{12} in the ileum is treated by monthly B_{12} injections.

In severe disease with considerable weight loss, special high-calorie liquid products are sometimes used to boost nutrition. A small number of patients with severely inflamed intestines, or who cannot absorb enough nutrition from food, may need temporary intravenous feeding.

Women with Crohn's also need to watch their diet, avoiding foods that irritate the bowel, such as spicy foods or high-fiber foods.

Disease Activity in Crohn's

The following classifications have been developed by the American College of Gastroenterology (ACG) and are used to help determine or adjust treatment. Your doctor may also use the Crohn's Disease Activity Index (CDAI) to monitor your condition.

Mild to moderate disease: You are able to eat normally without pain, abdominal tenderness, painful intestinal masses (or obstruction), fever, or dehydration.

Moderate to severe disease: You have failed treatments for mild to moderate disease, or you have prominent symptoms like fever, weight loss (more than 10 percent of your body weight), abdominal pain and tenderness, periodic nausea or vomiting (without bowel obstructions), or anemia.

Severe (or fulminant) disease: Symptoms persist despite treatment with corticosteroids or other immunosuppressant drugs, or you present to your doctor with high fever, persistent vomiting, abdominal tenderness, severe weight loss, evidence of an abscess or obstruction.

Remission: This is defined as the absence of symptoms or signs of inflammation. It includes women who have undergone acute treatment or surgery.

Surgery

If symptoms don't respond to drugs, or there are repeated blockages or bleeding in the intestine, surgery may be the next step. While surgery to remove a damaged section of intestine can help Crohn's disease, it doesn't cure it.

Unfortunately, inflammation tends to recur right next to the resected area of intestine.

In severe cases where Crohn's has damaged the large intestine, some women may need to have their entire colon removed. The procedure, called *colectomy*, brings the end of the ileum to the surface of the lower right side of the abdomen, with an opening the size of a quarter (stoma), to allow waste to exit into an external pouch (which is emptied as needed). In some cases, women can avoid a colectomy, having only the diseased section of intestine removed and the two ends reconnected (*anastomosis*), with no stoma or bag needed. However, this procedure has a higher risk of disease recurrence. (Smoking also increases the risk of recurrence after surgery.)

Mesalamine, 6-MP, and *Imuran* are all being tested to see whether they can prevent recurrences after surgery. If your Crohn's is severe, you need to discuss the pros and cons of surgery with your physician.

Small bowel transplants may also be helpful. According to the CCFA, transplants of a small section of healthy intestine from a donor can reverse intestinal failure. As with any transplant, lifelong immunosuppressant treatment is needed.

What's Next?

New biologic therapies being researched for Crohn's including other TNFα inhibitors, additional drugs that target alpha 4 integrin, and agents to suppress inflammatory cytokines such as interleukin-12 (IL-12) *semapimod*[14] and interferon gamma (*fontolizumab*).[15] IL-10 is a cytokine that suppresses (rather than produces) inflammation and studies are underway into a synthetic form of IL-10 for treating Crohn's disease.

Drugs approved for other autoimmune diseases are also being tested in Crohn's such as the *Janus kinase (JAK)* inhibitor *tofacitinib (Xeljanz)*[16] and the IL-6 inhibitor *tocilizumab (Actemra)* both used to treat RA.[17] The psoriasis drug *ustekinumab (Stelara)*, which targets IL-12, may help people with Crohn's resistant to TNF-blockers.[18]

One experimental therapy is designed to produce "oral tolerance"—using an oral agent to induce the immune system to tolerate specific antigens—with an extract called *Alequel*, derived from a mixture of colon-extracted proteins from the patient's own gut. The therapy could be individually tailored and it appears to be safe.[19]

Antibiotics are now used to treat the bacterial infections that often accompany Crohn's disease but some research suggests that they might also be useful as a primary treatment for active Crohn's and for fistulas.

Thalidomide (Thalomide) has been used with some success in Crohn's and is being tested in ulcerative colitis (see page 81).[20] And the use of stem cell transplants to treat severe Crohn's is also being investigated.[21]

Janine's story continues:

I always had worse symptoms around my periods . . . I would have increased bowel activity, going to the bathroom a lot more during that time of the month. I went on birth control pills for other reasons—I actually was having ovarian cysts and they were concerned about that. But after I started on them I didn't fluctuate, even on my off week. My doctor was kind of reluctant to put me on the pill, so he put me on a low-dose pill because he thought maybe the hormones would cause my Crohn's to flare. But I've never had a problem with it. The only non-GI symptoms my doctor ever asks about are joint pain. But we never discussed my susceptibility to other autoimmune diseases. And I'm not sure if it's just because he's a gastroenterologist and he's not thinking about it because he's only interested in my Crohn's. But aside from arthritis concerns, they don't monitor me for thyroid or anything else.

Crohn's Disease Clusters

If, like Janine's, your gastroenterologist is mainly focused on GI symptoms, you need to be aware of the other diseases that can cluster with Crohn's.

Ankylosing spondylitis (AS) is an inflammatory disease that affects the spine and nearby structures and progresses to a fusing of the bones of the spine (*ankylosis*). It mostly affects men, but can occur in women with Crohn's. Symptoms can include stiffness and pain in the spine, neck, shoulder, and hips.

Other autoimmune diseases that can cluster with Crohn's include:

- Rheumatoid arthritis
- Thyroid disease
- Primary sclerosing cholangitis

How Crohn's Disease Can Affect You Over Your Lifetime

Crohn's can create special problems for women. Ulcerations and pain in the perineal area can cause painful sex (leading some women to avoid sexual contact), and some may develop a negative body image. "Women worry about having children, being attractive to the opposite sex, feeling that they are somehow ugly, and scarred, that they will be alone in their lives with this diagnosis," comments the Mayo Clinic's Dr. Sunanda Kane. "There are also intimacy issues and worries about sexual performance. Crohn's disease can be a very disfiguring disease, especially when we are talking about deep ulcers and fistulas, around the perianal area and in the vagina."

Other issues that can interfere with relationships include diarrhea, sleep disturbances, and fatigue. Women may also have more problems with fecal incontinence, before and after surgery for Crohn's, or after injury to the anal sphincter during childbirth.

Menstruation

If inflammatory bowel disease begins during childhood or adolescence, it may lead to a delayed puberty, and women may get their first menstrual period later than usual. There are also reports that women experience more severe symptoms around the time of their menstrual periods. There are no clinical studies of premenstrual flares, but a survey of women with irritable bowel and inflammatory bowel disease done by Dr. Kane and colleagues at the University of Chicago found that women with IBD seemed to have more symptoms of PMS. "They polled a group of healthy women, and then compared that to a group of women with inflammatory bowel disease and a group with irritable bowel. The healthy women had premenstrual symptoms, and the group with ulcerative colitis and IBS had the same symptoms but in higher percentages. Of the women with Crohn's disease, 100 percent had premenstrual symptoms," remarks Dr. Kane.

Fertility and Pregnancy

Fertility seems to be unaffected when Crohn's disease is inactive, but if your disease is active you may have some trouble getting pregnant. There are also reports that fertility may be decreased if you've had surgery for Crohn's.

"Two-thirds of women with inactive disease at the time they conceive will do just fine, but perhaps a third may get worse," says Dr. Kane. "Among women who have active disease at the time of conception, one-third will stay the same, one-third will have worsened disease activity, and one-third will actually get better. We simply don't know which group a woman will fall into, even if it's a second or third pregnancy." Women with severe, active disease of the terminal ileum may have a harder time with pregnancy, she adds.

The goal is to maintain a remission during pregnancy, and most treatments do not pose a risk. So you need to stick with medication. Sulfasalazine can cause nausea, which may worsen morning sickness in the first trimester and may exacerbate heartburn in the later part of pregnancy. "Sulfasalazine does not carry a risk of fetal malformation. It does cross the placenta, but is only minimally found in breast milk. Sulfasalazine does interfere with folic acid metabolism, so we give women an extra milligram of folic acid a day," says Dr. Kane. Folic acid protects against neural tube defects. "Mesalamine, our first-line medication for both ulcerative colitis and Crohn's, is a topical anti-inflammatory, and we have not seen any increased risk in pregnant women." The dose of prednisone should be reduced in nursing mothers, if possible.

Ulcerations in the genital area are a concern seldom discussed. "I have seen a patient who developed a rectovaginal fistula after an episiotomy. What happens is the rectal tissue is inflamed, it doesn't heal, and a tract starts forming between the vagina and rectum. For women with IBD, episiotomy should not be taken lightly," adds Dr. Frissora.

Although no harms have been seen for Remicade and Enbrel, risk during pregnancy can't be ruled out (see page 51). Immunosuppressants like azathioprine and 5-ASA drugs should be avoided during pregnancy. (See pages 251 to 252 for details.)

Crohn's may worsen during the first trimester and after delivery, but this may be because women go off their medications in order to breast-feed, remarks Dr. Kane. IBD may also occur for the first time during pregnancy or in the postpartum period.

While the course of pregnancy and delivery is usually not affected in most women with Crohn's disease, you need to have a thorough discussion with your doctors before you start trying to conceive.

Remicade or other biologics can be continued in pregnancy until at least week 20. "We then assess whether disease activity dictates continued therapy, since this is when they start to cross the placenta," says Dr. Kane.

Colonoscopy and x-ray procedures should be avoided, particularly during the first trimester; sigmoidoscopy can be done to track disease activity, however.

Inflammatory bowel disease is not "inherited" in the same way as a disease like cystic fibrosis (in which inheriting two copies of a defective gene, one from each parent, means you will develop the disease). There are multiple genes involved. Still, not enough is known to predict how many children of women with IBD will be predisposed to Crohn's (or ulcerative colitis).

Menopause and Beyond

Crohn's disease that develops in midlife and beyond seems to affect more women than men. Women with Crohn's who have severe menopausal symptoms can consider hormone replacement therapy, says Dr. Kane. "The risks and benefits are the same as for other women."

Osteoporosis is a major concern for all women after menopause, and especially so for women with Crohn's. "Since Crohn's causes osteoporosis, we encourage weight-bearing exercise and tell women to take calcium. Some women may need bone-building drugs, depending on how severe the bone loss is," adds Dr. Kane.

Perhaps 15 percent of patients with inflammatory bowel disease first develop symptoms after age 65. Although the symptoms and course of the disease are similar to that in younger patients, there's slightly more colon involvement when Crohn's affects older people. Conditions that can mimic IBD in older age include diverticular disease, colitis caused by medications (especially nonsteroidal anti-inflammatory drugs), infections, cancer, and other diseases. However, medical and treatment options are not different from those for younger women.

Janine's story continues:
I had started to have severe back pain, and I was lucky to find a really smart orthopedist, who looked beyond just the bones. This doctor really looked at my history. He sees a 46-year-old woman who had a hysterectomy, who has Crohn's disease, who took prednisone for many years, who is not on estrogen, who has a small frame and is suffering severe back pain. He said it could be osteoporosis and asked me when my last bone density screening was, and

I hadn't had one yet. I was first put on Fosamax, but it irritated my esophagus, so I was put on Evista. But after years of prednisone the osteoporosis is pretty severe. Now they think about it as soon as they put you on steroids. But years ago they didn't. And if any woman is on steroids and her doctor doesn't mention her bones, she should make sure she's being protected.

Ulcerative Colitis

In contrast to Crohn's, *ulcerative colitis* affects only the top layers of the mucus membrane that lines the colon and the rectum, producing inflammation and ulcerations. But the effects of inflammation are the same: the colon empties frequently, causing diarrhea. UC can be difficult to diagnose because the symptoms are similar to irritable bowel syndrome and to Crohn's. It develops most often between ages 15 and 40 (although children and older people can have it, too). The incidence of UC may be 20 percent higher in men, and it seems to run in families.

What Causes Ulcerative Colitis?

Many of the same theories as to what causes Crohn's disease also apply to ulcerative colitis (see pages 241 to 243). It seems likely that in vulnerable people, a reaction to a virus or a bacterium causes ongoing inflammation. Those bacteria could be among those normally found in the gut. Although emotional stress and sensitivities to certain types of food may trigger symptoms, they do not cause the disease itself.

Multiple genes are also likely to be involved in ulcerative colitis. It does tend to run in families; as many as 20 percent of patients have a close relative with ulcerative colitis or, less often, Crohn's disease. But again, genes tell only part of the story.

Symptoms of Ulcerative Colitis

The most common symptoms of UC are abdominal pain and bloody diarrhea. You may also experience fatigue, weight loss and loss of appetite, dehydration, and rectal bleeding.

One of the first signs that you may have UC is stools that are looser and softer than usual, often with blood mixed in. You may also feel an intense urge to defecate (called *tenesmus*), and this may result in the accidental passage of a small amount of stool, soiling your underwear. This is due to inflammation of the rectum usually present at the onset of UC and one of the signs that distinguishes it from Crohn's. Moving your bowels relieves this urge only temporarily, another key sign of UC. You can experience this problem during the night, causing sleep disturbances. Crampy abdominal pain is also common (caused by inflammation in other areas of the bowel). Half of women with UC have only mild symptoms; that's common if the disease is confined to the lower (*sigmoid*) colon and the rectum.

When inflammation is confined to the rectum, it's called *ulcerative proctitis*. This may only produce blood and mucus in the stool, and tenesmus. If your disease is more severe and involves large areas of the colon, the symptoms will be more severe and likely to include anemia (from bleeding), weakness, fever, and weight loss.

Because of its inflammatory component, ulcerative colitis may also cause arthritis, eye inflammation, fatty deposits in the liver, and liver disease such as *chronic hepatitis*, *cirrhosis*, and *primary sclerosing cholangitis* (a disease more common in men).

Ankylosing spondylitis, a form of inflammatory arthritis affecting the lower back and spine, affects 2 to 6 percent of people with ulcerative colitis, causing lower back pain, morning stiffness, and sometimes a stooped posture. You may also experience skin rashes, anemia, and kidney stones. Large, circular ulcers called *pyoderma gangrenosa* that eat away at the skin and soft tissues can occur in UC (and, less commonly, in Crohn's). As with Crohn's, osteoporosis is a frequent complication. Many of the inflammatory symptoms subside when UC is treated.

Diagnosing Ulcerative Colitis

Tests You May Need and What They Mean

Ulcerative colitis is also a clinical diagnosis, requiring a thorough physical exam and two key diagnostic tests: *sigmoidoscopy* and a barium enema.

Colonoscopy and proctosigmoidoscopy are needed to determine the extent of the disease and the mucosal changes common in UC, including ulcerations. (For details on colonoscopy and sigmoidoscopy, see pages 247 to 249.) Proctosigmoidoscopy examines the rectum using the same fiber-optic scope.

Sigmoidoscopy can often easily distinguish ulcerative colitis from Crohn's; UC is not patchy, and there will be continuous areas of inflammation and ulcerations. In ulcerative proctitis, there will be a clear separation between red, inflamed tissue and normal bowel above it.

During periods of remission, ulcerations in the lining of the colon may heal to such an extent that the colon will appear close to normal during sigmoidoscopy or a barium x-ray.

Stool testing can reveal bleeding or infection in the colon or rectum. Since rectal bleeding or blood in the stool can also be a sign of colon cancer, further tests may be needed (such as colonoscopy with a biopsy).

Stool tests can also find infections such as *Clostridium difficile (C. difficile)*, which is increasing among patients with UC, and *Escherichia coli (E. coli)*, both of which can cause severe diarrhea. *Infectious colitis* can also produce bloody diarrhea, as can parasites. A mucosal biopsy may be needed to distinguish this from ulcerative colitis.

A **complete blood count (CBC,** see page 33) can pick up anemia, which can be a sign of bleeding in the colon or rectum. A high white blood cell count is a sign of inflammation.

Erythrocyte sedimentation rate (SED rate) will be normal in mild to moderate UC, and elevated in severe disease. (For a complete explanation of a SED rate, see page 32.)

Treating Ulcerative Colitis

The following disease activity classifications were updated in 2010 by the American College of Gastroenterology (ACG) and are used to help select or adjust treatment.

These classifications, based on clinical and endoscopic findings, do not take into account symptoms including abdominal pain, nighttime bowel movements, urgency, or "the dreadful fear of episodes of incontinence, which are often the patients' greatest concerns," the ACG notes in its Practice Guidelines.[22]

- **Mild disease:** Patients have four or fewer bowel movements a day, with or without small amounts of blood present, no systemic signs of toxicity (such as fever or anemia), and a normal SED rate.
- **Moderate disease:** Patients have four or more bowel movements a day (usually bloody), with only minimal signs of toxicity.
- **Severe disease:** Patients have six or more bloody bowel movements a day and fever, anemia, rapid heartbeat (*tachycardia*), or an elevated *SED* rate.
- **Fulminant disease:** In this case, UC patients experience more than 10 bowel movements daily, continuous bleeding, toxicity, abdominal tenderness and distension, and may need a blood transfusion and colonic dilation on abdominal plain X-rays.

Unless your disease is very severe, it's likely you'll be given medication. In many cases, medications can bring about long periods of remission, from months to years, where the mucosal lining of the colon heals and virtually returns to normal. Unfortunately, your symptoms are likely to return eventually. If the disease is severe, you may need to have the entire colon removed.

In cases of severe symptoms, such as extensive bleeding or diarrhea causing dehydration, you may need to be hospitalized. In that event, you'll be given medications to stop the diarrhea and bleeding and replace lost fluids and electrolytes. If the colon is severely inflamed, you may need a special diet or intravenous feeding.

Ulcerative colitis is a chronic disease (the only cure is radical surgery) that requires long-term medical care, and you need to be followed closely by a gastroenterologist.

According to ACG guidelines, patients with mild to moderate distal colitis may be treated with oral aminosalicylates, topical mesalamine, or topical steroids, depending on the patient's preference, since both types of therapies are effective.[17]

Aminosalicylates are given orally or rectally (or both) to suppress inflammation in the rectum and colon. Oral medications include *sulfasalazine* and *5-aminosalicylic acid (5-ASA)* drugs (*mesalamine*, *olsalazine*, and *balsalazide*), which are generally used in mild to moderate ulcerative colitis, and as maintenance therapy once remission is achieved. In cases of extensive but mild disease, only oral sulfasalazine or 5-ASA medications are used. If disease is moderate and extensive, azathioprine or 6-MP may be added.

Side effects of oral 5-ASA drugs include nausea, vomiting, heartburn, diarrhea, and headache (see page 251 for more about sulfasalazine and 5-ASA drugs). Topical 5-ASA agents in suppository form or suspension *enemas (Rowasa)* can cause hemorrhoids, itching, and allergic reactions (rashes) in some people. They can also stain your clothing.

Combining oral and topical aminosalicylates is more effective than either alone. In patients who don't respond to oral aminosalicylates or topical corticosteroids, mesalamine enemas or suppositories may still be effective. In rare cases where there's no improvement with all of those therapies, or if there's a systemic illness, patients may need oral *corticosteroids* such as prednisone or *infliximab (Remicade).*

Sulfasalazine, 5-ASA drugs, and infliximab are used in patients with more extensive mild to moderate UC.

Prednisone and other corticosteroids like *methylprednisolone (Medrol, Depo-Medrol)* can be given orally, intravenously, through an enema, or in suppository form, depending on where the inflammation is located. These medications are used in UC patients with moderate to severe disease. Systemic corticosteroids carry a risk of osteoporosis and can cause side effects like weight gain, acne, facial hair, mood swings, high blood pressure, diabetes, and an increased risk of infection.

Immunosuppressants used to treat ulcerative colitis include *azathioprine (Imuran), 6-mercaptopurine (6-MP)*, and *cyclosporine (Neoral).* These drugs dampen immune activity and keep immune cells from provoking inflammation. They are usually given orally to patients who have not responded to aminosalicylates or corticosteroids. Azathioprine or 6-MP may also be used in combination with corticosteroids (they also allow lower doses to be used) in moderate and extensive disease. It can take up to three months before benefits are seen with these drugs. Intravenous cyclosporine may be given for severe disease. The oral immunomodulator *tacrolimus (Prograf)*, used in transplant patients, is also approved to treat UC.[23]

The first-line therapy is still the 5-ASA drugs. If the disease involves only the rectum or the rectum and the sigmoid colon, we use topical agents such as 5-ASA enema or, in some cases, cortisone enemas. And that can control distal disease. For mild disease, usually the oral 5-ASAs are effective. For flares, steroids are used a little more often, but we try to avoid their use, or use them only for very short periods. As with Crohn's disease, other drugs may be given to relieve pain, diarrhea, or infection (see pages 254 to 255).

Golimumab (Simponi) is a newer *TNFα* blocker approved for treating adults with moderate to severe UC who've have become dependent on corticosteroids or who have had an inadequate response (or can't tolerate) oral aminosalicylates, corticosteroids, azathioprine, or 6-MP. Golimumab improves the mucosal lining of the colon and helps achieve and maintain remission.

An initial subcutaneous injection of 200 mg is followed by a 100 mg at week 2 and then 100 mg every month afterward. You can learn to inject it yourself (or have a family member learn) at home.[24]

Two other *TNFα* drugs used for Crohn's disease, *infliximab (Remicade)* and *adalimumab (Humira)* are also approved for treating UC. Infliximab is given to patients with severe UC. (See pages 252 to 253.)[8]

The integrin receptor antagonist *vedolizumab (Entyvio)* is also approved to treat people with moderate to severe ulcerative colitis who have not responded adequately to corticosteroids, immunomodulators, or *TNFα* blockers.[10]

Recent studies suggest that biologics are safer, more effective, and have more sustained benefits as maintenance therapy than the immunomodulators tacrolimus or 6-MP.[25]

Surgery

If the disease cannot be controlled with medication, or if there's extensive bleeding, rupture, or the threat of colon cancer, surgery may be recommended.

Until recently, radical surgery to remove the entire colon and rectum (*colectomy*), with an *ileostomy* and an external bag to collect solid waste, had been the only "cure" for ulcerative colitis. However, newer surgical techniques allow for the colon to be removed without the need for an ileostomy.

The *ileoanal anastomosis* (commonly called a pull-through operation) preserves part of the rectum and allows patients to have normal bowel movements. In this procedure, the diseased part of the colon and the inside of the rectum are removed, leaving the outer muscles of the rectum intact. The ileum is attached to the inside of the rectum and the anus, creating a pouch that stores waste, which is passed in the usual manner. Inflammation of the pouch and more frequent, watery bowel movements are possible complications.

The type of surgery depends on the severity and extent of the disease; you need to get as much information as possible to make an informed decision.

What's Next?

A number of new treatment approaches for ulcerative colitis are now in clinical trials.

Epithelial growth factors are being tested; they may speed healing of the colon lining and prevent infiltration of inflammatory cells.

Another experimental drug being used is an antibody to a molecule dubbed *alpha4beta7* that has been shown to contribute to inflammation in IBD. Preliminary clinical trials involving 28 patients found the drug LDP-20 induced remissions in 40 percent of patients, compared to those on a placebo. Further clinical trials are under way in ulcerative colitis and in Crohn's.

Thalidomide (Thalomid), a once-banned drug, has found a new use in fighting IBD. Thalidomide was given as an antinausea drug to pregnant women and caused catastrophic birth defects; it was banned in the 1960s. But in recent years, it has been tested against ulcerative colitis, Crohn's, and other diseases.[26] Side effects include sedation, numbness, and dry skin.

Tests are also being conducted of other forms of thalidomide called *selective cytokine inhibitory drugs*, which inhibit an enzyme that spurs production of tumor necrosis factor. These drugs seem to be more potent at dampening inflammation than thalidomide, and animal tests have not shown any birth defects.

It's an odd occurrence that smoking seems to be protective in ulcerative colitis, so nicotine is being studied as a potential therapy, mostly in nicotine patches. But it has not been approved as a therapy for UC.

Your Risk of Colon Cancer

About 5 percent of people with UC develop colorectal cancer, and the risk increases the longer you have UC and with the extent and location of the disease. For example, if the entire colon is involved, your risk of cancer may be as high as 32 times the norm; if UC involves only the lower colon and rectum, your risks are not higher than normal.

Ulcerative colitis can lead to precancerous changes called dysplasia in the cells lining the colon. Signs of dysplasia can be picked up during colonoscopy and biopsy.

Guidelines for colon cancer screening (endorsed by the American Cancer Society, the American College of Gastroenterology, the American Society of Colon and Rectal Surgeons, and the Crohn's & Colitis Foundation of America) advise that people who have had IBD throughout their colon for at least eight years, and those who have had IBD in only the left colon for at least 15 years, should have a colonoscopy every one to two years to check for dysplasia. Recent studies show that colonoscopy is the most effective way of finding colon cancer in its earliest, most curable stage.

How Ulcerative Colitis Can Affect You Over Your Lifetime

As with Crohn's disease, ulcerative colitis can affect women during their reproductive years.

Reproduction

Fertility among women with ulcerative colitis seems to be unaffected by the disease itself. However, women who undergo removal of their colon may have trouble conceiving after the surgery. A study from Denmark compared fertility rates of women with UC to women without the condition. Those women who had not undergone colectomy had an equal or higher fertility rate compared with women without ulcerative colitis. Those women who underwent colectomy had a significantly lower fertility rate and an increased use of in vitro fertilization.[27] Another study found that women who had anal ileal pouch anastomosis had three times the risk of infertility after the procedure.[28]

Around a third of women with active ulcerative colitis who become pregnant will improve, and a third will worsen, notes the Mayo Clinic's

Dr. Sunanda Kane. UC can also occur during pregnancy and the postpartum period. However, sulfasalazine is safe to use during pregnancy, and the 5-ASA agents also appear safe.

Midlife and Beyond

Osteoporosis is a major concern for women taking corticosteroids, especially later in life. Corticosteroids tend to complicate and worsen diabetes, high blood pressure, and other age-related diseases. Women with UC may need antiresorptive agents called bisphosphonates, such as *alendronate (Fosamax)* or *risedronate (Actonel)* to stem bone loss. (For more on these drugs, see page 58.)

One form of colon inflammation, called *ischemic colitis*, can occur in later life and is caused by poor circulation and can mimic the symptoms of IBD. One study found that 75 percent of people with colitis after the age of 50 actually had ischemic colitis, and neither form of IBD. Older women may also develop an antibiotic-associated colitis.

> *I was diagnosed with celiac disease as a child. Apparently it runs in my family. My grandmother later told me one of her sisters died of diarrhea and dehydration as a baby; they thought it was colic. But I thought it was something you outgrew. . . . I found out by accident that you don't really outgrow it. I never had a digestive system that worked properly, from what I can tell. Once every few weeks, I'd have what they called a "stomach virus." I thought I was just susceptible to that. No matter how much I ate, I felt full. If I didn't eat, I'd drop five pounds. If I looked at my stool, I'd see whole pieces of undigested food, and globs of fat. I'd think, "I'm not digesting my food."*
>
> *I didn't know anything about celiac. Except they made you live on nothing when you were a kid, then they thought you outgrew it and you were fine. I made an appointment with an internist and told him I don't know that much about celiac disease, but maybe there's a relationship between that and what's going on with my digestive system. I said, "I think you need to do a stool analysis because I'm not digesting my food." And he said no. Celiac disease has nothing to do with it. This was in 1975 when this happened. I was 18 or 19. I thought I was being completely logical. But he dismissed it.*

He gave me a blood test of some kind, which showed nothing. So I figured celiac had nothing to do with it, and I gave up. I didn't pursue it until much later on.

Ronnie, 45

Celiac Disease

Celiac disease is an autoimmune disease that damages the small intestine and interferes with absorption of nutrients. In celiac disease, the immune system mounts an inflammatory reaction against *gluten*, a protein found in wheat (similar proteins are found in rye and barley), in the process destroying the numerous tiny *villi* in the lining of the small intestine and establishing a state of chronic inflammation in the intestine.

You'll recall that villi absorb nutrients from food; without villi you become malnourished, no matter how much you eat. Celiac disease can affect the entire small intestine or localized areas, such as where iron and calcium are absorbed. So most people with celiac have iron-deficiency anemia and bone loss. The disease also destroys cells in the intestinal lining containing the receptors for vitamins A, D, E, K, and B_{12}. Vitamin B_{12} deficiency results in another form of anemia, macrocytic anemia (in which abnormally enlarged red blood cells crowd out normal cells).

Celiac disease runs in families, and genes play a role. It was once thought to be relatively rare in this country compared to Ireland and Italy, but recent research indicates it is much more common, affecting as many as one percent of people in Western countries, and is on the rise in Asia, where wheat products are replacing rice as a dietary staple.[29] In the United States there is a very low rate of diagnosis, only 17 percent of that one percent, partly because some physicians may not be aware of celiac and because the symptoms are so varied.

While men and women are affected, women are diagnosed three times more often than men, partly because the symptoms are similar to irritable bowel syndrome and partly because women tend to visit doctors more often, so there's more opportunity for a diagnosis.

Celiac disease is associated with a tenfold increased chance of acquiring other autoimmune disorders. Some autoimmune diseases share a very high

Warning Signs of Celiac Disease

- Recurrent abdominal bloating and pain
- Chronic diarrhea
- Weight loss
- Anemia
- Gas
- Bone loss
- Muscle cramps
- Fatigue and depression
- Joint pain
- Tingling and numbness in the legs (neuropathy)
- Mouth sores
- Painful blistering skin rash (dermatitis herpetiformis)
- Discolored teeth; loss of enamel
- Missed menstrual periods

rate of being associated with celiac disease. These include type 1 diabetes, Sjögren's syndrome, and primary biliary cirrhosis.

Celiac typically arises during early childhood, but it can also be triggered (or become active for the first time) after surgery, pregnancy, childbirth, viral infections, or even severe emotional stress. Like Ronnie, people were once thought to "outgrow" celiac disease. But we now know that's not true. And untreated celiac disease can have serious complications, including an increased risk of certain types of cancers.

What Causes Celiac Disease?

Unlike other autoimmune diseases, in celiac the immune system doesn't attack self-antigens. The attack is actually directed against water-insoluble proteins, or *prolamins*, in grains as they pass through the digestive system. Toxic peptides found in these proteins—*gliadin* (found in wheat), *secalin* (from rye), and *hordein* (contained in barley)—trigger an inflammatory reaction in the small intestines of genetically susceptible individuals.

When the immune system senses a prolamin, it sends white blood cells to attack it. These lymphocytes infiltrate the lining of the small intestine, and the resulting inflammation causes overgrowth of the valleys (*crypts*) between the villi, and eventually the destruction of the villi themselves.

"It's not a case of mistaken identity or molecular mimicry. The villi are not the targets; they are innocent bystanders," remarks Peter H. R. Green, MD, the Phyllis and Ivan Seidenberg Professor of Medicine and director of the Celiac Disease Research Center at Columbia University. "Celiac disease is a unique autoimmune disease because we know what the environmental antigen is." What isn't known is why any individual may lose his or her tolerance to gluten. In people who are genetically susceptible to celiac disease, "tolerance" to gluten is lost.

Technically, all the foods we eat are "foreign" antigens. But as we gradually start eating solid foods as babies, the immune system becomes programmed to tolerate them. The immune system has to reach a certain maturity before it can do this, however. That's one reason breast-feeding is beneficial. Breast milk not only contains a perfect balance of proteins, carbohydrates, and fat to nourish an infant, but because these nutrient antigens come from the mother, they are less likely to set off an immune reaction. Breast milk also contains many important antibodies that help an infant fight off infections, and it creates a protective environment in the intestines. Baby formulas contain cow's milk that's been altered to closely resemble human milk (but it lacks the key antibodies). In families where food allergies or lactose intolerance is common, soy baby formula is used. In the case of milk allergies, babies are fed protein *hydrolysate* formulas, which contain cow's milk proteins broken down in a way that mimics digestion and is less likely to provoke allergic reactions. (Allergic reactions also involve the immune system and often occur in people with autoimmune disease.) The first solid food babies eat is rice cereal, which does not contain gluten.

Recent large placebo-controlled European studies of the role of breast-feeding and timing of gluten introduction have debunked current thinking. These two studies of around 1,500 children, who were at high risk of developing celiac disease because of having family members with celiac disease, show that breast-feeding was not protective against developing celiac. In addition, giving small amounts of gluten between four to six months, as is the recommended practice (at least in Europe) did not provide protection against celiac.

Neither was delaying gluten introduction to after the child was a year old. Their only risk factor: the number of at-risk genes.[30]

A majority of people with celiac disease produce antibodies against gliadin, the product in the toxic grains, and other antibodies, setting off a process that leads to production of autoantibodies. These include *anti-gliadin peptide tissue transglutaminase antibodies (tTG)* and *antiendomysium antibodies (EMAs)*, which react against components of smooth muscle tissue in the esophagus and the upper part of the small intestine *(jejunum)*.

Celiac disease is closely associated with other autoimmune diseases, including type 1 diabetes, thyroid disease, and Sjögren's syndrome, which are often the initial diagnosis in adults with celiac. "It's thought that you get the celiac disease first, then you get these autoantibodies to other organs, and then you get the other organ disease, and much later the celiac gets diagnosed," explains Dr. Green. "If you take a bunch of kids with celiac disease, they will often have autoantibodies to the pancreas or to the thyroid. If you put them on a gluten-free diet, those autoantibodies go away. So maybe if you can diagnose celiac early enough, you may prevent these other autoimmune diseases."

Genes also play a major role in celiac disease. Among identical twins (who share identical genes), if one twin has celiac there's only a 70 percent chance the other twin will have it too. Among nonidentical twins, this concordance rate is 40 percent. In the study of high-risk children fed gluten before six months of age or later, the deciding factor for developing celiac seemed to be genes rather than when they were exposed to gluten.

However, sharing the same *human leukocyte antigens (HLAs)* may not be the only factor that predisposes people to celiac disease. Environmental causes can play a role, as well.

"We now know that there are about 40 different genes associated with the development of celiac disease. Celiac is associated with specific HLA genes, but they are also common in the general population," observes Dr. Green.

It's not clear whether female (or male) hormones play a role in celiac disease. "We have looked at male-female differences in celiac disease, and men seem to have more severe manifestations than women. Men have lower bone density and lower total cholesterol, suggesting more malabsorption. But more women get it than men," remarks Dr. Green. "Hormones have not been looked at closely in women with celiac disease, but in men you have low testosterone levels. There's a circulation of estrogen within the liver that gets secreted in bile and then reabsorbed. So potentially, you don't get reabsorption of secreted estrogen. Women may well have lowered testosterone, too. But it hasn't been studied."

Ronnie's story continues:

I actually learned about celiac disease from a free magazine I got in a health food store . . . the article talked about all the symptoms I had been having for years. It mentioned a book, and I ordered it. It told you what to eat and not to eat. So I tried eliminating all the gluten in my diet. I went to a bookstore that had a medical text section and found two books that had something on celiac and took notes. That's how I learned everything . . . the tests that diagnose it, which does include a stool analysis to look for evidence of undigested fat . . . and they described all the damage to the villi. I did go to see another doctor who didn't want to hear about anything I had learned. She just wanted to run tests. She got very huffy and said, "You think you know so much . . . I'm the doctor." I have other problems along with the celiac. I've had chronic fatigue . . . I had fibromyalgia . . . on both sides of my family there's diabetes, and I am very prone to hypoglycemia. But aside from avoiding gluten and fat, I figured there was nothing the medical profession could really do for me.

Symptoms of Celiac Disease

Celiac disease affects each person differently. You may have more diarrhea and abdominal pain, while another woman may have anemia or bone loss as signs of malabsorption. Some women may have no symptoms at all; the undamaged parts of their small intestine are able to absorb enough nutrients to prevent GI problems or malabsorption. This hidden (*occult*) disease may contribute to the notion that celiac disease is rare in this country, says Dr. Green. It's estimated that 17 percent of Americans with celiac aren't even aware they have it.

But even people with no symptoms are at risk for complications, including certain cancers (see page 282).

The classic symptoms of celiac include diarrhea, flatulence, weight loss, and fatigue. If celiac is severe and involves most of the small intestine, fat absorption will also be impaired, and fat goblets may appear in stool (*steatorrhea*) and there may be oil floating in the toilet. Some people may experience constipation with celiac.

Manifestations of celiac can also depend on specific areas of the intestine that are affected. When the duodenum and nearby parts of the small intestine are involved, iron is poorly absorbed, leading to iron-deficiency anemia. This is also the area where fat-soluble vitamins—A, D, E, and K—are taken in, and celiac disease may cause them to be poorly absorbed as well. Vitamin B_{12} is absorbed in the furthest part of the small intestine (the ileum), which is less frequently involved in celiac disease. But if the disease causes a deficiency of vitamin B_{12}, it can lead to macrocytic anemia. Poor absorption of calcium and vitamin D leads to bone loss. In serious, untreated celiac disease, women can develop severe malnutrition, osteoporosis, and even malignant tumors of the small intestine (see page 282).

"The classical presentation is uncommon in this country, and many people might be misdiagnosed with irritable bowel syndrome. One study from London found that one in 20 people diagnosed with IBS might actually have celiac disease. Iron-deficiency anemia may be blamed on menstrual blood loss when some women might have celiac disease," remarks Dr. Green. "With women there may be a delay in diagnosis because they are seen as a complaining patient, they're told, 'It's all in your head' or 'It's irritable bowel syndrome.' Gastroenterologists are taught that IBS is the most common diagnosis, and if they see a woman with altered bowel habits and all the other manifestations, they may not think of celiac disease."

Celiac disease can manifest at any time in life. "Kids can get diagnosed and they go on a gluten-free diet, and many years ago people were told they 'grew out of it.' But that was because during adolescence they tolerated going back to gluten. Then later on in life they get rediagnosed and may present with osteoporosis or a malignancy. So making this diagnosis is important," says Dr. Green.

You may develop a rash as a consequence of gluten intolerance. The itchy, blistering rash—dermatitis herpetiformis—affects the arms, legs, trunk, and scalp. Less commonly, there may be leg ulcerations.

Some people are *allergic* to wheat and have classic allergy symptoms within minutes or hours of eating wheat products, including a runny nose (*allergic rhinitis*), an itchy rash (*contact urticaria*), asthma-like wheezing (*baker's asthma*), and in severe cases, *anaphylaxis*, a potentially deadly reaction where the throat swells and blocks breathing.

Other people are not allergic to wheat but are *intolerant* to gluten, and have the same symptoms as celiac but without the intestinal damage or the antibodies. This is called *non-celiac gluten sensitivity (NCGS)*, which, like wheat allergy, is among a spectrum of gluten-related disorders.[20] "However, it's not clear that gluten that is causing the problem," remarks Dr. Green. Some studies suggest that NCGS stems from an *innate* immune response, one that's built into some people's immune systems, rather than an *adaptive* immune response to foreign antigens, as in autoimmune disease.

Diagnosing Celiac Disease

Diagnosing celiac disease can be difficult because some symptoms are similar to irritable bowel syndrome, NCGS, Crohn's disease, ulcerative colitis, diverticular disease, intestinal infections, chronic fatigue syndrome, and depression. Some of those diseases, such as IBS, may also coexist in women with celiac.

The longer you remain undiagnosed and untreated, the greater the chance of developing malnutrition and other complications. In Italy, where celiac disease is common, screening is routine, says Dr. Green. In the United States, where celiac has been considered rare, the time between the first symptoms and a diagnosis averages about 10 years.

"It's actually an easy diagnosis to make. Most people with celiac test positive for antibodies to gliadin, which is the part of wheat that people mount the immunological reaction to. Then you test for tissue autoantigens. Those tests are widely available. If they are positive, the next step is a small intestinal biopsy done with endoscopy," explains Dr. Green. Because celiac disease is hereditary, first-degree family members—your parents, siblings, and children—should also be tested, he adds.

Additional tests are done to detect complications of celiac, such as anemia and osteoporosis.

Tests You May Need and What They Mean

Antigliadin antibodies are present in up to 40 percent of people with celiac disease, but they are not specific to celiac; they can also be found in people with small-bowel Crohn's disease and, in low amounts, in the general population. However, antigliadin antibody tests are no longer available and have been replaced by the following more specific tests.

According to the 2013 guidelines from the American College of Gastroenterology (ACG),[31] a confirmed diagnosis of CD should be based on a combination of a medical history, physical exam, blood tests, and examination and biopsies of the upper part of the digestive tract.

Anti-tissue transglutaminase antibody immunoglobulin A (tTG IgA) is the most sensitive and specific blood test for celiac test, especially in people at high risk. Tests for tTG IgA can also be used to monitor the disease. TTG levels should fall if you stick to a gluten-free diet.

Deamidated gliadin peptide antibodies (anti-DGP) may be positive in some people with celiac who test negative for anti-tTG (especially children younger than two).

Antiendomysium (EMA) antibodies recognize parts of smooth muscle tissue in the esophagus and the upper part of the small intestine and are considered specific for celiac disease.

Upper endoscopy with small bowel biopsy is considered the gold standard for diagnosing celiac disease. Under sedation (to make you more comfortable and quiet your gag reflex) a long, thin hollow tube called an endoscope is passed through the mouth, esophagus, and stomach into the small intestine. Small samples of tissue from the upper area of the small intestine (duodenum) are taken with instruments passed through the endoscope. In celiac disease the biopsy will reveal atrophy of the villi. The test takes about 10 minutes, and no special preparation is needed. Small-intestine biopsy is also done to test the effectiveness of a gluten-free diet; damage to the small intestine is often healed if the diet is followed carefully.

New guidelines in Europe propose making a diagnosis in children without a biopsy. Under these guidelines, children must have symptoms, plus a tTG IgA antibody level over 10 times normal and, on a second blood draw, show positive tests for EMA and celiac-related genes. This approach has yet to be validated in children or adults.[31]

A complete blood count (CBC) includes a count of the iron-carrying red blood cells (RBCs) and *hemoglobin*, the component in red blood cells that transports iron. A low red blood cell count and low hemoglobin diagnose iron-deficiency anemia, caused by malabsorption of iron from the small intestine. Women normally have lower levels of hemoglobin than men, between 12 and 16 grams of hemoglobin per deciliter of blood (g/dL). In *macrocytic anemia*, caused by malabsorption of vitamin B_{12}, red blood cells will become enlarged and crowd out normal RBCs. Borderline deficiency of vitamin B_{12} is considered to be 258 picomoles per liter of blood (pmol/L); clinical deficiency is a B_{12} level of 148 pmol/L or below.

Dual-energy x-ray absorptiometry (DEXA) measures bone density and can detect osteoporosis, a frequent complication of celiac disease. DEXA is a painless test that uses very low doses of radiation. You lie on a table with your legs elevated while a special x-ray device slowly moves up and down above you, taking pictures of your hips and spine to measure bone density at key areas, including the vertebrae in the lower spine and the upper part of the thigh (femur) inside the hip joint. The test takes around 20 minutes.

You get DEXA results in two numbers: the T-score and the Z-score. The Z-score compares your *bone mineral density (BMD)* to that of women in your age and ethnic group (or men, as the case may be), and a T-score compares your BMD to the average for Caucasians between the age of 25 and 35, when bone density is at its peak. These scores are reported as standard deviations (SD) from the norm in each group, which is set at zero. You can be above or below, plus or minus, the mean. The more important reading is the T-score. You're considered to have osteoporosis if your BMD is 2.5 standard deviations below the mean for young adult women; a T-score between –1 and –2.5 standard deviations below the peak bone mass is considered to be mild bone loss.[32]

Treating Celiac Disease

The only real treatment for celiac disease is a gluten-free diet. Technically, "gluten" is a mixture of proteins that occur naturally in wheat, rye, barley, and crossbreeds of these grains.

So a "gluten-free" diet means avoiding foods that contain wheat (including *Kamut*, also called khorasan; *spelt*, an older form of wheat; and *triticale*, a blend of rye and wheat), rye, and barley—that includes most grains, pastas, cereals, and breads, as well as foods containing fillers made from grain.

Instead, choose whole grain foods that list whole grains, such as brown rice, whole corn, millet, sorghum, wild rice, teff, amaranth, quinoa, or gluten-free oats and buckwheat, as the first ingredient.

You need to follow this diet even if you don't have GI symptoms, since damage may be occurring silently.

Within days of starting a gluten-free diet, your symptoms start to ease and the condition of the small intestine begins to improve. Within three to six months, the small intestine is usually completely healed—meaning the villi are intact and working (in older adults, this may take up to two years). An endoscopic small-intestine biopsy can determine whether you're responding to the diet.

These days, gluten-free products are easily found in most grocery stores, and restaurants increasingly offer gluten-free menu choices, even pizza.

Many gluten-free products (including breads, pastas, crackers, and the like) are made with corn, rice, soy, sorghum, or chestnut flower.

By law, *packaged foods* must contain less than 20 ppm (parts per million) of gluten to be labeled "gluten-free."[33] That's the lowest level that can be detected by current technology.

A "gluten-free" product cannot contain *any* type of wheat, rye, barley, or crossbreeds of these grains (like *triticale*), or an ingredient derived from these grains that has not been processed to remove gluten. Even if an ingredient *has* been processed to eliminate gluten, it must still meet the 20 ppm cutoff. That goes for any product that claims to be "free of gluten," "without gluten," or "contains no gluten." Foods such as bottled spring water, fruits and vegetables, and eggs can also be labeled "gluten-free" if they inherently don't have any gluten in them, the FDA explains.

But you still need to read ingredient lists carefully.

Ingredients derived from grain may not always be obvious. For example, *malt* is a common ingredient used to give foods flavor; you may not know it's made from barley. Another common ingredient, *hydrolyzed vegetable protein*, is actually made from grain. On the other hand, *buckwheat* may have wheat in its name, but it's a grain that doesn't contain gluten.

Gluten can even be found in medications. The bulk of a pill or capsule is filler, or binder, usually cornstarch or wheat starch. So people with celiac are advised to check labels on over-the-counter and prescription drugs, as well as supplements (which are regulated as foods not drugs). Gluten can lurk anywhere, notes Dr. Green. "A surprising source of gluten is communion wafers." Many over-the-counter medication labels now specify if the preparation is gluten free.

What about "take-out" food or restaurant meals?

This gets a bit tricky. While the FDA rule only applies to packaged foods, which may also be sold for take-out, restaurants that make gluten-free claims on their menus should be consistent with the FDA's definition of "gluten-free."

Before ordering anything, you'll need to ask servers at each restaurant what they *mean* when they say "gluten-free." (For example, is a food just "wheat-free"?) You also need to ask what's in a particular dish and how it's prepared.

Eating even the smallest amount of gluten could trigger damage to the small intestine. So if you have celiac disease, you'll need to educate yourself about safe food ingredients.

It is essential to see a dietitian after diagnosis of celiac disease and establish an ongoing relationship.

For one thing, it's not only important to know what *not* to eat—but also *what to eat.* A gluten-free diet can be low in fiber, vitamins, and minerals. So read the Nutrition Facts label to choose gluten-free foods that have the most grams of fiber per serving. Choose gluten-free refined grain-based products that are enriched or fortified with iron and B vitamins, and make sure you eat foods that are good sources of calcium, such as low-fat milk (or calcium fortified gluten-free soy milk), nonfat yogurt, and calcium processed tofu. A nutritionist can also keep you up to date about issues such as potential toxins in rice and corn.

In addition to a gluten-free diet, you may also need added pancreatic enzymes to aid digestion. "When you eat, the gut secretes hormones that stimulate the pancreas to produce enzymes needed for digestion. If you have celiac disease you don't secrete these hormones, and therefore the pancreas doesn't respond well when you eat. So if people are feeling unwell at diagnosis, we give them pancreatic enzymes," explains Dr. Green.

A small percentage of people with celiac don't respond to a gluten-free diet; their small intestines may be so damaged that they can't heal. Some people with celiac develop an associated autoimmune disease, *lymphocytic colitis.* "The intestine looks normal endoscopically, but on biopsy is found to have lymphocytic infiltration. And that's a cause of failure to respond to a gluten-free diet," says Dr. Green. Other people may have such severe intestinal damage that they can't absorb enough nutrients to maintain health and may need intravenous supplementation. "Some patients have refractory, nonresponsive celiac disease, and they may require steroids or immunosuppressants. These include prednisone or azathioprine," he adds.

Many Americans believe gluten-free foods are healthier and claim they feel better and lose weight on such a diet. If you don't have celiac disease, gluten allergies, or sensitivity, there's no evidence that a gluten-free diet can benefit people in the general population, according to the American Academy of Nutrition and Dietetics.[34] The academy does note that there are some data to suggest that a gluten-free diet can help ease gastrointestinal symptoms of other autoimmune diseases, such as lupus, type 1 diabetes, and thyroiditis.

Related disorders include *collagenous sprue*, which resembles celiac disease, but a thick layer of collagen is deposited beneath the inner lining of the intestines. This condition may not respond to a gluten-free diet and may require immunosuppressants.

A small number of people with celiac disease develop *mucosal ulcerations*. If this occurs in the duodenum, it can be mistaken for peptic ulcers; if it occurs farther down in the small intestine, it may be mistaken for Crohn's disease. The condition, called *ulcerative jejunitis*, is more common in the elderly.

Celiac Disease Clusters

Celiac disease is associated with a number of autoimmune diseases, especially type 1 diabetes. Take a look at the chapters on the diseases that cluster with celiac, since early diagnosis of celiac could well prevent or aid in diagnosing other diseases.

- Type 1 diabetes
- Thyroid disease
- Sjögren's syndrome
- Primary biliary cirrhosis
- Myasthenia gravis
- Pernicious anemia

Celiac disease is associated with an increased risk of certain kinds of cancers, including *non-Hodgkin's lymphoma*, *intestinal T-cell lymphoma*, small bowel and esophageal cancer, and melanoma. "However, it's been shown in Europe that once you put people on a gluten-free diet, the risk of developing these cancers eventually goes back to that of the general population. So this makes it especially urgent for people to be diagnosed as early as possible," says Dr. Green.

How Celiac Disease Can Affect You Over Your Lifetime

Celiac disease can cause special complications for women, including delayed puberty and menarche, menstrual irregularities, miscarriages, infertility, and premature menopause. In childhood, the complications are due to delayed development, but it's not clear how celiac can cause reproductive problems, says Dr. Green.

While celiac can show itself at any time, diagnosis in adults seems to peak around age 50. And the irritability and depression of celiac may even be mistaken for symptoms of menopause.

Celiac poses the threat of osteoporosis for women of all ages. But if a woman is diagnosed with low bone density during her forties or fifties, the underlying cause is often assumed to be estrogen loss, and the standard treatment of bisphosphonates (*Fosamax, Actonel*) to prevent bone resorption may create problems. "Potentially, if the osteoporosis is due to malabsorption of calcium, and a woman is actually maintaining a normal serum calcium, the calcium is being leached out of bones because it is not being absorbed from the gut," he explains. "If people have osteoporosis due to celiac disease and are just put on Fosamax, the body would not be able to remove calcium from the bones, and serum calcium could potentially drop to dangerous levels. So we don't recommend that people with osteoporosis and celiac disease be put straight on Fosamax, because we have to increase their calcium absorption first. And that must be done through a gluten-free diet."

Malabsorption of calcium can also lead to *secondary hyperparathyroidism*; about 20 percent of women with osteoporosis and celiac disease will develop this problem. The four tiny parathyroid glands are buried in the thyroid and produce *parathyroid hormone (PTH)*, needed along with calcitonin (produced by the thyroid gland) and vitamin D to regulate the balance of calcium in the body. If there's too little calcium in the blood, the parathyroid glands secrete more PTH, taking calcium from the bones to correct the imbalance. In celiac disease, calcium isn't properly absorbed and passes out of the body. Vitamin D isn't being absorbed, either. So the parathyroid produces more PTH. Chronic low levels of calcium can cause the gland to become overactive, causing even more calcium to be removed from the bones.

Hyperparathyroidism is diagnosed by measuring levels of PTH, urinary calcium, and vitamin D. In hyperparathyroidism, PTH is elevated, as is one form of vitamin D (1,25-dihydroxy vitamin D), and urinary calcium is high (signaling malabsorption). Hyperparathyroidism is treated by surgically removing abnormal parathyroid tissue and giving oral calcium and *1,25-dihydroxy vitamin D* supplements (*Calcitriol*) to normalize calcium.

Pernicious Anemia

An autoimmune disease common in women over age 60 is *pernicious anemia.* It results from an autoimmune attack on the parietal cells lining the stomach, which secrete a chemical called *intrinsic factor (IF)* that binds to vitamin B_{12} and helps it absorb in the small intestine. The destruction of the parietal cells impairs production of intrinsic factor, and autoantibodies against IF prevent it from binding to vitamin B_{12}, so the vitamin can't be absorbed.

The resulting vitamin deficiency can cause atrophy of the surface of the tongue (*atrophic glossitis*), producing a red, smooth appearance; diarrhea; and nerve damage (*peripheral neuropathy*) that leads to tingling and numbness. Nerve damage is a result of lesions caused by autoantibodies, and in severe cases lesions can develop in the brain, leading to memory loss and even psychosis (in some cases, it may even be mistaken for Alzheimer's disease). It can also occur in women with celiac disease and other autoimmune diseases.

Pernicious anemia is diagnosed with blood tests to measure vitamin B_{12} and levels of *folate*, another B vitamin. Red blood cells become enlarged in pernicious anemia (they're called *megaloblasts*). More than 90 percent of women will have autoantibodies to parietal cells; nearly half of patients have autoantibodies to intrinsic factor.

The treatment is simple: monthly injections of 100 micrograms (mcg) of vitamin B_{12}. This remedies the anemia and, in many cases, corrects the nerve-related complications.

In some elderly people, the lining of the stomach may atrophy, and a daily supplement of 25 micrograms of vitamin B_{12} is recommended to prevent deficiency.

Notes

1. Crohn's and Colitis Foundation of America (CCFA), 2014. http://www.ccfa.org/what-are-crohns-and-colitis/what-is-crohns-disease/.
2. Ogura Y, Bonen DK, Inohara N, et al. A frameshift mutation in NOD2 associated with susceptibility to Crohn's disease. *Nature.* 2001;411(6837):603–606.
3. Glas J, Martin K, Brünnler G, et al. MICA, MICB and C1_4_1 polymorphism in Crohn's disease and ulcerative colitis. *Tissue Antigens.* 2001;58(4):243–249. doi:10.1034/j.1399-0039.2001.580404.
4. Kawamoto S, Maruya M, Kato LM, et al. Foxp3+ T cells regulate immunoglobulin a selection and facilitate diversification of bacterial species responsible for immune homeostasis. *Immunity.* 2014. doi:10.1016/j.immuni.2014.05.016.
5. Paget SA. The microbiome, autoimmunity, and arthritis: cause and effect: an historical perspective. *Trans Am Clin Climatol Assoc.* 2012;123:257–267.
6. Ott C, Takses A, Obermeier F, Schnoy E, Müller M. Smoking increases the risk of extraintestinal manifestations in Crohn's disease. *World J Gastroenterol.* 2014;20(34):12269–12276. doi:10.3748/wjg.v20.i34.12269.
7. Sources: American Society for Gastrointestinal Endoscopy. Understanding capsule endoscopy. http://www.asge.org/patients/patients.aspx?id=390. Retrieved May 22, 2014. American Gastroenterological Association Patient Center. Preparing for capsule endoscopy. http://www.gastro.org/patient-center/procedures/capsule-endoscopy. Retrieved May 22, 2014.
8. Crohn's and Colitis Foundation of America (CCFA). Biologic therapies. 2014. http://www.ccfa.org/resources/biologic-therapies.html.
9. Osterman MT, Haynes K, Delzell E, et al. Comparative effectiveness of infliximab and adalimumab for Crohn's disease. *Clin Gastroenterol Hepatol.* 2014;12:811–817.
10. Patient Information on Entyvio. https://www.entyvio.com/.
11. US Food & Drug Administration (FDA). FDA approves Takeda's Entyvio™ (vedolizumab) for the treatment of adults with moderately to severely active ulcerative colitis or Crohn's disease. May 21, 2014. http://www.takeda.com/news/2014/20140521_6573.html.
12. Mozaffari S, Nikfar S, Abdolghaffari AH, Abdollahi M. New biologic therapeutics for ulcerative colitis and Crohn's disease. *Expert Opinion on Biol Ther.* 2014;14(5):583–600. doi:10.1517/14712598.2014.885945).

13. http://enteragam.com/assets/lib/EnteraGam-full-prescribing-info.pdf.
14. Dotan I, Rachmilewitz D, Schreiber S (Semapimod-CD04/CD05 Investigators), et al. Randomised placebo-controlled multicentre trial of intravenous semapimod HCl for moderate to severe Crohn's disease. *Gut.* 2010;59(6):760.
15. Reinisch W, de Villiers W, Bene L, et al. Fontolizumab in moderate to severe Crohn's disease: a phase 2, randomized, double-blind, placebo-controlled, multiple-dose study. *Inflamm Bowel Dis.* 2010;16(2):233.
16. Sandborn WJ, Ghosh S, Panes J. Phase 2 study of tofacitinib, an oral Janus kinase inhibitor, in patients with Crohn's disease. *Clin Gastroenterol Hepatol.* 2014; 12(9):1485.
17. G Dwivedi, L Fitz, M Hegen, et al. A multiscale model of interleukin-6–mediated immune regulation in Crohn's disease and its application in drug discovery and development. *CPT Pharmacometrics Syst Pharmacol.* 2014;3:e89; doi:10.1038/psp.2013.64.
18. Sandborn WJ, Gasink C, Gao LL, et al. Ustekinumab induction and maintenance therapy in refractory Crohn's disease. *N Engl J Med.* 2012;367(16):1519–1528.
19. Israeli E, Yaron I. Oral administration of Alequel, a mixture of autologous colon-extracted proteins for the treatment of Crohn's disease. *Therap Adv Gastroenterol.* 2010; 3(1):23–30. doi:10.1177/1756283X09351733.
20. Lazzerini M, Martelossi S, Magazzù G, et al. Effect of thalidomide on clinical remission in children and adolescents with refractory Crohn disease: a randomized clinical trial. *JAMA.* 2013;310(20):2164–2173.
21. Hasselblatt P, Drognitz K, Potthoff K, et al. Remission of refractory Crohn's disease by high-dose cyclophosphamide and autologous peripheral blood stem cell transplantation. *Aliment Pharmacol Ther.* 2012;36(8):725–735. Doi:10.1111/apt.12032.
22. Kornbluth A, Sachar DB. Ulcerative colitis practice guidelines in adults: American College of Gastroenterology, Practice Parameters Committee. *Am J Gastroenterol.* 2010;105:501–523; doi:10.1038/ajg.2009.727.
23. http://www.nlm.nih.gov/medlineplus/druginfo/meds/a601117.html.
24. http://www.simponi.com/ulcerative-colitis-hcp/.
25. Shah ED, Siegel CA, Chong K, Melmed GY. The comparative effectiveness of biologics and immunomodulators for the treatment of ulcerative colitis. *Gastroenterology.* 2014;146(5)(suppl 1):S-2. doi:http://dx.doi.org/10.1016/S0016-5085(14)60005-6.
26. Srinivasan R, Akobeng AK. Thalidomide and thalidomide analogues for induction of remission in Crohn's disease. *Cochrane Database Syst Rev.* 2009;2. doi: 10.1002/ 14651858.CD007350.pub2.
27. Ording Olsen K, Juul S, Berndtsson I, et al. Ulcerative colitis: female fecundity before diagnosis, during disease, and after surgery compared with a population sample. *Gastroenterology.* 2002;122:15–19.
28. Waljee A, Waljee J, Morris AM, et al. Threefold increased risk of infertility: a meta-analysis of infertility after ileal pouch anal anastomosis in ulcerative colitis. *Gut.* 2006;55:1575–1580.

29. Sapone A, Bai JC, Ciacci C, et al. Spectrum of gluten-related disorders: consensus on new nomenclature and classification. *BMC Med.* 2012;10:13. http://www.biomedcentral.com/1741-7015/10/13.
30. Lionetti E, Castellaneta S, Francavilla R, et al. Introduction of gluten, HLA status, and the risk of celiac disease in children. *N Engl J Med.* 2014;371(14):1295–1303. doi:10.1056/NEJMoa1400697.
31. Rubio-Tapa A, Hill ID, Kelly CP, et al. Diagnosis and management of celiac disease. *Am J Gastroenterol.* 2013;108:656–676. doi:10.1038/ajg.2013.79. Advance online publication Apr 23, 2013.
32. Florence R, Allen S, Benedict L, et al. Diagnosis and treatment of osteoporosis. Bloomington, MN: Institute for Clinical Systems Improvement (ICSI). July 2013. http://www.guideline.gov/content.aspx?id=47543.
33. US Food and Drug Administration. Questions and answers: gluten-free food labeling final rule. Aug 5, 2014. http://www.fda.gov/Food/GuidanceRegulation/GuidanceDocumentsRegulatoryInformation/Allergens/ucm362880.htm.
34. Gaesser GA, Angadi SS. Gluten-free diet: imprudent dietary advice for the general population? *J Am Acad Nutr Diet.* 2012;112(9):1330–1333. doi:http://dx.doi.org/10.1016/j.jand.2012.06.009.

9

An Attack of Nerves—Multiple Sclerosis

When I was told I had multiple sclerosis in 1999 it knocked me for a loop . . . it was like being blown across the room. I couldn't quite believe it. I was just in my late 40's. It was so unexpected. I tried to be very calm when I got the results of the tests, but one night I just sat down and decided that I would let it all out, and cried hysterically. But my dog got so upset, I had to calm myself down. I still haven't quite gotten used to it. Every time I get a cold, it seems to flare. It seems like it's there all the time. My greatest fear is ending up in a wheelchair. Even though my doctor reassures me that won't happen, I still worry about it. I guess the worry will never leave.

Ana, 68

If you can imagine an electrical cord with insulation that's frayed and worn away in places, causing a short in the wire and then shorting out the electrical system, then you can visualize *multiple sclerosis (MS)*.

In MS, autoantibodies, immune cells, and inflammation damage the "insulation" (called *myelin*) wrapped around nerve cell fibers in the brain and spinal cord that carry messages to the rest of the body, causing a variety of symptoms, from vision problems to limb weakness.

According to the National Multiple Sclerosis Society, MS is believed to affect more than 2.3 million people around the world.[1] Two-thirds of the 400,000 Americans with MS are women, and the number of new cases among women is rising. The reasons why are unclear; it may be due to better diagnosis or a real increase.

Warning Signs of MS

- Fatigue
- Vision problems—blurred or double vision
- Tingling, numbness, burning sensations in the arms or legs
- Muscle weakness, especially in the legs
- Muscle stiffness or spasticity
- Problems with balance or coordination
- Problems with short-term memory
- Dizziness or vertigo
- Slowed or slurred speech
- Change in bladder or bowel function

MS typically appears between the ages of 20 and 50, but it can arise at any age. More people are now being diagnosed at an earlier stage in the disease and started on disease-modifying drug treatments that can slow the progression of MS. Once MS meant disability and confinement to a wheelchair, but these new treatments are reducing long-term disability and allowing many people to live fairly normal lives.

What Causes MS?

Myelin is usually compared to the insulation around electrical wires that helps electrical transmission and protects the wires from being damaged and shorting out. But it's not really like the single, smooth layer of rubber found on electrical wires. The *myelin sheath* is a membrane made up of layers of a fatty substance manufactured by specialized cells called *oligodendrocytes* that coils around nerve fibers (*axons*), more like multiple wrappings of electrical tape. *Myelinated axons* are commonly called white matter.

Both myelin and oligodendrocytes find themselves under attack in MS. Autoantibodies reacting to proteins in myelin (including *myelin basic protein*) and other toxic products of immune cells eat away one or more layers of the

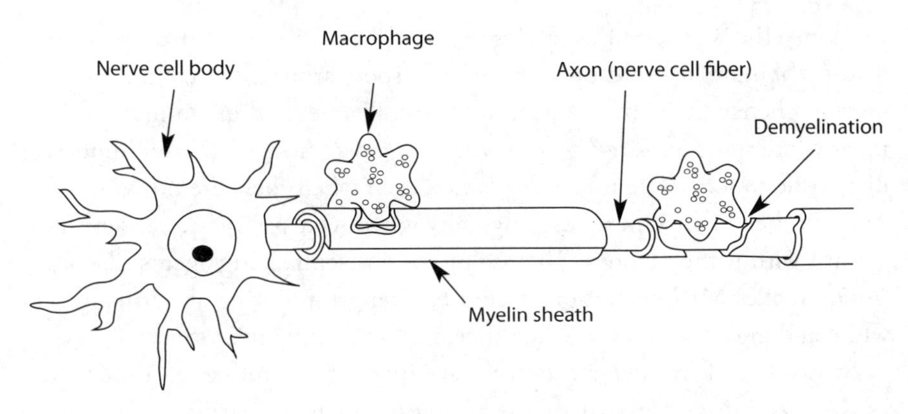

How MS Affects Nerve Cells

myelin sheath and the cells producing it. MS also damages nerve cell bodies, found in the brain's "gray matter."[2]

Since a single oligodendrocyte may spin out myelin for 50 to 100 axons, an attack on one of these cells can result in problems for multiple axons, notes Anthony T. Reder, MD, professor of neurology at the University of Chicago and director of the Neurology and Inflammatory Disease Infusion Center at UC.

However, because there are so many layers of myelin, it may take a while for the damage to produce symptoms. And myelin may regenerate over a period of months in the beginning (the brain may even reorganize some of its circuits to compensate for minor damage). But the new myelin is not as stable, and eventually spots along the sheath are totally eaten away (*demyelination*). Inflammation of the sheath at areas of demyelination, which may come in cycles or bursts of activity, is believed to be responsible for MS flares. Immune attacks and inflammation can occur in any area of the *central nervous system (CNS)*—the brain, the spinal cord, or the optic nerve—but early on, most of this damage may occur silently.

As myelin is eaten away, messages between nerve cells are increasingly disrupted. When the axon is exposed, it can become damaged or even severed. Accumulated damage to axons can be widespread, eventually leading to irreversible loss of function and permanent disability. It's now known that brain atrophy can occur early in the disease process.[3]

As myelin is stripped away, it's replaced by scar (*sclerotic*) tissue, which forms *plaques* that build up at numerous spots around the central nervous system—hence the name multiple sclerosis. Plaques and inflammation show up as white spots on *magnetic resonance imaging (MRI)*. MRI is an important diagnostic tool because it reveals plaques even when there are no symptoms. The number of myelin-producing cells is reduced (or they're absent altogether) within the plaques. The use of contrast-enhancing agents like *gadolinium* makes MRI even more accurate, often pinpointing abnormalities in white and gray matter even when there's no focal inflammation.[3]

Symptoms of MS depend on the severity of the immune reaction as well as the location and extent of the plaques, which primarily appear in the brain stem, cerebellum, spinal cord, optic nerves, and the white matter of the brain around the brain *ventricles* (fluid-filled spaces inside of the brain).[2]

One theory that generated a lot of attention involves a condition dubbed *chronic cerebrospinal venous insufficiency (CCSVI)*. The idea, first put forth by an Italian researcher in 2009, is that obstructions in the *cerebrospinal veins* (located in the head and neck) cause iron deposits that may lead to MS. However, imaging studies of these veins done with ultrasound and *magnetic resonance venography* show that CCSVI does not appear to be related to MS.[4] And small clinical trials of *percutaneous transluminal venous angioplasty* to surgically improve blood flow had no significant benefits.[5] While the Italian Multiple Sclerosis Society and others have dismissed CCSVI, some research continues.

For all of the newfound knowledge about the underlying process of MS damage, it's still unclear what triggers it in the first place.

Faulty genes may predispose people to the most common form of MS. Up to 20 percent of MS patients have at least one relative with the disease. While there's no evidence that MS itself can be inherited, having certain genes may also make people vulnerable to environmental toxins or viruses. Some MS experts believe female hormones may protect nerve cells to some extent.

The agents of destruction in MS are thought to be cell-killing (*cytotoxic*) T cells, activated as if to rout a foreign invader, along with hordes of scavenger macrophages attracted by chemicals released by the activated T cells. In fact, there may be an invader hidden in the nerves themselves. Some viruses can infect the body and then remain dormant in nerve trunks. To T cells, those viruses may look similar to proteins in myelin (*molecular mimicry*). There are dozens of suspects—including *Epstein-Barr virus* (*EBV*, which causes infectious mononucleosis), the respiratory virus *Haemophilus influenzae*, the mumps and measles viruses, and a herpes virus that causes the childhood illness *roseola*. We've all been exposed to them, but it's unclear whether they actually trigger the initial MS attack.[6]

Antibodies to these viruses (evidence the body has reacted to an infection) are elevated in people with MS; antibodies have also been found in *cerebral spinal fluid (CSF)*.

Evidence of viral infections in the central nervous system and in MS plaques has also been detected. EBV antibodies are increased in MS, and during MS exacerbations, notes Dr. Reder. "One out of every three upper respiratory viruses triggers an MS attack, probably caused by the activation of the immune system." Respiratory infections are known to prompt MS relapses (probably through a reaction in "memory cells" programmed by a previous encounter with a virus). But so far there's no direct evidence that viruses actually cause MS.

Almost all of us have been exposed to EBV at some point, so other factors must be involved in MS, such as genetic predisposition, the age at which a woman is infected, or even infection with other microbes, the researchers speculate.

But how would the destructive T cells get through the blood-brain barrier that protects our brain from toxins? New research indicates that cells in the tough brain membrane (*endothelial cells* in the veins of the brain) somehow become activated and secrete chemicals that attract T cells, then literally pull them through the cells, crossing the normally impervious barrier, says Dr. Reder.

These chemicals are called *adhesion molecules*, because they act like glue. Once inside the brain, myelin-reactive T cells multiply and likely release chemicals that bring more inflammatory cells into the area to cause damage.[6]

MS is more common in people who live in northern climates farthest from the equator, such as Scandinavia, where there's less (and less intense) year-round ultraviolet light from the sun to manufacture natural vitamin D in the skin. So many scientists believe that low vitamin D levels may be related to the development and disease progression in MS. This appears to be especially true in people who lived in such areas until age 15.[7]

Animal research suggests vitamin D may prevent formation of adhesion molecules, which allow immune cells to cross the blood-brain barrier.[8] Recent research shows vitamin D levels may be lower in those with progressive MS than in *relapsing-remitting MS (RRMS)*.[6]

A relationship has also been found between vitamin D levels and the degree of disability in a subgroup of people with RRMS. In patients in one drug study, as vitamin D levels decreased, the number of new, active MS lesions increased, and this held true even in those considered to have adequate levels of vitamin D.[7, 9]

A five-year international study later analyzed by researchers from Harvard suggests that blood concentration of *25-hydroxyvitamin D*, abbreviated *25(OH)D*, a marker of vitamin D status, is associated with disease activity in MS. The study used *magnetic resonance imaging* to follow 465 patients being treated after an initial episode suggestive of MS. Increases in vitamin D levels within the first year were associated with a 57 percent lower risk of new active brain lesions on MRI and a 57 percent lower risk of relapse.[9]

These studies, intriguing as they are, are not conclusive. So consult your doctor before you start taking extra vitamin D.

The first symptom I had was actually vision loss in one eye. I went to an ophthalmologist who suspected that I had MS and wrote in my file that he suspected nerve damage, but he told me it was "only optic neuritis" and that it would go away. I immediately went and looked up optic neuritis in the encyclopedia, and it scared me because it said it was inflammation of nerves. And that led me to believe it wasn't going to stop. And I became very frightened and thought I was going to be completely blind, but I decided to ignore it.

I went on for about six years with various symptoms that were not really conclusive enough to make a diagnosis, which I know now . . . I didn't realize that fatigue was a part of MS, and I had other symptoms as well . . . like problems with my bladder, and dizziness if I sat down and stood up too fast. But the symptoms of MS are things everyone has at one time or another, but they're just more magnified and chronic. Everyone has the tingling hand or the limb that falls asleep, everyone's been tired and fatigued.

So I could easily chalk up all of my symptoms to other problems. I didn't even think about pulling all this together. I was in my early twenties, I was going to college, I had a lot going on, and I chose to ignore it. I saw various doctors, but no one could make a definitive diagnosis.

Mariana, 39

Symptoms of MS

MS can be sneaky—the first symptoms can come and go, and like Marianna you might not pay much attention to them. A mild tingling in one leg, a little trouble with your eyes. Perhaps some fatigue, joint pain, or trouble remembering things. Sometimes these symptoms last a few days and may include balance problems, slurred speech, and stiffness. Symptoms can resemble other conditions, including Lyme disease, which may also delay a diagnosis.

The most common symptom is actually fatigue, reported by up to 92 percent of MS patients.[3] "MS fatigue is very distinctive. It's not a function of physical disability, or of not sleeping, but if you don't sleep well that can aggravate it. These women sleep eight hours and wake up feeling like they are just drained. It's generally made worse with heat, and generally gets worse later in the day," says Barbara S. Giesser, MD, a professor of neurology and clinical director of the MS Program at the David Geffen School of Medicine at the University of California, Los Angeles.

Unlike other autoimmune diseases, *chronic fatigue syndrome (CFS)*, and *fibromyalgia* are not usually fellow travelers with MS. "However, I certainly have had patients who were initially erroneously diagnosed with fibromyalgia or CFS and turned out to have MS," Dr. Giesser adds.

Depression is actually the second most common symptom of MS, reported by 50 to 70 percent of patients at some point during the course of their illness.[3] One study suggests that depression may be more common among African Americans and Latinas with MS than among Caucasian women.[10]

Some women may experience wide mood swings, unprovoked and uncontrollable euphoria followed by extreme depression. In fact, Dr. Reder speculates that sometimes these mood swings, which may be attributed to *bipolar depression* (also called *manic depression*), could be an early symptom of MS. No brain lesions are found in manic depression, but they can be seen in early MS.

Depression in MS may be due to brain lesions or immune dysregulation; depression may also induce abnormalities of immune function that may contribute to MS. One recent study found that treating depression is accompanied by a reduction in *interferon-gamma* production, one of the inflammatory proteins associated with MS.[11]

Vision problems are very common, especially *optic neuritis*. This can take the form of blurred or hazy vision, usually in the central area, or even a complete loss of vision. Problems can come on gradually or suddenly, and resolve quickly. Pain around the eyes may precede loss of vision, sometimes by a few hours, sometimes by a few days. An eye exam may reveal paleness at the back of the eye, indicating optic nerve damage.

Motor symptoms can include a vague feeling of weakness or heaviness in the legs (one leg may tend to drag), as well as a tendency to trip or fall. Five percent of MS patients present with a tremor, while 2 percent may suffer from nerve pain that affects the jaw called *trigeminal neuralgia*, notes Dr. Reder. Some women may have trouble swallowing or experience facial twitches or intense itching.

The most common cognitive changes are slowed thinking and visual tracking and memory retrieval, especially short-term memory. Corresponding brain changes may even be seen, such as thinning of the *corpus callosum*, which connects the two hemispheres of the brain, caused by degeneration of nerve fibers.

Some of the sensory changes experienced in MS include tingling, numbness, or feelings similar to small electrical shocks in the limbs or other areas of the body. Some women may experience vertigo or clumsiness. Five percent of women may initially experience bladder problems, a sense of urinary urgency along with more frequent urination, or incontinence. In some women, the bladder may not empty completely, and they may have frequent urinary tract infections. Bladder or urinary problems may be the only initial symptoms of MS. Heat can cause a worsening of symptoms, making it even harder for damaged neurons to communicate.

The four types of multiple sclerosis are based on general patterns of symptoms[12]:

- **Relapsing-remitting MS (RRMS).** This is the most common type of MS, in which symptoms flare and then go into remission. This respite may be due to bursts of inflammation that subside or to the regeneration of myelin. That inflammation can be seen on MRI using a special contrast agent. Up to 75 percent of people with MS have the relapsing-remitting type.
- **Primary progressive MS (PPMS).** In this type of MS, there are continual attacks on nerves and inflammation with no remissions, causing increasing disability; about 10 percent of patients

have primary progressive MS. (This is actually more common in men.)

- **Secondary progressive MS (SPMS).** About two-thirds of people with the milder relapsing-remitting MS evolve into a secondary progressive form. This can occur with or without occasional flares, minor remissions, and even long plateaus of stability in the disease. But eventually the disease keeps worsening, with a progressive loss of axons.
- **Progressive-relapsing (PRMS).** This is relatively rare, occurring in about 5 percent of patients. In this type of MS, there's a steady worsening of disease from the start, but with distinct flare-ups that may or may not get better. There's continued disease progression in between flare-ups.

Ana's story continues:
I'd had a cold and sinus infection the winter before I was diagnosed. It seemed like it would never go away. And I had started to feel dizzy. I felt dizzy all the time. I figured it was from the sinus infection, so I went to see an ear, nose, and throat doctor. I was tested for Lyme disease, which came back negative. I had all kinds of other tests, but nothing showed up. The doctor was concerned about the dizziness, and sent me to a balance function center. I went through a whole set of tests. But they couldn't determine what was wrong. I was eventually sent for a brain scan, and that's when they saw small lesions. I also had a spinal tap. That's when I was told I probably had MS for some time. I was lucky to be diagnosed so quickly.

Diagnosing MS

The National Multiple Sclerosis Society (NMSS) issued revised criteria for diagnosing MS, which include the use of MRI and other tools to determine the amount of nerve damage and make a diagnosis more specific after an MS attack.[12]

An "MS attack" is defined as a "neurological disturbance typical of those seen in MS, either reported by the patient or observed by the physician," lasting at least 24 hours. A single episode of muscle weakness wouldn't qualify, but multiple episodes would.

There are three basic diagnostic categories: MS, "possible MS," and "not MS."

MS is diagnosed after finding evidence on MRI of damage in at least two separate areas of the central nervous system (the brain, spinal cord and optic nerves) occurring at least one month apart. All other possible diagnoses must be ruled out, stresses the NMSS.

Clinically isolated syndrome (CIS) is defined as a single attack (or one or more symptoms characteristic of MS) with a very high risk of developing MS, when no other diseases or causes can be found.[12]

Several subtypes of MS have also been recognized, and you may hear these terms mentioned:

- **Radiologically isolated syndrome (RIS)** is an incidental finding of typical MS lesions on MRI without evidence of clinical disease. This is sometimes called asymptomatic or preclinical MS.[12]
- **Malignant (fulminant) MS** is a rare form of MS with very fast progression, leading to significant disability or even death in a relatively short period of time.[12]
- **Single-attack progressive MS** is another a rare condition in which a single initial MS attack is followed by a progressive phase.[12]
- **Transitional MS** is considered to be a gradual transition phase between RRMS and SPMS.[12]
- **Benign MS** is a concept where an MS patient remains fully functional in all neurologic systems 15 years after an initial attack.

The new guidelines keep the older threshold of two separate attacks (or evidence of damage in two areas of the CNS) for a formal diagnosis of MS. But since MRI is so accurate, there's no longer any need to wait for a second attack to start treatment.

The two attacks needed to make a formal MS diagnosis must be at least 30 days apart. A clinical evaluation and sometimes three tests—MRI, analysis of cerebrospinal fluid (CSF), and analysis of visual evoked potentials (VEPs)—are used to confirm a second attack. The clinical guidelines also allow for the diagnosis of people who've had only one attack, so they can be started on medication if needed. Evidence of a second attack must be seen on MRI.

There are also people who've had no obvious MS attacks, but have had steady progression of disability. For those people, the diagnostic criteria require a positive CSF test, plus multiple lesions in the brain or spinal cord seen on MRI, or an abnormal VEP with fewer brain and spinal cord lesions.

Depending on the symptoms, the neurologist must also exclude other conditions that mimic MS. Blood tests may be needed to rule out other autoimmune diseases or Lyme disease; those tests usually turn out normal in MS patients.

Tests You May Need and What They Mean

Magnetic resonance imaging (MRI) of the brain is the most frequently used test for multiple sclerosis, clearly showing the white plaques characteristic of MS. The addition of a contrast agent (*gadolinium*) can "light up" areas where inflammatory cells have crossed into the brain, causing demyelination.

Plaque that is seen in certain areas of the brain, such as the optic nerve, can be correlated with symptoms. The amount and location of plaques are taken into account in assessing the stage, severity, and progression of the disease. White matter makes up most of the brain and gets its name from the color of the myelin insulation. Gray matter makes up the cerebral cortex, the multifold outer layer of the brain where most information processing occurs. To be diagnosed with MS with an MRI, separate scans must find at least one *gadolinium-enhanced* lesion (or a new lesion suggesting inflammation), plus plaques in characteristic areas of the brain or in the spinal cord.[12]

MRI scans may be able to pick up the earliest signs of the disease in people who have only mild, intermittent symptoms, so they can be put on medication as soon as possible.

Evoked potentials (EPs) are noninvasive tests that can reveal problems in myelin conduction. During a VEP test, you look at a checkerboard pattern or series of flashing lights while being monitored by a device that measures the conduction of visual images from the eyes to the brain. A delay or prolongation of conduction signals (or weaker conduction) is seen when there's demyelination. EPs are especially useful in confirming a diagnosis of MS, because they can often detect lesions not seen on MRI.

Lumbar puncture (spinal tap) tests a sample of cerebrospinal fluid for antibodies and proteins that result from the breakdown of myelin. Under local anesthesia, a hollow needle is inserted into the spine to withdraw a small sample of the fluid bathing the spinal cord and brain. The fluid is then examined for the presence of abnormal levels of immunoglobulins (which are occasionally autoantibodies), fragments of myelin basic protein produced by inflammation, and immune cells. This helps to distinguish MS from other nervous system diseases. A spinal tap is usually done when an MRI is inconclusive.

The severity of MS is scored using a numerical scale. **The Extended Disability Status Score (EDSS)** measures vision, sensation, coordination, strength, and walking ability. For example, a score of 0 indicates a normal neurological exam. A score of 1.0 to 1.5 indicates an abnormal neurological exam, but no disability. A score of 2.0 to 2.5 shows mild disability, while a score of 3.0 to 3.5 shows mild to moderate disability. By the time patients have a score of 6.0, they need a cane to help them walk.

Some clinical signs can also provide helpful clues to potential neurological damage. For example, women who present with optic neuritis show paleness in the back of the eye after symptoms resolve; the paleness indicates a lesion on the optic nerve that caused demyelination, says Dr. Reder. Some women may show an impaired response to a pinprick, heat, or light touch in areas that correlate to areas of nerve damage. Clumsiness and an impaired ability to sense vibrations can be signs of demyelination that can sometimes be correlated with an MRI (however, often MRIs do not correlate with symptoms).

MS Clusters

The problems that often cluster with MS are not all autoimmune. But the fatigue and depression of an underactive thyroid may not be apparent if you're having similar symptoms from your MS. So it's important to be aware of anything that occurs in addition to MS symptoms.

- Hypothyroidism
- Fibromyalgia and arthritis pain
- Epilepsy (may occur in 5 percent of patients)
- Ulcerative colitis
- Interstitial cystitis

Ana's story continues:

I recall that years ago when I was trying to get pregnant and was losing each pregnancy after a few weeks, I was told I had some kind of "autoimmune" problem. I didn't pay much attention to it at the time. I was seeing a fertility specialist and she took some blood tests. I was told I had IgG antibodies, and that my body was rejecting the pregnancy. I was put on heparin, this blood thinner, and they wanted to put me on prednisone and put me in some kind of clinical trial. But I wouldn't take it. Eventually I decided to adopt. But I think now there must have been some kind of autoimmune thing going on even then.

The Female Factor

Over the years, there have been hints that female hormones may play a role in MS. For one thing, there are fewer MS relapses during pregnancy, when estrogen levels are increased. This may be partly due to pregnancy-associated elevations of a weaker form of estrogen called *estriol*, normally produced in small amounts in fatty tissues. Lower levels of estrogen that are usually present in the body may not be enough to protect against MS. Animal studies also show that *testosterone* may be protective, and this may be one reason men get MS less frequently (and later in life when testosterone levels decline).

"There are all sorts of immunosuppressant substances produced during pregnancy. When you look at women with relapsing-remitting MS who become pregnant, the relapse rate during the nine months of pregnancy goes dramatically down, especially in the third trimester, compared to prepregnancy levels," says UCLA's Dr. Giesser. "There's an increase in the relapse rate immediately postpartum, in the three to six months after delivery, and then the relapse rate returns to prepregnancy levels." She cites one study that included MRIs of pregnant women with MS. "Two women who were in a study protocol happened to get pregnant, and they elected to stay in the study. They were given MRIs during pregnancy, and lesion activity went down during pregnancy and rebounded after they delivered."

Studies that have followed women with MS for long periods of time after pregnancy have found that they do not have increased long-term disability compared to women who have not been pregnant. "And there are a couple of studies to suggest that pregnancy may even have kind of a protective effect, that women who became pregnant may have a little longer time before increased disability, or the onset of things may be delayed," she adds. Again, it's not clear if that's due to hormones.

"A lot of the sex differences in MS may be due to the protective effects of testosterone, and pregnancy-associated levels of estriol. But that's probably not the whole story. Sex chromosomes may also have a role in making the disease better or worse," says Rhonda Voskuhl, MD, a professor of neurology and the Jack H. Skirball Chair for Multiple Sclerosis at the University of California, Los Angeles.

Relapsing-remitting MS is largely inflammatory, and estrogen may act as an anti-inflammatory agent, observes Dr. Voskuhl, who is also director of the UCLA Multiple Sclerosis Program. When female mice, engineered to develop an MS-like disease, *experimental autoimmune encephalomyelitis (EAE)*, are given estrogen, they produce higher levels of an anti-inflammatory cytokine. And the effects of estrogen during pregnancy also dampen inflammation in the immune system, she notes.

Dr. Voskuhl initially studied the effects of estriol in mice with EAE and found that they had fewer exacerbations, less disability, and improved health compared to mice not treated with the hormone.[13] Based on these results, she conducted a small pilot study of estriol among 12 women, six of whom had relapsing-remitting MS and the other six with secondary progressive disease. "We saw a beneficial effect on the immune system, and on MRI we saw a reduction in gadolinium enhancing lesions, a marker of inflammation in the brain. Secondary progressive patients with a less inflammatory stage of MS did not show these changes," she says. That early research has led to two clinical trials of estriol in MS. One, a phase II trial of an estriol preparation (*Trimesta*) given with *glatiramer acetate (Copaxone)* in relapsing-remitting MS showed a reduction in relapses among the estriol group versus those given placebo.[14] The second clinical trial, involving estriol taken in combination with standard MS anti-inflammatory drugs is ongoing. It is investigating whether estriol treatment can improve cognitive testing compared to placebo in either relapsing or progressive types of MS who have some evidence of cognitive disability at baseline.[15]

Oral contraceptives don't seem to affect the risk or the course of MS, although research has been very sparse.[16] Some studies have suggested that women who get their periods at an earlier age may have an increased risk of MS, but this has never been proven conclusively. The same can be said of the effect of having children or not having children.

Another sex difference may be due to inflammatory cytokines. During pregnancy, levels of *interferon gamma* (a damaging inflammatory cytokine associated with MS) are lower. One small study at the Cleveland Clinic Foundation revealed that when T cells from women with MS were stimulated with a myelin protein, they produced higher levels of interferon gamma compared to men. At the same time, women with MS produced none of a regulatory cytokine that may dampen the disease process. It's not clear what role, if any, sex hormones may play in this response.

However, the inflammatory immune response does switch to a regulatory response during pregnancy (so the body doesn't reject the fetus), and MS typically improves during pregnancy, when estrogen and estriol levels are high. Researchers at the Cleveland Clinic Foundation say a possible new direction in MS therapy would be stimulating that regulatory response.

One of the ways estrogen suppresses EAE in mice is by changing the action of T cells and the activity of brain cells called *microglia*, which can produce toxic molecules that attack myelin-producing cells.

However, Dr. Giesser believes that estrogen—either in birth control pills or in hormone replacement therapy—can be safely used by women with MS, as long as they're being followed by a gynecologist.

Ana's story continues:

I had a hard time getting used to the Avonex. They had to put me on half doses, and then took me off it. I was then put on Copaxone for a while, and felt great. But then they noticed that I had an allergic reaction at the injection site, and I had to go back on Avonex. And that was rough. So I started with tiny doses and gradually increased the dose until I could get acclimated to the drug. You learn to live with a lot. I had to learn to give myself injections. That was difficult. What is wonderful is that these drugs are shipped right to your home, and there are nurses you can call with questions. And that makes it easier. For example, the nurses told me to drink a lot of water the day I get the injection and the day after, to keep me hydrated. You use every piece of information they give you, and it all makes you feel that much better.

I was also fortunate to have a gynecologist who works with my neurologist, and when I started to have hot flashes she said I should absolutely be on estrogen. Since heat can make MS feel worse, I thought it was a good thing to do. Menopausal symptoms are just one more thing I don't want to worry about.

Treating Multiple Sclerosis

Under the new diagnostic criteria, a woman who experiences a single MS attack can be started right away on injectable or oral medications that have been shown to slow the progression of the disease—in many cases preventing permanent disability. Early treatment also benefits patients with CIS, who have a very high risk of developing MS.

Interferon beta-1b (Betaseron), The first disease-modifying drug for MS, was approved by the FDA back in 1993, and there are now a dozen more approved for treating relapsing-remitting MS, secondary progressive MS, and progressive-relapsing disease.

Betaseron works like natural human interferon to inhibit immune system activity and reduces MS relapses by about 30 percent in active MS and by 50 percent in patients treated at the onset of their first symptoms. It is injected under the skin every other day. Betaseron slows the progression of physical disability and reduces exacerbations in relapsing-remitting MS and in CIS.[17]

Interferon beta-1a (Avonex) also works like natural human interferon to dampen immune system activity. It is also given after a single MS attack and reduces the frequency and severity of exacerbations in people with relapsing-remitting MS. The drug is given by self-administered injection (using either a prefilled syringe or an auto-injector pen) once a week into the large muscles of the thigh (or the hip or upper arm muscle). Avonex reduces relapses by about 18 percent, slows MS progression, and studies show it may help cognitive impairment in relapsing MS.

Avonex can cause liver damage, so liver enzymes must be monitored carefully.[18]

Avonex and Betaseron both can cause menstrual irregularities in about 15 percent of women.

Extavia (interferon beta-1b) is identical to Betaseron but delivered by a different company (made in the same plant). It's administered by subcutaneous injection every other day to treat relapsing MS and individuals with CIS. The side effects and safety profile of Extavia are also identical to Betaseron.[19]

Interferon beta-1a (Rebif) reduces the frequency of MS exacerbations, reduces disease activity seen on MRI, and slows progression of disability. A study comparing Rebif to Avonex showed it produced a 32 percent reduction in relapses compared to Avonex. Another trial showed Rebif could delay MS development after a first MS-like attack.[20]

Rebif is prescribed in prefilled syringes and given by self-injection three days a week at the same time of day, with each injection 48 hours apart. There can be reactions at the injection site (soreness, redness, pain, bruising), so you're advised to pick a different spot each time to lessen the chance of an infection or other problem.

Plegridy (PEGylated interferon beta-1a) is a new interferon drug for relapsing forms of MS. *PEGylation* is a chemical alteration of the interferon beta-1a molecule that allows the drug to be given under the skin with a prefilled autoinjector every two weeks, rather than the more frequent injections required by other interferons. In clinical trials, Plegridy reduced relapses by about 36 percent and new brain lesions by 67 compared to a placebo after a year.[21]

Betaseron and other interferon drugs cause flu-like symptoms (fatigue, fever, chills, muscle aches), which lessen after a while. (Note: Influenza infections cause the body to produce interferons, which causes those "flu-like" symptoms.) In addition, interferon drugs may cause elevated liver enzymes and low red and white blood cell counts that can increase the risk of infection, changes in thyroid function, and allergic reactions. Periodic blood testing is needed to monitor liver or blood changes. There can also be reactions at the site of the subcutaneous injections, which can be serious and require medical attention in about 5 percent of cases.

These medications cannot be used during pregnancy.

Glatiramer acetate (Copaxone) is a synthetic protein that looks like myelin to the immune system. It seems to block attacks on myelin by T cells, apparently acting as a decoy for myelin, but it may also change the immune system to suppress inflammation. Copaxone is approved for relapsing-remitting MS. A 12-year clinical trial among patients with relapsing-remitting MS found that most of those who stayed on Copaxone had an improvement in their neurological status or remained unchanged. Another study found that Copaxone stopped new brain lesions caused by MS flares and reduced the amount of damaged brain tissue over time, with the protective effects appearing three to four months after treatment began.[22]

Copaxone is available in prefilled syringes and given by injection once a day. It can cause reactions at the injection site. In rare cases, there may be anxiety, chest tightness, shortness of breath, and flushing right after an injection, but there do not seem to be any long-term consequences.[23] A generic version of *glatiramer acetate* is also available.

"I like to think that these drugs give the brain a 'breather,' allowing more of the normal remyelination to occur," says Dr. Reder, who also serves as director of clinical neurology trials at the University of Chicago.

Natalizumab (Tysabri) is one of a new class of therapeutics called *alpha 4 integrin inhibitors*. It's a monoclonal antibody designed to prevent the migration of inflammatory cells from the blood to other sites in the body. (In MS, it would block adhesion molecules that attach T cells to cells lining the blood vessels in the brain pulling them across the blood-brain barrier.)

According to the Multiple Sclerosis Association of America (MSAA), recent data also suggest that it may also enhance remyelination and stabilize damage to the myelin sheath.[7] Studies show it slows relapse rates by as much as 66 percent, reduces lesions seen on MRI by 80 percent, and produces sustained improvement in disability in patients with RRMS. (It's also approved for Crohn's disease.)

Like other drugs in this class, Tysabri carries a "black box" warning that it can cause *progressive multifocal leukoencephalopathy* (*PML*, see page 254), a potentially fatal viral infection, so it's only available only through a "restricted distribution" program for physicians (the TOUCH® Prescribing Program, see Appendix A).[24]

There are now three oral disease-modifying MS drugs: *fingolimod (Gilenya), teriflunomide (Aubagio)*, and *dimethyl fumarate (Tecfidera)*, all in capsule form.

Gilenya (fingolimod) is the first of a new class of drugs called *sphingosine 1-phosphate (S1P) receptor modulators*. It keeps potentially damaging T cells from exiting lymph nodes, so there are fewer of them in blood and tissues. By doing so, it may reduce damage to the central nervous system (CNS) and allow or enhance nerve repair within the brain and spinal cord; Gilenya may also have neuroprotective effects.

Gilenya capsules are taken once a day, with or without food. The adverse side effects include an initial reduction in heart rate; infrequent changes in the conduction of electricity in the heart (*atrioventricular [AV] block*); macular edema (swelling behind the eye, which can affect vision); and infections, including reactivation of herpes infections.

FDA labeling recommends that all patients have an *electrocardiogram (ECG)* before taking their first dose of the drug and a second ECG six hours after the first dose. New patients also are advised to take the drug in their doctor's office the first time with hourly blood pressure and heart rate checks during a six-hour monitoring period.[25]

Aubagio (teriflunomide) is a pyrimidine synthesis inhibitor, related to the rheumatoid arthritis drug leflunomide. It inhibits a key enzyme needed by activated lymphocytes to make DNA. This helps reduce proliferation of T and B immune cells that are active in MS and also blocks T cells from producing immune messenger chemicals. Clinical trials data indicate it reduces relapse rates by more than 30 percent in RRMS[26] and reduces the size of MS brain lesions.[27] The higher dose (14 mg/day) tested in the trials lessens disability. Aubagio capsules are taken in one (7 mg or 14 mg) dose, once a day with or without food.

Side effects include elevations in liver enzymes and severe liver problems (including liver failure). Women taking the drug need monthly blood tests for the first six months to monitor their liver enzymes and additional testing if symptoms of liver problems arise (such as nausea, vomiting, abdominal pain, unusual fatigue, loss of appetite, and yellowing of the skin or whites of the eyes). Aubagio can cause numbness and/or pain in the hands or feet (peripheral neuropathy) and transient elevations in blood potassium that can lead to kidney failure, so women must be monitored for both, as well as for high blood pressure. Aubagio can also trigger severe skin reactions.[28]

Aubagio cannot be taken during pregnancy, by women (or men) who want to conceive a child, or even by women of childbearing age who aren't using an effective contraceptive method, since animal data indicate that it may cause significant birth defects.

In addition, Aubagio remains in the blood for an average of eight months after it is stopped and may even linger in the blood for up to two years after the last dose is taken. If you become pregnant while taking the drug, it must be discontinued immediately and an accelerated elimination procedure will be needed to decrease Aubagio to a safe level in the blood (less than 0.02 mg/L), according to the FDA. The medication can be eliminated from the body in 11 days with cholestyramine or active charcoal.[28]

Tecfidera is approved for people with relapsing forms of MS. The starting dose is a 120 mg capsule twice a day. After a week, the dose is increased to 240 mg twice a day, a maintenance dose. While it can be taken with or without food, taking the capsules with a meal may reduce flushing (warmth, redness, itching, and/or burning sensation), a common side effect of the drug. Other side effects can include gastrointestinal upsets, such as nausea, vomiting, diarrhea, abdominal pain, and indigestion.[29]

Because it can lead to decreased white blood cell (*lymphocyte*) counts, it's recommended that before starting the drug a complete blood count be done to detect preexisting lymphopenia.

Animal studies show adverse effects on a fetus during pregnancy and lactation, but there are few well-controlled studies in pregnant women. So the FDA recommends that Tecfidera be used during pregnancy only if the potential benefits outweigh potential risks to the fetus.[29] The drug label also carries a warning about *PML*.[30]

Alemtuzumab (Lemtrada), another injectable medication is a new MS drug. It's a humanized monoclonal antibody (note the suffix *mab*) directed at CD52, a protein that sits on the surface of immune cells, of unknown function. The drug reduces suppressor T cells and increased autoreactive B cells. Because of these effects, it can trigger other autoimmune diseases.

Lemtrada is given by intravenous infusion for five consecutive days initially and for three consecutive days after 12 months. The Lemtrada label includes a boxed warning about a potential 30 percent risk of thyroid disease, immune thrombocytopenia, serious infusion reactions within 24 hours, and malignancies, including thyroid cancer and melanoma.[31] It's only available from certified prescribers, and all patients must be enrolled in a "Risk Evaluation and Mitigation Strategy (REMS)" program so potential side effects can be periodically monitored and any adverse effects reported back to the FDA.[32]

More common side effects include rash, headache, dizziness, fever, nasal congestion, nausea, diarrhea, urinary tract infections, fatigue, insomnia, upper respiratory tract and fungal infections, herpes infections, hives, itching, and joint and back pain.[32]

Clinical trials reported in 2012, comparing Lemtrada with Rebif in patients not previously given any MS disease-modifying therapy (including Rebif), found a majority of those treated with Lemtrada were free of new brain lesions, had significant reductions in disease activity seen on MRI, and remained relapse-free for two years.[32] The drug also slowed the loss of brain volume.[33]

Mitoxantrone (Novantrone) is an anticancer drug that suppresses T cell, B cell, and macrophage activity and seems to lessen attacks on myelin. It is usually given intravenously every three months for up to two years (or up to a specific cumulative lifetime dose). A 2002 study from France, where it has been used for more than two decades, found that an initial "induction" course of more intense mitoxantrone therapy for six months significantly reduced relapse rates, and kept 43 percent of patients relapse free for a five-year period. More recent studies also suggest that combining Novantrone with Betaseron may reduce disease progression in people with aggressive relapsing-remitting disease, or with secondary progressive disease when MS isn't well-controlled by Betaseron.[34]

Novantrone can affect the heart, raising the risk of congestive heart failure. So you must have normal heart function to take the drug, and tests of cardiac function are necessary before and during treatment. Novantrone also imparts an increased risk of developing leukemia and can cause permanent sterility. It is being used much less to treat MS currently with the advent of newer and safer medications.

All of these new MS drugs can be very costly, especially the oral medications. The wholesale price of Gilenya (with no discount) is a hefty $60,000 a year, Tecfidera costs almost $55,000 a year, and the annual price tag for Aubagio is $45,000. Out-of-pocket costs will depend on your insurance; some states have drug assistance programs, and drug manufacturers also have programs to provide MS medications at low or no cost (see Appendix A).

Other treatments target MS symptoms such as pain, tremor, bladder or bowel dysfunction, and fatigue.

"Up to 85 percent of MS patients have fatigue, and it may be the single most disabling symptom," remarks Dr. Giesser. An antiviral medication called *amantadine* is widely used to treat MS-related fatigue.

Some patients benefit from a stimulant used for hyperactivity, *methylphenidate hydrochloride (Ritalin)*. Wakefulness promoting agents used for sleep disorders, *modafinil (Provigil)* and *armodafinil (Nuvigil)* are also effective against MS-related fatigue. "Activating" antidepressants such as *fluoxetine (Prozac)* may also help fatigue.

Physical, occupational, and/or cognitive therapy may sometimes be recommended, and studies show aerobic exercise produces many physical and emotional benefits for MS patients, including improved bowel and bladder control and reduced fatigue.

Most MS patients are sensitive to increases in body heat, so exercising in an air-conditioned room is highly recommended. Dehydration can exacerbate fatigue, but many women with MS don't drink enough water because of bladder incontinence. However, getting enough water during exercise is extremely important.

Antiseizure medications like *gabapentin (Neurontin)* and *carbamazepine (Tegretol)* help nerve pain. Other drugs used for MS-related pain include the tricyclic antidepressants *amitriptyline (Elavil)* and *imipramine (Tofranil)*, which interfere with pain signals from nerves, and a newer antidepressant, *duloxetine (Cymbalta)*, is also FDA indicated for pain. Antispasmodic drugs, such as *baclofen (Lioresal)* or *tizanidine (Zanaflex)* can help leg or back spasms. Prednisone may be given for optic neuritis.

MS patients have specific bladder problems. "In MS, the bladder often doesn't store urine properly. So instead of holding a normal volume of urine, around two or three cups, before you have the urge to go or before you empty reflexively, a patient's bladder may hold only a cup or so. The result is urgency, a spastic, nervous bladder that wants to go all the time," says Dr. Giesser. "Or, MS patients may have a bladder that doesn't empty itself completely, so when you void there's still urine in the bladder, which leads to urinary tract infections, urine reflux (it can theoretically back up into the kidneys), and kidney disease. And there are women who have a 'mixed' bladder problem, a bladder that wants to empty all the time, but doesn't empty well."

For a purely spastic bladder that doesn't store urine well, patients are prescribed *anticholinergic* agents, drugs that relax the bladder and allow it to hold more urine. In some cases, women are taught how to use urinary catheters. "For 'mixed' bladders we may use medication along with self-catheterization. It's very individual." A newer procedure, *sacral nerve stimulation*, a kind of "pacemaker" that helps eliminate abnormal nerve signals to the bladder, may work for some women with MS, she adds.

Another common problem is constipation. "Women who are less mobile are more prone to constipation. Some of the drugs we give cause constipation. A lot of women with bladder problems self-treat by restricting liquids and become dehydrated, which contributes to constipation. And MS probably has some effect on gut motility, as well," says Dr. Giesser. In general, women with MS are advised to increase fiber intake, take bulking agents, keep well hydrated, and eliminate on a schedule to help keep regular.

Studies conducted by the National Multiple Sclerosis Society (NMSS) show that two out of three people with MS will remain ambulatory 20 years after diagnosis, and those numbers should improve as more people are treated earlier for the disease. Again, just because you're not experiencing a relapse doesn't mean there's no disease progression. So medication is needed.

What's Next?

There is a great deal of research going on in MS, and many scientists are hopeful, especially about new drug treatments.

Among these new drugs is *Ocrelizumab*, which is being tested in relapsing MS. Late-stage trials show it is more effective than Rebif at reducing MS lesions in the brain, lessening relapses and the progression of disability. Ocrelizumab, a relative of rituximab, reduces the number of CD20-positive B cells, thought to be a key player in the myelin destruction.[35]

Also in the pipeline is *Laquinimod*, a once-daily oral immunomodulator being tested for the treatment of RRMS. Laquinimod also increases levels of a molecule called brain-derived neurotrophic factor (BDNF), which may help protect nerves and myelin. In one large clinical trial, laquinimod significantly reduced atrophy of gray matter and white matter in the brain. Other large studies show laquinimod lessened relapses, disability, and problems walking for some patients.[7]

Daclizumab (also known as *Zenapax*) is an intravenous drug that's also being studied in subcutaneous injections for RRMS and secondary-progressive MS. It's a humanized monoclonal antibody (a "smart bomb" that zeros in on interleukin-2 receptors) and appears to inhibits disease activity by increasing the number of natural killer T cells (NK cells), autoreactive cells that play a key role in MS.[36]

A large clinical trial comparing monthly infusions of daclizumab to weekly subcutaneous injections of Avonex showed daclizumab produced a 45 percent reduction in relapses and reductions of around 60 percent in brain lesions. Risks associated with daclizumab treatment included infections, rash, and liver enzyme abnormalities. Side effects associated with daclizumab include respiratory and urinary tract infections, skin reactions, and elevated liver enzymes.[7]

Some studies suggest that stem cell transplants might put many MS patients in long-term remission or even regrow myelin.[7]

One technique, *hematopoietic stem-cell transplantation* (*HSCT*, see page 142) aspirates the patient's own blood-forming cells from the bone marrow. First, the immune system is wiped out with high-dose chemotherapy (destroying the stem cells and the bone marrow), then the stem cells are infused back into the patient in hopes of "resetting" the entire immune system.

Another approach uses transplanted *mesenchymal stem cells (MSCs)*, which can be extracted from other tissues without the need to destroy the bone marrow. Animal studies indicate that, under the right conditions, MSCs can mature into myelin-producing cells, which may be a potential way to stop or even reverse myelin loss. In early clinical trials, MSC transplants had no major adverse side effects and showed some promise.[37]

A third technique would harvest stem cells from bone marrow and infuse them back into cerebral spinal fluid, in hopes they will go into the central nervous system and perhaps help nerve cells regrow lost myelin.

Scientists are also investigating the possibility of using inactivated myelin-reactive T cells from a patient's blood then injected back into the patient. The idea is that the body's immune system may potentially protect the myelin. While it didn't reduce brain lesions seen on MRI, in a one-year study the relapse rate was reduced among patients with a previous relapse who hadn't been exposed to other MS therapies. In addition, "vaccine" treated patients remained relapse-free for a year. The vaccine, called *Tcelna*, is undergoing further study.[7]

The American Academy of Neurology has endorsed plasma exchange (*plasmapheresis*) to treat severe exacerbations of relapsing-remitting MS. In plasma exchange the liquid part of your blood (the plasma) is replaced with plasma from a donor. In MS, plasma could contain immune factors that are attacking the myelin and nervous system. By swapping out the plasma, these factors are eliminated and symptoms of an MS flare may improve. It's kind of like kidney dialysis in that it "cleans" the blood. Plasma exchange is an outpatient procedure, done in a hospital or outpatient facility, much like a chemotherapy infusion. Each exchange can last two to four hours, and you may need two or three treatments a week for several weeks.[38]

Ritonavir (Norvir), a drug used to treat *human immunodeficiency virus (HIV)*, has shown potential benefits in preliminary animal studies. Ritonavir is a protease inhibitor, which affects an enzyme (called a proteasome enzyme) thought to play a role in the activation of lymphocytes that attack the myelin sheath in MS. Daily doses of ritonavir prevented clinical symptoms in the animal model of MS in such a way that researchers feel it may have a protective effect when given early in the disease. Drugs used in Alzheimer's disease are also being tested to see whether they can slow cognitive decline in MS. Preliminary indications are that *donepezil (Aricept)* slightly improved cognitive function in the small group of patients who have tried it, Dr. Reder reports, but definitive data will have to come from large clinical trials. Newer drugs such as *galantamine (Reminyl)* may be even more effective.

Mariana's story continues:
I was formally diagnosed when I was 30, when I started to have my first problems with walking. Then it was completely undeniable that I had MS, there was no way I could ignore it. I found myself a good neurologist . . . and my husband dragged me to my first support group, which scared me to death. Because there were a lot of people there who were worse off than I was. And that frightened me. I'd been told for years it could be MS. But I hadn't accepted it in my mind until that point. I finally came to grips with it . . . I didn't go back to the support group until later and I ended up being the program coordinator because I didn't like the way it was being run; everyone would just sit around and complain. So we started getting people to come in to talk to us about MS and things to do to take charge of your life. And we also talked about touchy subjects like sexual dysfunction. For me, it was the emotional issues that were hardest. For example, it was hard to get my groceries in and out of the house and it was good to find out how to make that easier. But how does it make me feel as a person that I can't do that anymore, that I have to ask neighbors to help me? That was the hardest part for me. To me, it's a sign of weakness. You make yourself vulnerable and indebted to them. Some people like to do for others, do community service. But I had no way to "pay them back." I felt very inadequate. That was an emotional stumbling block I had to get over.

How MS Can Affect You Over Your Lifetime

While MS flares and relapses seem to be affected by hormones in younger women, there's little research on the subject, and menopause is largely uncharted territory.

Premenstrual Flares

Women with MS often report that symptoms get worse in the days before their periods, but there have been only a few studies of this.

"We published the first abstract in 1990 on premenstrual fluctuations. We surveyed 149 women, who completed a questionnaire that asked, 'Do you ever notice an increase in your symptoms during your menstrual cycle? If so, when?' Seventy percent said they had changes in their symptoms every month, most of them saying this occurred during the week prior to menses," said Dr. Giesser.

"About 40 percent noticed exacerbations—different than symptom fluctuation—came at a particular time during their cycle. Since then, there have been several other reports, self-report questionnaire samples that have also reported this. There have also been three small studies that reported some changes in MRIs correlated with different phases of the menstrual cycle. So we have uncontrolled, preliminary data in very small samples of women that yes, there seems to be an association with neurological symptoms and the premenstrual period. But we don't know what is causing it."

It's not clear whether this is related to a temporary worsening of preexisting symptoms or disease exacerbation, comments Dr. Voskuhl. "These are very different. If you are getting a relapse, this could be an indication of inflammation and new demyelination. In contrast, when a woman is exposed to heat, her symptoms get worse, but it doesn't mean her disease is worsening," she points out. Menstrual changes fit best with a temporary worsening of symptoms, not a relapse of MS.

According to Dr. Giesser, the most common symptoms that worsen premenstrually are fatigue, imbalance, difficulty walking, and spasticity. Specific symptoms can be individually treated (see page 307). It's not known whether there are menstrual cycle changes in the metabolism of various medications.

Pregnancy/Postpartum

The good news is that MS doesn't seem to hamper a woman's ability to get pregnant and carry to term, and MS symptoms get better during pregnancy. Some studies suggest pregnancy may even slow the progression of the disease.[39]

This is thought to be partly due to high estrogen levels (especially *estriol*), which appear to reduce immune system activity and reduce the frequency of MS attacks. The relapse rate seems to be lowest in the third trimester, and spikes in the three to six months after delivery as hormones return to normal levels (depending on whether or not a woman breast-feeds).

The American College of Obstetricians and Gynecologists (ACOG) reassures women with MS that they can "safely choose to become pregnant, give birth, and breastfeed children."[40]

A recent ACOG review notes there may be an increased risk of MS relapses after undergoing IVF or other assisted reproductive techniques, but "there does not appear to be a major increase in adverse outcomes in newborns of mothers with MS."[40] This includes early miscarriage, stillbirth, birth defects and low-birthweight babies, says ACOG.

If you want to become pregnant, it's advisable to discontinue any disease-modifying therapies under the supervision of your doctors. Since it may take longer to become pregnant, there's a risk of relapse.[41] In this case, monthly intravenous steroids may be given (but only after a negative pregnancy test).

While pregnancy does have positive effects on MS, there's no guarantee you'll totally avoid a relapse. If your doctor feels there's a high risk of relapse, ACOG says monthly *intravenous immunoglobulin (IVIG)* or steroids after the first trimester can be considered, although the safety data are limited.[40] And if your MS is severe or highly active, the risks of treatment have to be weighed with the still unknown risks to the baby.

The Multiple Sclerosis Association of America stresses that "because disease-modifying therapies (DMTs) are not tested in pregnant women, information about the potential risks of fetal exposure is not available to guide decision-making by women who are pregnant or wish to become pregnant."[42]

While recent data from a small number of women who became pregnant on MS drugs did not find abnormalities in their babies, this should not suggest that getting pregnant is considered safe while taking DMTs, says the MSAA.

The good news is that, for the most part, MS drugs are not needed because of pregnancy's favorable effects. "Women should be off any one of these drugs for different periods of time depending upon the drugs' metabolism before they try to get pregnant," advises Dr. Giesser. "There are a lot of reports about women who happened to become pregnant while they were on these drugs, stopped the drugs, and had perfectly healthy babies. But we prefer to be cautious."

During pregnancy, standard urine and blood tests are done to monitor for preeclampsia and other problems. A neurological exam would be given once or twice over the course of the pregnancy.

The decision on whether to resume disease-modifying therapy after delivery, especially if a woman is planning to breast-feed, is an individual one; a woman should discuss this with her neurologist, says Dr. Giesser. Because of a lack of safety data, Avonex, Betaseron, Copaxone, Rebif, and other interferon drugs can't be used during breast-feeding.

Because the FDA has changed its labeling of medications during pregnancy and lactation (see page 18), check with your neurologist about specific MS drugs.

Aside from a spike in the relapse rate after delivery (as estrogen levels return to normal), women who breast-feed do not seem to have more relapses than women who don't. "It's not clear why there is a relapse rebound after delivery. It could be the effects of all the hormones returning to normal levels. All the immunosuppressant chemicals do, too. There's an increase in prolactin during lactation, but I don't think you can hang it on any one hormone," says Dr. Giesser.

Some studies of women who exclusively breast-feed their babies suggest it may reduce the risk of relapses.

A German study presented at the triennial joint conference of ACTRIMS (Americas Committee for Treatment and Research in Multiple Sclerosis) and ECTRIMS (European Committee for Treatment and Research in MS) in 2014, found that women with MS who exclusively breast-fed their newborns for two months did not experience more postpartum relapses than those who bottle-fed or used supplemental feedings.[8] However, a 10-year study of all pregnancies at one Spanish hospital presented at the conference found no difference in the course of MS between women who chose to breast-feed and those who bottle-fed their babies and restarted their treatment sooner.[7]

If you choose to breast-feed, your doctor may prescribe monthly intravenous corticosteroids or IVIG to prevent relapses.[40] The biggest problem for many women who decide to become pregnant is fatigue and caring for their children in the event of a relapse. Strong support is needed from family members to share the load. To keep sleep disruption at a minimum, ACOG suggests scheduled naps during the day, pumping and storing breast milk on a schedule for others to feed to the baby while you nap. If you can, get outside help with household chores and consult your neurologist about potential relapse triggers.

Almost 20 percent of women experience postpartum depression (PPD) in the six months after giving birth. ACOG notes that women with MS may be at increased risk of PPD because of the increased incidence of depression in MS and possible worsening of symptoms.[40]

Menopause and Beyond

It's not known whether the wide shifts in hormones during perimenopause or the decline in estrogen after menopause affect the course of MS.

There's also little information on the effects of menopause and hormone therapy on symptoms. A 2006 study found that 40 percent of women reported a worsening of MS symptoms at the time of menopause, 56 percent said they'd had no change, and 5 percent even reported an improvement.[43] A study back in 1992 reported that 75 percent of women who used hormone therapy had an improvement in their symptoms.[44]

"A woman in her late forties or early fifties probably has had MS for 20 to 30 years, and she may stop having defined relapses as her disease becomes secondary progressive. So there are fewer relapses in menopause, but it may be for reasons that have nothing to do with hormones and more to do with the natural history of the disease," remarks Dr. Giesser.

Menopause may have some effects on the symptoms of MS. For example, hot flashes raise body heat, which can worsen fatigue and other symptoms.[45] Menopause itself may not have any effect on the inflammatory process that underlies MS. However, there's simply not enough information on the effect of hormone replacement on MS. "Right now, we have no data to suggest that it's good for them, although it may be, we certainly don't have any data to suggest that it's bad. So if a woman's gynecologist or internist thinks she should be on hormone replacement for any kind of medical or gynecological reason, I tell them go ahead," says Dr. Giesser.

Dr. Voskuhl concurs. "I think if a woman wants to take hormone replacement, there's no reason not to. However, I don't think very-low-dose estrogens will be very helpful." Cooling vests can help dampen symptoms in hot weather and they may also be helpful to women experiencing hot flashes.

Some women may want to investigate branded herbal remedies like black cohosh (*Remifemin*) or red clover (*Promensil*) for menopausal symptoms.

Corticosteroids cause bone loss, but interferon drugs do not. So bone-building drugs are needed if a woman is taking steroids for MS attacks.

Throughout life, women are twice as likely as men to suffer from depression—and it's also a more common symptom in people with MS. One small study found that the antidepressants known as *selective serotonin reuptake inhibitors (SSRIs)* not only help relieved depression, but also significantly reduce levels of gamma interferon. The researchers suggest that treating depression could also be an important factor in downregulating autoreactive T cells.[46] So it's possible that treating depression may benefit women with MS.

Ana's story, a postscript, 2015:

Developing MS is the toughest thing that has ever happened to me. I had to give up a 30-year career that I loved and that defined me. It utterly changed the assumptions about myself that I'd had my entire life—what my strengths are, how my brain works, and how I would live the rest of my life. My doctor said that none of his patients ever reconcile themselves to having this illness. And he's right. I hate it.

That's probably a healthy way to look at chronic illness. You have to think about those things that are important in your life and fight for them.

I was lucky to have access to aggressive treatment early on. It's necessary to push for the best treatment and advice you can get, even if you have to travel for it. There is such a wide range of symptoms in MS that it's important to find a doctor with lots of experience and many patients.

Because an illness like this is so isolating, volunteer work has become important to me. It gets me out with people, doing something of value, out of my own thoughts, and makes me use my brain.

I always said kiddingly that everyone with MS should have a dog (mine worked as a therapy dog). Having a dog is a social activity; you have to go out, walk, and you end up talking to people.

Most importantly, my life has found balance again. It has definitely changed. But there is life after diagnosis.

Notes

1. National Multiple Sclerosis Society, Who gets MS? (epidemiology). http://www.nationalmssociety.org/What-is-MS/Who-Gets-MS#section-0.
2. Multiple sclerosis: hope through research: National Institute of Neurological Disorders and Stroke (NINDS). http://www.ninds.nih.gov/disorders/multiple_sclerosis/detail_multiple_sclerosis.htm#264603215.
3. The use of disease-modifying therapies in multiple sclerosis: principles and current evidence. A consensus paper by the Multiple Sclerosis Coalition, July 2014. National Multiple Sclerosis Society. http://www.nationalmssociety.org/getmedia/5ca284d3-fc7c-4ba5-b005-ab537d495c3c/DMT_Consensus_MS_Coalition_color.
4. Traboulse AL, Katherine B, Knox KB, Machan L, et al. Prevalence of extracranial venous narrowing on catheter venography in people with multiple sclerosis, their siblings, and unrelated healthy controls: a blinded, case-control study. *Lancet*. 2013. doi:10.1016/S0140-6736(13)61747-X.
5. Siddiqui A, Zivadinov R, Weinstock-Guttman B, et al. Percutaneous transluminal venous angioplasty (PTVA) is ineffective in correcting chronic cerebrospinal venous insufficiency (CCSVI) and may increase multiple sclerosis (MS) disease activity in the short term: safety and efficacy results of the 6-month, double-blinded, sham-controlled, prospective, randomized endovascular therapy in MS (PREMiSe) trial. American Academy of Neurology Annual Meeting (AAN) 2013: Abstract P04.273.
6. Milo R, Miller A. Revised diagnostic criteria of multiple sclerosis. *Autoimmun Rev*. 2014; 13(4–5):518–524. doi:10.1016/j.autrev.2014.01.012. Epub 2014 Jan 12.
7. Krieger S, Schneider D, McCormick MM. MS research update, 2014. Multiple Sclerosis Association of America (MSAA), February 2014. http://www.mymsaa.org/publications/msresearch-update-2014/.
8. Multiple Sclerosis Association of American (MSAA). Highlights from the 2014 Joint ACTRIMS-ECTRIMS Meeting. http://www.mymsaa.org/news-msaa/1178-actrims-ectrims-2014-highlights.
9. Acherio A, Munger KL, White R, et al. Vitamin D as an early predictor of multiple sclerosis activity and progression. *JAMA Neurol*. 2014;71(3):306–314. doi:10.1001/jamaneurol.2013.5993.
10. Buchanan RJ, Zuniga MA, Carrillo-Zuniga G, et al. Comparisons of Latinos, African Americans, and Caucasians with multiple sclerosis. *Ethnicity Dis*. 2010;20:451–457.

11. Mohr DC, Goodkin DE, Islar J, Hauser SL, Genain CP. Treatment of depression is associated with suppression of nonspecific and antigen-specific T(H)1 responses in multiple sclerosis. *Arch Neurol.* 2001;58(7):1081–1086.
12. Polman CH, Reingold SC, Banwell B, et al. Diagnostic criteria for multiple sclerosis: 2010 Revisions to the McDonald criteria. *Ann Neurol.* 2011;69(2):292–302. doi:10.1002/ana.22366.
13. Soldan SS, Alvarez Retuerto A, Sicotte WL, Voskuhl RR. Immune modulation in multiple sclerosis patients treated with pregnancy hormone estriol. *J Immunol.* 2003; 171(11)6267–6274. doi:10.4049/jimmunol.171.11.6267.
14. Voskuhl RR, Wang H, Jackson Wu TC, et al. Estriol combined with glatiramer acetate for women with relapsing-remitting multiple sclerosis: a randomised, placebo-controlled, phase 2 trial. *Lancet Neurol.* 2016;15(1):35–46. Doi:http://dx.doi.org/10.1016/S1474-4422(15)00322-1.
15. Estriol treatment in multiple sclerosis (MS): effect on cognition. https://clinicaltrials.gov/ct2/show/NCT01466114.
16. D'hooghe MB, Haentjens P, Nagels G, D'Hooghe T, De Keyser J. Menarche, oral contraceptives, pregnancy and progression of disability in relapsing onset and progressive onset multiple sclerosis. *J Neurol.* 2012;259:855–861.
17. Betaseron® (interferon beta-1b) [prescribing information]. Whippany, NJ: Bayer HealthCare Pharmaceuticals Inc.; 2014. http://labeling.bayerhealthcare.com/html/products/pi/Betaseron_PI.pdf.
18. Avonex® (interferon beta-1a) [prescribing information]. Cambridge, MA: Biogen Idec, Inc.; 2014. http://www.avonex.com/pdfs/guides/Avonex_Prescribing_Information.pdf.
19. Extavia® (interferon beta-1b) [prescribing information]. East Hanover, NJ: Novartis Pharmaceuticals Corporation; 2012. http://www.pharma.us.novartis.com/product/pi/pdf/extavia.pdf.
20. Rebif® (interferon beta-1a) [medication guide]. Rockland, MA: EMD Serono, Inc.; New York, NY: Pfizer, Inc.; 2014. http://emdserono.com/cmg.emdserono_us/en/images/Rebif%20PI_Jun2014_tcm115_19765.pdf?Version.
21. National MS Society. FDA approves plegridy (pegylated interferon beta) for relapsing MS, August 15, 2014. http://www.nationalmssociety.org/About-the-Society/News/FDA-Approves-Plegridy-(Pegylated-Interferon-Beta).
22. Company announces positive results from clinical trial of a generic glatiramer acetate in relapsing-remitting MS, National Multiple Sclerosis Society News Release, March 27, 2014. http://www.nationalmssociety.org/About-the-Society/News/Company-Announces-Positive-Results-from-Clinical-T.
23. Copaxone® (glatiramer acetate) [prescribing information]. Overland Park, KS: Teva Neuroscience, Inc.; 2014. https://www.copaxone.com/Resources/pdfs/PrescribingInformation.pdf.
24. Tysabri® (natalizumab) [medication guide]. Cambridge, MA: Biogen Idec, Inc.; 2013. http://www.tysabri.com/pdfs/I61061-13_PI.pdf.

25. Gilenya® (fingolimod) [prescribing information]. East Hanover, NJ: Novartis Pharmaceuticals Corporation; 2014. http://www.pharma.us.novartis.com/product/pi/pdf/gilenya.pdf.
26. Miller A, O'Connor P, Wolinsky JS, et al. Clinical and MRI outcomes from a phase III trial (TEMSO) of oral teriflunomide in multiple sclerosis with relapses. *Neurology*. 2011;76:A545.
27. Wolinsky J, et al. A placebo-controlled phase III trial (TEMSO) of oral teriflunomide in multiple sclerosis with relapses: additional magnetic resonance imaging (MRI) outcomes. *Neurology*. 2011;76:A545–A546.
28. Aubagio® (teriflunomide) [prescribing information]. Cambridge, MA: Genzyme Corporation; October 2014. http://products.sanofi.us/aubagio/aubagio.pdf.
29. http://www.accessdata.fda.gov/drugsatfda_docs/label/2013/204063lbl.pdf.
30. FDA Drug safety communication: FDA warns about case of rare brain infection PML with MS drug Tecfidera (dimethyl fumarate), November 25, 2014. http://www.fda.gov/Drugs/DrugSafety/ucm424625.htm.
31. Lemtrada prescribing information, US Food and Drug Administration (FDA); November 2014. http://www.accessdata.fda.gov/drugsatfda_docs/label/2014/103948s5139lbl.pdf.
32. National MS Society. FDA approves Lemtrada (alemtuzumab) for relapsing MS, update December 18, 2014. http://www.nationalmssociety.org/About-the-Society/News/FDA-Approves-Lemtrada (alemtuzumab)-for-Relapsing MS.
33. Coles AJ, Twyman CL, Arnold DL, et al. Alemtuzumab for patients with relapsing multiple sclerosis after disease-modifying therapy: a randomised controlled phase 3 trial. *Lancet*. 2012;380(9866):1829–1839.
34. National MS Society. Treating MS: medications. Novantrone. http://www.nationalmssociety.org/Treating-MS/Medications/Novantrone.
35. http://www.msdiscovery.org/research-resources/drug-pipeline/550-ocrelizumab.
36. Milo R. The efficacy and safety of daclizumab and its potential role in the treatment of multiple sclerosis. *Ther Adv Neurol Disord*. 2014;7(1):7–21. doi:10.1177/1756285613504021.
37. Connick P, Kolappan M, Crawley C, et al. Autologous mesenchymal stem cells for the treatment of secondary progressive multiple sclerosis: an open-label phase 2a proof-of-concept study. *Lancet Neurol*. 2012;11(2):150–156.
38. American Academy of Neurology (AAN). Using plasma exchange to treat neurologic conditions. AAN summary of evidence-based guideline for patients and their families, 2011. https://www.aan.com/Guidelines/home/GetGuidelineContent/472.
39. Karp I, Manganas A, Sylvestre MP, Ho A, Roger E, Duquette P. Does pregnancy alter the long-term course of multiple sclerosis? *Ann Epidemiol*. 2014;24:504–508.e2.
40. Bove R, Alwan S, Friedman JM, et al. Management of multiple sclerosis during pregnancy and the reproductive years: a systematic review. *Obstet Gynecol*. 2014;124(6):1157–1168. doi:10.1097/AOG.0000000000000541.

41. Alwan S, Yee IM, Dybalski M, et al. Reproductive decision making after the diagnosis of multiple sclerosis (MS). *Multiple Sclerosis.* 2013;19:351–358.
42. Krieger S. MS research update 2015. Multiple Sclerosis Association of America, April 2015. http://www.mymsaa.org/publications/msresearch-update-2015/.
43. Holmqvist P, Wallberg M, Hammar M, et al. Symptoms of multiple sclerosis in women in relation to sex steroid exposure. *Maturitas.* 2006;54:149–153.
44. Smith R, Studd JW. A pilot study of the effect upon multiple sclerosis of the menopause, hormone replacement therapy and the menstrual cycle. *J R Soc Med.* 1992;85:612–613.
45. Bove R, Chitnis T, Houtchens M. Menopause in multiple sclerosis: therapeutic considerations. *J Neurol.* 2014;261(7):1257–1268. doi:10.1007/s00415-013-7131-8. Epub 2013 Oct 8.
46. Mohr DC, Goodkin DE, Islar J, et al. Treatment of depression is associated with suppression of nonspecific and antigen-specific T_H1 responses in multiple sclerosis. *Arch Neurol.* 2001;58:1081–1086.

10

Weak in the Knees—Myasthenia Gravis

There were signs that there was something wrong for a while. My husband and some of my friends had thought I was taking prescription tranquilizers, because my voice would start slurring. And my secretary said it had gotten to the point that I would dictate a letter to Mr. Smith and say Mr. Jones. I would forget phone numbers. I was clumsy; I would step wrong and fall . . . I couldn't put the backs on earrings. Or use a little calculator. Little things like that. But because I'm such a Type-A person, I masked the symptoms. Then I collapsed in church on July 4, 1999 . . . after the service, I walked over to hug a friend, and suddenly I didn't know where I was. And my legs were like real rubbery. My husband got me out of there, got me in the car, and drove to the emergency room. The neurologist thought maybe it was a TIA or an aneurysm and was going to send me to a larger hospital, but the doctor on call said it was stress: "Stress does funny things to you," he said. They did a bunch of tests but couldn't find anything, so they sent me home. The following morning, after my husband left for work, I went to brush my teeth and choked. And I panicked. I crawled upstairs to the phone and paged him, and then we went back to the hospital. They did the blood test and they did the Tensilon test. It was unreal. When they gave me the Tensilon, all of my symptoms disappeared. And we cried because we knew what was facing me. I started on medication that day.

Jackie, 64

Myasthenia gravis (MG) involves miscommunication between nerves and muscles. It results from an autoantibody attack on the receptors for a chemical that carries signals between the nervous system and voluntary muscles—the muscles we have direct control over.

Up to 60,000 people in the United States may be affected by MG, three to four times more women than men up until the age of 40. In older age, more men than women are affected. Symptoms usually appear after age 50.[1]

Once considered a fatal disease, MG can now be controlled successfully, and a majority of people with MG live productive lives.

Warning Signs of Myasthenia Gravis

- Weakness or drooping of eyelids in one or both lids
- Double vision
- Eye closing can be weak
- Difficulty chewing, swallowing, or speaking
- Regurgitating fluid up the nose
- Difficulty with facial muscles, smiling
- Weakness in upper limbs
- Difficulty breathing

What Causes MG?

When we pick up a pencil or take a walk, we may not be conscious of directing specific muscles, but our brain has to tell those muscles to move. That message is sent by a chemical called *acetylcholine (ACh)*, released at the *neuromuscular junction*, the spot where the motor nerve terminal meets a folded muscle membrane called the *end plate*. When the brain stimulates the motor nerve, acetylcholine is sent out in little packets (*vesicles*) that cross the space between the muscle and nerve (the *synapse*) and binds to receptors concentrated on the peaks of each end-plate fold. When the vesicles bind to *acetylcholine receptors (AChR)*, it stimulates the muscle to contract. We couldn't pick up that pencil without ACh.

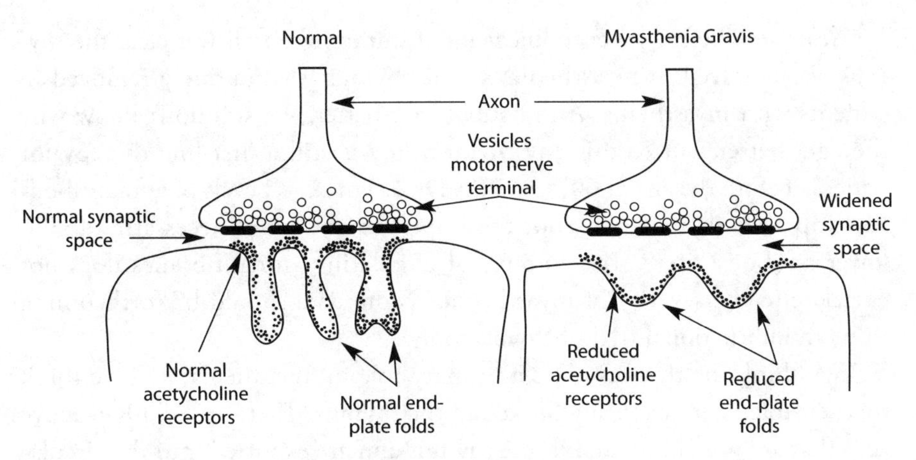

The Neuromuscular Junction

In autoimmune myasthenia gravis, antibodies to proteins on *ACh receptors (anti-AChR antibodies)* cause the loss of those receptors, so that fewer remain.[2] The muscle end plate also loses its folded shape, further reducing the number of ACh receptors and widening the space between muscle and nerve. Anti-AChR antibodies also trigger the deposit of proteins called *complement* at the neuromuscular junction, further increasing receptor loss.[3,4] The upshot: while there's plenty of ACh, there are fewer receptors to pick it up, and the membrane becomes less sensitive.

The effects of ACh are reduced, so there's less chance that a nerve impulse will provoke a muscle contraction, leading to muscle weakness, explains Arnold I. Levinson, MD, emeritus professor of medicine and neurology associate dean for research, Perelman School of Medicine, who has been researching the origins of MG.

"The hallmark of the disease is a marked reduction in the number of receptors but a normal amount of acetylcholine. There is also actual destruction of the muscle end plate by the autoantibodies and complement," says Dr. Levinson. The fewer the ACh receptors the worse the symptoms of MG.

Abnormal cell growth in the thymus may lead to production of autoantibodies. Ten percent of people with MG have small, benign tumors in the thymus (called *thymomas*); 60 to 70 percent have abnormal development of B-cell-enriched areas (*germinal center hyperplasia*) in the thymus, says Dr. Levinson. Thymic abnormalities may result in sensitization of B cells to produce anti-AChR autoantibodies.[5] Defective Treg cells also play a role.[6]

"Years ago, before we even knew about immune cells, it was clear the thymus was involved in myasthenia, so the thymus was routinely removed in patients with myasthenia. And patients got better. We still don't know why they get better, but to this day thymectomy is still a first-line therapy for patients before the age of 60," remarks Dr. Levinson. "Levels of autoantibodies drop after thymectomy, but the improvement is not necessarily due to lower antibody titers. The amount of circulating autoantibodies does not correlate to the severity of myasthenia." More data should be forthcoming from an international trial of thymectomy.

"We think the thymus plays a primary role in myasthenia, and we think that self-tolerance is actually broken in the thymus. There are AChR-reactive cells that are not eliminated in the thymus and are exported into the circulation. We're testing the hypothesis in animals that some inflammatory event allows these T cells, which react with acetylcholine receptors, to travel back to the thymus, where they're activated by locally expressed AChR in people with myasthenia," says Dr. Levinson.

Some research suggests that molecular mimicry may play a role in autoimmune myasthenia gravis, with immune cells mistaking ACh receptors for a virus (possibly a *herpes simplex* virus) or bacteria.[7]

MG may also have a genetic component, since a variety of autoimmune diseases are associated with myasthenia (in both patients and their family members—see "MG Clusters," page 330). It's possible that an inherited defect in immune regulation may predispose people to myasthenia gravis.

Genetic defects also cause *congenital myasthenia syndrome (CMS)*—a group of disorders where abnormalities of the neuromuscular junction cause muscle weakness. However, CMS is not considered autoimmune, and the autoantibodies that attack the neuromuscular junction in MG are not found. CMS is relatively rare and appears in childhood.

Jackie's story continues:

I was lucky I was diagnosed quickly. And I think it was because I had a female doctor . . . I knew, and my husband Joe knew, that I wasn't crazy. But you feel that way when doctors dismiss you and say, "Oh, it's just stress." Even one of my best friends said to me, "Maybe you just need to chill out and take some time off." And really, the symptoms were deceptive. Now we look back and we know what was going on. But I was extremely fortunate.

I've heard horror stories from other women with this disease going two and three years and even more before they're diagnosed. Going from doctor to doctor, and all of them saying it's all in their heads. After I was diagnosed with MG, the doctor who told me it was stress came into my room and I told him, "I'm going to make you a better doctor. You blew off my symptoms as stress, and embarrassed me in front of my family and friends. You have to start to think about your attitude." He needed to know that. And he did change the way he treats his patients. But he wasn't unusual. Many doctors tell a woman who has complaints he can't pin down, "Oh, it's in your head," when he would start doing every kind of test if it was a man. And it shouldn't be that way.

Symptoms of MG

The first symptom of MG is usually droopy eyelids (*ptosis*). Muscle weakness around the eyes (*ocular muscles*) and/or the development of double vision (*diplopia*) are usually what bring women to see their doctor. According to the Myasthenia Gravis Foundation of America (MGFA), two-thirds of patients experience one or both symptoms at first.[1] Eyes may not close completely, and eye movements may be difficult or tiring. For example, looking upward and trying to hold the eyes open may result in eyelid drooping that gets progressively worse.

There can be problems with the bulbar muscles around the mouth and throat, causing problems speaking, chewing, swallowing, and even smiling. Such problems are the initial symptoms in around one-sixth of patients.[1]

Women can also experience weakness in the arms or legs (this is less common as a first symptom of MG, occurring in only around 10 percent of cases).[1] Usually, muscle weakness is less severe in the morning and worsens as the day goes on, especially if the affected muscles are used for long periods of time.

While MG is a progressive disease, it doesn't always cause rapid deterioration. In 10 to 15 percent of cases, weakness is restricted to the eye muscles. Many women will have some progressive weakness during the first year or two involving the mouth and throat (*oropharyngeal*) muscles and/or the limb muscles. But the disease can stabilize over time. "If myasthenia doesn't become severe early on, it may stay on a plateau. For example, if muscle weakness is restricted to the eyes for the first three years, it's likely to remain there in 90 percent of cases. It's unusual for the disease to be mild for 10 years and then start progressing," remarks Janice M. Massey, MD, Professor of Neurology and Chief of the Division of Neuromuscular Diseases at Duke University Medical Center.

Often a woman may have mild weakness and not attach much importance to it, and up to 25 percent of people may see some remission of initial symptoms. So it can be a while before she sees a doctor, especially if she doesn't have classical symptoms such as drooping eyes or double vision. Mild symptoms also may not be constant; ptosis may get worse toward the end of the day, or with exercise, and improve after rest. "In fact, it's not unusual for patients not to realize the degree of weakness they have had until it's improved by treatment," adds Dr. Massey.

Conversely, if MG worsens rapidly over days to weeks, especially in the muscles involving speaking, chewing, or swallowing, that can indicate a case that needs swift and aggressive treatment, says Dr. Massey. "In rare cases we see a patient whose symptoms have been stable for over 10 years get the flu or another illness, something that activates the immune system, and their disease can progress to a more serious level."

In mild cases, a diagnosis may be delayed until symptoms start to worsen, sometimes by coexisting thyroid disease. An overactive thyroid (*hyperthyroidism*) or an underactive thyroid (*hypothyroidism*) can cause muscle weakness, and *Graves' disease* may mimic the eye muscle weakness of MG. In women with myasthenia, mild symptoms that had not caused concern previously may worsen with the onset of thyroid disease to the point where a woman may finally seek medical attention. "Changes in thyroid function, either hypo- or hyperthyroidism, can produce true worsening of disease activity," comments Dr. Massey.

Myasthenic symptoms can be worsened by medications. The most common drugs that affect myasthenia are antibiotics, particularly mycin drugs (like *streptomycin*), *fluoroquinolone* (like *ciprofloxacin*), *macrolide* antibiotics (like *azithromycin*), *botulinum toxins*, *beta-blockers*, and other cardiac drugs, which have a direct effect on neuromuscular transmission. Even nonprescription drugs can exacerbate symptoms of MG—for example, milk of magnesia, because magnesium affects the neuromuscular junction. A partial list of medications that exacerbate myasthenia appears on page 337.

Myasthenic symptoms can also be worsened temporarily by illness (particularly respiratory viral infections), increases in body temperature in hot weather (especially in high humidity), stress, emotional upsets, and pregnancy. "Women can become profoundly weak after walking in the heat or working in the garden. After they cool off and rest, within a day or so they completely recuperate. That exacerbation doesn't indicate a worsening of disease," Dr. Massey emphasizes.

"If a patient comes in whose symptoms have gotten worse out of the blue, I will ask her if she's had a recent viral infection, if she has been put on any new medications, or if she is pregnant. I will also check her thyroid function. Sorting out the causes of symptoms and what may be causing them can be complicated, since there are many factors that could contribute."

Fifteen percent of myasthenia patients will present with thymoma, although this is more common in men. In this case, removal of the tumor and the residual thymus tissue (*thymoma/thymectomy*) can cure the disease.

Diagnosing MG

While muscle weakness is a primary symptom of MG, it's not specific to myasthenia gravis. Again, muscle problems, especially around the eyes, can be caused by congenital myasthenia syndrome or Hashimoto's thyroiditis or Graves' disease, and medications may produce or exacerbate muscle weakness. So other causes must be definitively ruled out.

"A good clinical evaluation with a thorough history is really at the heart of making a diagnosis of myasthenia. Lab tests can be useful, but are not as useful as a good clinical evaluation," stresses Dr. Massey.

Among the tests that can help confirm a diagnosis is a test for antibodies to the acetylcholine receptor and tests that involve electrically stimulating muscle fibers, either a single muscle fiber or repetitively stimulating specific groups of muscle fibers. "We may have to do other routine electrophysiological studies to verify key abnormalities we see on these tests, or to make sure there's no other underlying problem causing the muscle weakness," explains Dr. Massey.

Tests You May Need and What They Mean

Acetylcholine receptor (AChR) antibodies are among several types of antibodies are found in the majority of patients with myasthenia gravis. More than three-quarters of people with generalized MG and around half of those with ocular MG have antibodies directed against the acetylcholine receptor.

But unlike some markers of inflammation, the serum concentration of *anti-AChR antibodies* is not associated with the severity of disease (antibody levels can be low at the onset of MG and increase later on). AChR antibodies are also increased in women with lupus, *inflammatory neuropathy*, *amyotrophic lateral sclerosis (ALS)*, *thymoma*, in women with rheumatoid arthritis taking D-penicillamine, and even in healthy relatives of MG patients. You can even have a false-positive test if blood is drawn within 48 hours of a surgical procedure involving general anesthesia and muscle relaxants. But generally, elevated AChR antibodies—together with key clinical symptoms—confirm the diagnosis of myasthenia gravis, says Dr. Massey.

Anti-striational muscle antibodies (StrAbs) react with the contractile parts of skeletal muscle tissue. StrAbs are found in up to half of MG patients who test negative for AChR antibodies, as well as in older patients and in people with more severe MG. However, since StrAbs are rarely elevated in people who do not have AChR antibodies, the test is not useful for confirming a diagnosis of MG.

The test is useful in detecting and predicting thymomas. StrAbs are found in more than 90 percent of MG patients with thymomas (and in a third of people who have thymomas but don't have MG). Over half of people with an early onset of MG (before age 50) and thymomas also have elevated StrAbs.

Antibodies to muscle-specific receptor tyrosine kinase (MuSK) are found in up to half of people who test negative for AChR antibodies. MuSK is a protein essential in the development of the neuromuscular junction. Recent data suggests patterns of weakness in MG and the response to certain treatments may be different in people with MuSK antibodies.[1]

Ten percent of people with MG do not have detectable serum antibodies to either AChR or MuSK. In these "seronegative" patients, the diagnosis is based on their response to electrodiagnostic testing and cholinesterase inhibitors like Tensilon (see below).

Elevated AChR and MuSK antibodies can confirm a diagnosis of myasthenia gravis.[1]

Electromyography repetitive nerve stimulation (RNS) uses a harmless, low-frequency electrical signal to stimulate nerves, and the reaction in muscle is measured. In people with myasthenia, the muscle response becomes progressively weaker with each stimulation. Multiple muscle groups may be tested. This decreasing response is seen more often in facial muscles, arm muscles (*biceps, deltoids*), and shoulder muscles (*trapezius*). A significant decrease in response to repetitive stimulation in either a hand or shoulder muscle is found in about 60 percent of patients with myasthenia gravis. The response is not specific to MG, but an abnormal finding is a good predictor of the disease.

Single-fiber EMG (SFEMG) involves recordings that can be made from pairs of muscle fibers supplied by branches of a single nerve fiber. It's time consuming and difficult, and requires special expertise and equipment, but is the most sensitive diagnostic test of neuromuscular transmission abnormalities. However, in rare instances, it may not be specific for MG. What's seen is a "jitter" in some muscles in almost all patients with myasthenia gravis. Patients with mild or purely ocular muscle weakness may have increased "jitter" only in facial muscles.[8] The test is sensitive for MG in greater than 90 percent of cases.

The **edrophonium challenge test** is done if electrophysiological studies prove inconclusive or a patient has coexisting problems that may complicate her case. The test uses an intravenous infusion of a chemical called *edrophonium chloride (Tensilon)* to temporarily slow the breakdown of acetylcholine. Tensilon takes effect rapidly, in a minute or less, improving muscle weakness (such as ptosis) if it's caused by the abnormal neuromuscular transmission that occurs in MG. Tensilon's effects last only 5 to 10 minutes. If you have ptosis, and after the injection the ptosis goes away, that's a fairly good indication that you may have MG.

A small test dose is usually given to make sure there's no unusual sensitivity or side effects, such as a slowed heartbeat (a dose of atropine is kept on hand to counteract its effects). The test cannot be given to people with heart problems or the elderly.

The edrophonium test is not completely specific for MG; patients with other conditions may also show a response.

A similar drug, *neostigmine*, can be given as an intramuscular injection. Neostigmine takes effect more slowly and lasts longer, but has less potential for side effects. In some people, a trial of the drug *pyridostigmine (Mestinon)* may produce improvement in muscle weakness that can't be seen after only one dose of edrophonium chloride or neostigmine.

Because thyroid disease occurs so often with MG, thyroid function tests are needed to rule out Graves' disease, hyperthyroidism, or hypothyroidism as a cause of muscle weakness. These tests may include thyroid stimulating hormone (TSH) and thyroid antibody tests.

A CT scan of the chest is also needed to examine the thymus, since many women may have thymomas or thymus abnormalities.

MG Clusters

A variety of autoimmune diseases have been associated with myasthenia gravis (in both MG patients and their family members), ranging from endocrine to blood disorders, and symptoms may overlap. Thyroid disease occurs in up to 15 percent of people with MG.

- Graves' disease, Hashimoto's thyroiditis
- Type 1 diabetes
- Systemic lupus erythematosus
- Rheumatoid arthritis
- Sjögren's syndrome
- Pernicious anemia
- Alopecia areata
- Immune thrombocytopenia (formerly immune thrombocytopenic purpura)

Jackie's story continues:

I was diagnosed with pernicious anemia two years before I found out I had MG; I was told I had rheumatoid arthritis around the same time I was diagnosed with MG, in December. And over the years I had several falls and injured myself, and now we look back and almost all of it was clumsy behavior. So 1 probably had myasthenia for a long time, and probably these other illnesses, too. Now every six months I get tested with bloodwork for thyroid.

The Female Factor

Myasthenia gravis appears to affect more women than men at any age, particularly in their twenties and thirties. During the sixties and seventies the incidence among men increases from that seen in middle age. But things may not be that clear-cut.

"Presumably there's some hormonal relationship, but what that relationship may be is unknown. Some of the more recent statistics, especially with the aging of the population, give a more equal ratio between men and women after age 50," remarks Dr. Massey. As the over-50 population has increased, so has the prevalence of MG and the average age at diagnosis. As far as it's known, there are no sex differences in what occurs in the thymus or in the presentation of the disease, she adds. There may be some ethnic differences in the disease.[9]

However, gender does play a role in the way MG is treated, mostly in the choice of medications for women of childbearing age.

Treating Myasthenia Gravis

Because myasthenia gravis can be so varied and differs in each person, treatment is highly individualized according to the severity of disease, age, sex, and the degree of functional impairment. The major difficulty in treating MG is that a response may be difficult to measure; symptoms can improve spontaneously, or the disease can go into remission, especially early on.

For the majority of women with MG, treatment begins with drugs that slow the breakdown of acetylcholine and relieve symptoms. The second-line treatment is removal of the thymus (*thymectomy*) or immunosuppression. Sometimes they are combined. Newer treatments can provide sustained improvement in many patients.[10]

Cholinesterase inhibitors are the mainstay of treatment for symptoms of myasthenia gravis. *Anticholinesterase drugs* neutralize an enzyme that breaks down acetylcholine at the neuromuscular junction, increasing the amount of acetylcholine and giving it a better chance to be taken up by receptors, which have been reduced in number by the disease process. *Pyridostigmine bromide (Mestinon, Regonol)* and *neostigmine bromide (Prostigmin)* are the most commonly used oral medications, and may be given in combination. Prostigmin can be given by injection. *Ambenonium (Mytelase)* may be used in moderate to severe cases. *Edrophonium chloride (Tensilon)* may also be given intravenously.

"Cholinesterase inhibitors reduce muscle weakness, but do not affect the underlying disease that causes it," stresses Dr. Massey. "These drugs are usually given in conjunction with other treatments, particularly thymectomy in younger patients."

Some women can show substantial improvement with cholinesterase inhibitors, while there may be little to no effect in others. The need for medication can vary from day to day (even during the same day) in response to menstruation, emotional stress, infections, and hot weather. Various muscles may even respond differently; some may get stronger, some become weaker, and others show no change at all. Muscle strength rarely returns to normal with cholinesterase inhibitors, but people can be quite functional.

The side effects are due to the drugs' effects on receptors in smooth muscle, skeletal muscle, and certain glands. These can include: narrowing of the muscle of the iris in the eye, causing the pupil to become smaller; increased nasal and bronchial secretions; and increased salivation and urination. Gastrointestinal effects can include loose stools and diarrhea, queasiness or nausea, vomiting, and abdominal cramps. Cholinesterase inhibitors may also worsen urinary tract infections.

If you have problems with swallowing or breathing, the increased bronchial secretions and saliva can be a serious problem. If too much ACh accumulates at receptors in other muscle tissue (such as in smooth muscle), it can cause weakness and, in rare cases, respiratory failure.

Thymectomy, removal of the thymus, increases the frequency of remissions in MG, and is recommended for most patients, especially if they have thymomas.

The current evidence (at the time of publication) suggests that thymectomy seems to be most effective in people younger than 50, particularly those with early disease, and those with moderate to severe disease who have not responded to other treatments. Improvement in symptoms may not be seen immediately; it may take place gradually over several years. Data are expected soon from an international clinical trial of thymectomy.

Some studies suggest that African Americans may have somewhat less improvement after thymectomy, but not enough to advise avoiding the surgery. "Women, particularly those who have germinal center hyperplasia in the thymus or who were diagnosed in the previous two years, tend to do better after thymectomy," remarks Dr. Levinson.

Corticosteroid drugs, usually *prednisone*, decrease the buildup of antibodies to acetylcholine receptors and speed up the normal death *(apoptosis)* of the cells that produce the antibodies. Corticosteroids are used to prepare patients for thymectomy, and sometimes after the surgery, in people who fail to respond completely. More than 75 percent of patients show a marked improvement, or complete relief of symptoms, with prednisone (usually in the first six to eight weeks), often followed by a total remission. Afterward, some people may be able to take prednisone every other day at lower doses.

Around one-third of patients become temporarily weaker in the first week to 10 days after starting prednisone. While treatment can be started at a low dose to minimize the problem and slowly increased until there's improvement in muscle strength, it's hard to predict when the worsening from prednisone may take place, and it may be confusing. People with early MG usually respond best, but the severity of disease does not predict the ultimate improvement. Patients with thymoma have an excellent response to prednisone before or after removal of the tumor. The major disadvantages of corticosteroid therapy are the side effects (see pages 42 to 43).

For women, the major concern is the development of osteoporosis, and estrogen or bone-building drugs may be needed. "The fact that prednisone accelerates bone loss is something that, on occasion, would lead me to choose another medication over prednisone," comments Dr. Massey. "We do use bone-building drugs, such as alendronate, if there is significant osteoporosis as a complication of steroid therapy. This is something we would closely follow."

Immunosuppressant drugs dampen the activity of the immune system, and may be needed when a woman fails corticosteroid treatment, can't tolerate prednisone, or is unable to take steroids.

Azathioprine (Imuran) reverses symptoms in most women, but the effects may not be seen for four to eight months, and a woman may not achieve a full remission for one to two years. Once there's improvement in muscle strength, it will be maintained as long as the drug is taken; if azathioprine is discontinued, symptoms recur within two to three months. Some women may respond better to treatment with both prednisone and azathioprine than to either drug by itself. Both medications can be started simultaneously, and the dose of prednisone can be tapered once azathioprine becomes fully effective. Approximately one-third of patients have mild side effects (depending on the dose) that may require lowering their doses.

Cyclosporine A is sometimes helpful. It mostly inhibits the T cell–dependent immune responses. Most patients will see an improvement in muscle strength within one to two months after starting cyclosporine, but maximum benefits take six months. After achieving a maximum response, the dose of cyclosporine is gradually reduced to the lowest level that will maintain symptom improvement. Adverse effects include kidney damage and high blood pressure.

Cyclophosphamide (Cytoxan) is now used only infrequently to treat MG. It is used to treat some cancers and interferes with rapidly proliferating cells (including T cells and B cells) and reduces the production of autoantibodies. Cytoxan can be given intravenously or orally. More than half of patients become asymptomatic after one year on cyclophosphamide.

Side effects include nausea, vomiting, hair loss, appetite loss, anemia, thrombocytopenia, leukopenia, and infertility. Antinausea drugs (like *ondansetron*) given to chemotherapy patients can help relieve the nausea and vomiting. Cyclophosphamide also causes birth defects and is contraindicated in pregnancy. Infections are always a risk with any immunosuppressant drug. Life-threatening infections may occur in some people with invasive thymomas.

Mycophenolate mofetil (MMF, Cellcept) selectively inhibits proliferation of activated B and T cells and reduces formation of autoantibodies. It was initially used to prevent rejection of organ transplants but is now used in many autoimmune diseases. MMF is typically given in combination with cyclosporine and corticosteroids and to MG patients with severe disease who don't respond to corticosteroids and azathioprine.[11] A small study presented at the 2014 Scientific Sessions of the Myasthenia Gravis Foundation of America indicated that MMF, like azathioprine, may allow corticosteroid doses to be reduced in some MG patients.[12] Side effects can include an increased risk of infections and some cancers (see page 79).[13] MMF cannot be taken during pregnancy or by women who plan to become pregnant because it can cause birth defects and miscarriage. It can also decrease the effectiveness of oral contraceptives.

Tacrolimus (Prograf, Astagraf XL, Advagraf) is an oral T-cell immunomodulator that dampens inflammatory cytokines.[14] In MG it aids muscle contraction and strength and may enhance the effectiveness of corticosteroids. Like MMF, tacrolimus was originally approved to prevent rejection of transplanted organs and is used in other autoimmune disorders like lupus and RA.[15] It is taken in capsule form, starting with a low dose of 3 mg and slowly increased to 10 mg. Common side effects can include nausea, diarrhea, and constipation. Tacrolimus can lead to high blood pressure, changes in kidney and liver function, and gastrointestinal perforation, so it needs to be carefully monitored by a physician.[15]

Plasma exchange (plasmapheresis) is an exchange of the clear fluid component of the blood (plasma), which contains white blood cells and immune cells. The effect is to reduce the amount of damaging antibodies and immune complexes. Plasma exchange involves several treatments to exchange three to four liters of plasma over a two-week period. It produces rapid improvement, and is a short-term treatment for patients who experience a sudden worsening of symptoms (myasthenic "crisis") or in those rare cases where there's a rapid onset of disease involving the muscles of the mouth and throat (posing the threat of serious airway problems). It's also used to quickly improve muscle strength before surgery and as an intermittent therapy for patients who don't respond to other treatments.

Some women may improve right after the first treatment, or it may take as many as five to seven treatments to see an increase in muscle strength. Improvement can last for weeks or months, making it an effective short-term or stopgap therapy, says Dr. Massey. However, the temporary effect will be lost unless immunosuppressant drugs are given or the thymus is removed.

While most women who benefit from the initial plasma exchange will respond to subsequent exchanges, repeated treatments do not have a cumulative benefit. Plasma exchange is usually followed by thymectomy and/or immunosuppressant drugs.

Intravenous immunoglobulin (IVIG) can be used as an alternative to plasma exchange in cases of severe myasthenic exacerbation. IVIG is usually given over a period of two to five days. It's not clear how IVIG works; it may suppress the production of antibodies against acetylcholine receptors (see pages 370 to 371). Between 50 and 100 percent of patients show improvement, usually within a week, and the effects of IVIG can last for weeks or months. However, recent studies suggest IVIG is not as effective as plasma exchange. Side effects include a "sterile" meningitis (usually manifested as a headache) or, rarely, more serious events such as *deep vein thrombosis (DVTs)* (leg clots that can fragment and travel to the heart or lungs, which can be fatal), kidney failure, heart attack, or stroke.

Jackie's story continues:
Before I was diagnosed, I had planned to go skydiving with a group of people the next Saturday. They didn't think I would do it. But I did. I knew I was fixing to have major surgery . . . they had scheduled a thymectomy for the next Friday, and that's like open-heart surgery. So I said I'm going to do it. And I did. It was awesome.

At first, I was on high doses of Mestinon, but after the thymectomy they tapered it down. Now I'm on normal doses. And I can pretty much do what I want as long as I take my medicine and get plenty of sleep. And I have to take something to sleep, which I don't like. Before all this, give me four hours of sleep and I was ready to go. I went to law school when I was married with two kids . . . now, unfortunately, I'm in bed early. But I'm not complaining; I still get plenty of work done.

I have my ups and downs. When you have myasthenia, your muscles and ligaments are more susceptible to injury, and I've had a couple of knee injuries. I now have an electric muscle stimulator; it's a pad that you put on your legs or arms. You program it, and when it's on you tighten muscles, and when it's off you relax. It's a minute on and a minute off. And that helps to build muscle tone. I try to walk a little, even if it's only 10 minutes a day, three times a day. Recently I started to have hot flashes . . . that's not external heat, but it's heat and it affects you as much as external heat does. So my doctor put me on estrogen, Cenestin, and it keeps them pretty much under control. With the myasthenia, the more Mestinon you take, the more you sweat, especially at night. I woke up some nights just drenched in sweat. My doctor thought it was a combination of the Mestinon and the hot flashes. But if I have night sweats now, I think it's mostly from the Mestinon, and I hardly ever have them. That's one of the best things about my doctor; I could tell her anything. And she took my concerns seriously.

MG Crisis

A myasthenia crisis occurs when muscle weakness in the throat, chest, or diaphragm becomes so extreme that a person can't breathe. In some cases, it can be triggered by a respiratory infection, fever, stress, surgery, lack of MG medication, or an adverse reaction to other drugs, such as cholesterol-lowering statins. MG crisis is a medical emergency that can require artificial respiration.[16]

Drugs That Can Worsen MG

A number of medications, including antiarrhythmic drugs like beta-blockers and calcium channel blockers, as well as antibiotics, are reported to exacerbate symptoms of myasthenia because they block transmission at the neuromuscular junction. These may include:

- Tetracycline
- Streptomycin
- Neomycin (and other aminoglycoside antibiotics)
- Clindamycin
- Ampicillin
- Lithium
- Chloroquine (and other quinine derivatives)
- Cipro
- Propranolol
- Procainamide
- Statins

How Myasthenia Can Affect You Over Your Lifetime

As with other autoimmune diseases, there's a lack of research into how MG affects women at different times of their lives. Most of the information we have is anecdotal, gleaned from the experience of neurologists who treat women with myasthenia.

Premenstrual Fluctuations

Many women with MG report that their symptoms get worse during the premenstrual period. According to the Myasthenia Gravis Foundation of America, it's believed that progesterone is responsible for the worsening of muscle weakness during this period (especially since symptoms improve once a period begins and progesterone drops). However, it may be difficult to distinguish between possible hormonal effects, the effects of premenstrual syndrome, and a true exacerbation of symptoms.

"A small percentage of women report a worsening of myasthenia premenstrually. It's something that the literature has repeated over the years, but it's never been studied, to my knowledge," remarks Dr. Massey. "It really is unclear whether there's a worsening of symptoms or that women with premenstrual syndrome generally feel worse during that time, especially in terms of fatigue or stress, and that affects their myasthenia."

For example, fatigue is usually a product of muscle weakness rather than a symptom of the disease itself (as it is in RA or lupus), she notes. If PMS brings increased irritability and stress, that may worsen muscle weakness and fatigue. Women with myasthenia have to pace themselves and need to make extra accommodations during the premenstrual period, says Dr. Massey. Discomfort from symptoms that are clearly PMS related, such as bloating, breast tenderness, irritability, and mood swings, needs to be dealt with separately and in consultation with a gynecologist.

Pregnancy

Myasthenia itself does not affect your ability to become pregnant, and generally doesn't affect the normal growth and development of a fetus. (In rare cases, *arthrogryposis*, a congenital abnormality causing limb contractures, is seen in infants of MG mothers.)

There is a risk of the disease worsening and of the baby developing a temporary *neonatal myasthenia* (see pages 340 to 341).[17] MG can even be triggered by pregnancy.

"Some women initially present during the first trimester or immediately after delivery. The progression of symptoms can be fairly dramatic over a period of days or weeks. The immune system is markedly altered in pregnancy to allow a woman to carry a fetus, and that is partly hormonally driven," observes Dr. Massey.

However, having MG can—and does—affect decisions on whether or not to have children. A large survey conducted among women with MG found that half had decided not to have kids due to MG.[18] The majority (87 percent) said they were concerned about the possible influence of medications on an unborn child, especially women who were older and who'd had more intensive treatment.

So, prepregnancy counseling is extremely important. "We have no way of predicting how a particular woman will do during pregnancy. If we need to continue treatment, there are safety factors to consider. Women also need to know that they'll need more rest than usual to avoid symptom exacerbations," says Dr. Massey. "The course of myasthenia can be unpredictable during pregnancy. In general, it may worsen early in the pregnancy or right after delivery. However, after that exacerbation, the disease may stabilize again, as it does in MS." There's no way to predict which women will worsen after pregnancy, she adds.[19]

Cholinesterase inhibitors like *Mestinon* have not been shown to cause birth defects, but some muscle weakness has been reported in newborns whose mothers took the drugs. They cannot be given intravenously, since it can lead to premature labor. Prednisone carries minimal risks to the fetus and is used during pregnancy. MMF can cause birth defects and miscarriage. If you experience an exacerbation of MG during pregnancy, you can be admitted to the hospital, where you can undergo plasmapheresis or IVIg, and the baby can be monitored.

Late in pregnancy, the growing fetus can restrict the movement of the diaphragm, causing some shortness of breath. The drug *magnesium sulfate*, given to control *eclampsia* (high blood pressure in pregnancy), exacerbates MG, so other medications must be used to control blood pressure. In rare instances, a ventilator for respiratory support may be needed, says Dr. Massey.

While labor can be extra exhausting when you have MG, the disease doesn't affect the onset and duration of labor, since the uterus is smooth muscle. However, the voluntary and skeletal muscles can become weakened if labor is prolonged, and you can become extremely exhausted. Pain relief medication is given on an individualized basis. Muscle relaxants used during labor anesthesia may temporarily exacerbate muscle weakness. As in women without MG, Cesareans are done when indicated.

"Women with myasthenia need to be followed in a high-risk obstetrical facility, in conjunction with a neurologist, and there has to be close communication by the care team," stresses Dr. Massey. "We usually admit women for the last week or two prior to delivery, so they and their baby can be closely followed."

Breast-Feeding

There's no reason to avoid breast-feeding in MG, but you may find it extremely fatiguing. While antimyasthenics have not been reported to cause problems in nursing babies, Mytelase has not been rated for safety during lactation. The FDA advises caution with Prostigmin, since risk cannot be ruled out. Mestinon is excreted in breast milk, but since no effects have been reported in infants it can be used (however, newborns should be monitored). Steroids are excreted in low levels, and the risk to the baby is considered low, adds Dr. Massey. *Azathioprine*, *cyclosporine*, *mycophenolate*, and *cyclophosphamide* pass into breast milk and are not used in breast-feeding women.

AChR antibodies not only cross the placenta but can also be found in low levels in breast milk, which may discourage some women from breast-feeding.

"Getting up during the night to breast-feed may completely fatigue a woman with MG. It's difficult to deal with caring for a newborn and a chronic disease. Most of my patients opt not to breast-feed so that someone else can feed the baby at night, and because they are worried about medications and the antibody issue," says Dr. Massey.

Neonatal Myasthenia Gravis

Between 10 and 20 percent of children born to women with MG develop a temporary *neonatal myasthenia gravis*. However, having one child with neonatal MG does not necessarily mean subsequent children will have it.

As in neonatal lupus, neonatal MG is thought to be caused by autoantibodies that cross the placenta. Neonatal MG may occur from birth to 10 days after delivery (usually within the first 24 to 48 hours), with the baby showing poor sucking and generalized muscle weakness. Babies may also show eyelid drooping and have difficulty swallowing, and may not display facial expressions because of muscle weakness. In rare cases, some infants may have trouble breathing. Symptoms can be mild to severe, and they usually continue for three to five weeks, until the baby has cleared the mother's antibodies.

Treatment usually involves giving low doses of oral Mestinon every few hours, along with intensive monitoring and, in some cases, use of a respirator if breathing difficulties arise. Blood transfusions rather than plasma exchange may be done in rare instances, but severe cases may require plasma exchange. "Most babies recover completely from neonatal MG. Usually we are able to support and watch the child without aggressive treatment," adds Dr. Massey.

Children can also *develop juvenile myasthenia gravis*. The peak onset of the disease is between the ages of 1 and 4, and between ages 11 and 16. As with adults, other autoimmune diseases can cluster with juvenile MG, especially Graves' disease. The treatment is the same as for adult MG, with thymectomy usually performed after puberty. About 20 percent of all cases of myasthenia gravis develop during childhood; one-quarter of those children have complete remission with treatment.

Midlife and Beyond

While heat can exacerbate MG, hot flashes don't seem to make symptoms worse. "I've actually never had a patient tell me that her myasthenia got worse with hot flashes. No one likes hot flashes, but the heat is brief and may not be enough to truly exacerbate the myasthenia. The core temperature of the body may not really change with hot flashes, so it's more of a perception of heat," Dr. Massey remarks.

The decision to take *estrogen therapy (ET)* for menopausal symptoms is usually not based on having myasthenia. If a woman is taking prednisone, estrogen replacement would help prevent bone loss. "I would defer to a woman's gynecologist in this decision," Dr. Massey adds. In the case of corticosteroid use, other bone-building drugs may be used. "A family history or personal history of breast cancer would outweigh any other factor, for me, in the decision whether to take estrogen."

In later life, there's an increased risk of *pernicious anemia* (see pages 283 to 284), a condition in which vitamin B_{12} is not properly absorbed; this can be treated with supplements. Since it can also be related to aging, older women with MG need to be periodically checked for the condition.

Menopause can also affect the quality of sleep. "Sleep can be a big issue. If you haven't had a good night's sleep, it's hard to deal with your disease. If this becomes an issue, ET might be advised if hot flashes were interfering with sleep," remarks Dr. Massey. Sleep medications like *zaleplon (Sonata)* and *zolpidem (Ambien)* can be used for short periods, without daytime drowsiness.

What's in the Future?

A clinical trial of *eculizumab (Soliris)* among patients with refractory generalized MG (MG that doesn't respond to other treatments) is underway at multiple centers in North and South America. Eculizumab inhibits deposits of proteins called complement. In MG, complement deposits at the neuromuscular junction cause the loss of ACh receptors and the failure of nerve transmission. A small placebo-controlled clinical trial suggests the drug may be safe and effective in MG.[20] Eculizumab is approved for treating a rare condition called *paroxysmal nocturnal hemoglobinuria (PNH)*.

Since autoreactive B cells play a role in MG, the B cell depleting drug *rituximab (Rituxan)* is being tested in people who haven't responded to other MG treatments and seems particularly promising for people with MG who test positive for anti-MuSK (anti-muscle-specific receptor tyrosine kinase) antibodies. Anti-MuSK MG seems to predominantly affect women.[21] Results from early clinical trials suggest that it may produce a favorable response lasting up to two years.[22] Rituximab is given by intravenous infusion.

An experimental drug, *tirasemtiv*, a *skeletal muscle troponin activator*, has shown some promise in improving function and alleviating muscle fatigue in generalized MG.[23] The drug is also being developed to treat *amyotrophic lateral sclerosis (ALS)*, commonly called Lou Gehrig's disease.

According to the National Institute of Neurological Disorders and Stroke (NINDS),[24] other studies involve thymectomy in MG patients who do not have thymomas to see if there's any long-term benefit over medication. Investigators are also studying *autologous hematopoietic stem cell transplantation* (see pages 142 to 143) to treat refractory and severe MG.

Myositis

Myositis describes a group of inflammatory muscle diseases, thought to be autoimmune, that cause degeneration of skeletal muscle tissues, resulting in muscle weakness.

They are *polymyositis (PM)* (*myo* means "muscle," *itis* means "inflammation," and *poly* means multiple muscles are involved), *dermatomyositis (DM)* (which has a distinctive red facial rash), and *inclusion-body myositis (IBM)*.

Polymyositis affects the *proximal* muscles (those nearest to the trunk), including the arms, legs, and neck, and in rare cases the *distal* muscles (those farthest from the trunk, like the fingers); inclusion-body myositis involves both groups of muscles. As with myasthenia, muscle weakness comes on gradually in PM and IBM, sometimes over a period of years. Polymyositis affects more women than men; inclusion-body myositis occurs more frequently in men. Dermatomyositis is more common in women.

Symptoms of polymyositis can include difficulty swallowing or breathing; about a third of patients have muscle pain. In IBM, about half of patients have swallowing difficulties, and there can be weakness of the wrist and finger *flexor* muscles and *atrophy* (or shrinkage) of the forearm and *quadriceps* muscles. In contrast to the other myopathies, IBM often begins after age 50.

The rash of dermatomyositis is distinctive from the classic butterfly rash of lupus; it erupts over the eyelids, cheeks, and bridge of the nose and on the chest, knuckles, elbows, and knees. It's a reddish purple or dusky lilac in color, rather than bright red. People with DM may also develop hardened, calcified bumps under the skin. In contrast to the other myopathies, dermatomyositis can also come on suddenly over days or a period of months. The muscles of the trunk, hips, shoulders, and neck are usually involved. Polymyositis can be associated with malignancy.

These diseases are diagnosed through muscle biopsies, *electromyography* (see page 329), and blood tests. The treatment for PM and DM is high-dose prednisone and, sometimes, immunosuppressants like *azathioprine* (*Imuran*), and *methotrexate* (see page 38). Unfortunately, there's no effective treatment for IBM, although preliminary studies show some benefits for intravenous immunoglobulin (IVIG, see pages 370 to 373). IVIG also helps patients who don't respond to corticosteroids.

Jackie's story continues:

You just have to keep on going. Everything's good when I'm feeling good and my medicine is level; I can do pretty much what I want. But then I get up some mornings and it's all I can do to drag myself upstairs. In the last year, I have tried to put a self-imposed 24-hour limit on a pity party. I can go 24 hours, in my pajamas, lying around and whining "poor pitiful me" and I can cry, and then I make myself get up. There are some days I would rather stay in bed with the covers up. But you can't do that . . . self-pity is worse than any illness. And I'm lucky. Some people with this illness are in wheelchairs. I figure there are two things I can control: my faith and my attitude. The rest of it, you just have to play the hand you're dealt.

Notes

1. Howard JF. Clinical overview of MG, Myasthenia Gravis Foundation (MFA). 2010. http://www.myasthenia.org/HealthProfessionals/ClinicalOverviewofMG.aspx.
2. Mori S, Shigemoto K. Pathophysiology of myasthenia gravis with antibodies to the acetylcholine receptor, muscle-specific kinase and low-density lipoprotein receptor-related protein. Review article. *Autoimmunity Rev.* 2013;12(9):918–923.
3. Kusner LL, Henry J, Kaminski HJ, Soltys J. Effect of complement and its regulation on myasthenia gravis pathogenesis. *Expert Rev Clin Immunol.* 2008;4(1):43–52. doi:10.1586/1744666X.4.1.43.
4. Tüzün E, Christadoss P. Complement associated pathogenic mechanisms in myasthenia gravis. *Autoimmunity Rev.* 2013;12(9):904–911.
5. Nowak RJ, DiCapua DB, Zebardast N, et al. Response of patients with refractory myasthenia gravis to rituximab. A retrospective study. *Ther Adv Neurol Disorders.* 2011;4(5):259–266.
6. Alahgholi-Hajibehzad M, Kasapoglu P, Jafari R, Rezaei N. The role of T regulatory cells in immunopathogenesis of myasthenia gravis: implications for therapeutics. *Expert Rev Clin Immunol.* 2015;11(7):859–870. doi:10.1586/1744666X.2015.1047345. Epub 2015 May 14.
7. Im SH, Barchan D, Feferman T, et al. Protective molecular mimicry in experimental myasthenia gravis. *J Neuroimmunol.* 2002;126(1–2):99–106. doi:http://dx.doi.org/10.1016/S0165-5728(02)00069-3.
8. Chiou-Tan FY, Gilchrist JM. Repetitive nerve stimulation and single fiber EMG in the evaluation of patients with suspected myasthenia gravis or Lambert-Eaton myasthenic syndrome: review of recent literature. *Muscle Nerve.* 2015. doi:10.1002/mus.24745. Accepted article. [Epub ahead of print].

9. Abukhalil F, Mehta B, Saito E, et al. Gender and ethnicity based differences in clinical and laboratory features of myasthenia gravis. *Autoimmune Dis.* 2015. http://dx.doi.org/10.1155/2015/197893.
10. Li Y, Arora Y, Levin K. Myasthenia gravis: newer therapies offer sustained improvement. *Cleve Clin J Med.* Nov 2013;80(11):711–721.
11. Musilek K, Komloova M, Holas O, et al. Myasthenia gravis—current treatment standards and emerging drugs. In: Pruitt, JA, ed. *A Look into Myasthenia Gravis.* (Published online and in print, 2012.) InTech, ISBN: 978-953-307-821-2. http://www.intechopen.com/books/a-look-into-myasthenia-gravis/myasthenia-gravis-current-treatment standards-and-emerging-drug.
12. Myasthenia Gravis Foundation of America, 2014 Scientific Session, November 1, 2014, Savannah, GA. http://www.myasthenia.org/HealthProfessionals/ScientificSession.aspx.
13. Mycophenolate. Medline Plus drug information. http://www.nlm.nih.gov/medlineplus/druginfo/meds/a601081.html.
14. Gilhus NE, Jone F, Owe JF, Hoff JM, et al. Myasthenia gravis: a review of available treatment approaches. *Autoimmune Dis.* 2011. doi:10.4061/2011/847393.
15. Ponseti, JM, Gamez J, Azem J, López-Cano M, Vilallonga R. Tacrolimus for myasthenia gravis: a clinical study of 212 patients. *Ann N Y Acad Sci.* 2008;1132:254–263. doi:10.1196/annals.1405.000.
16. Kalita J, Kohat AK, Misra UK. Predictors of outcome of myasthenic crisis. *Neurol Sci.* 2014. [Epub ahead of print].
17. Norwood F, Dhanjal M, Hill M, et al. Myasthenia in pregnancy: best practice guidelines from a UK multispecialty working group. *J Neurol Neurosurg Psychiatry.* 2014;85:538–543. doi:10.1136/jnnp-2013-305572.
18. Ohlraun S, Hoffmann S, Klehmet J, et al. Impact of myasthenia gravis on family planning: how do women with myasthenia gravis decide and why? *Muscle Nerve.* 2014. doi:10.1002/mus.24556. [Epub ahead of print].
19. Massey JM, Jesus-DeCosta C. Continuum on neurology and pregnancy: myasthenia gravis and pregnancy. American Academy of Neurology, *Continuum* (Minneap Minn). 2014;20(1 Neurology of Pregnancy):115–127. doi:10.1212/01.CON.0000443840.33310.bd.
20. Howard JF Jr, Barohn RJ, Cutter GR, et al. A randomized, double-blind, placebo-controlled phase II study of eculizumab in patients with refractory generalized myasthenia gravis. *Muscle Nerve.* 2013;48(1):76–84. doi:10.1002/mus.23839. Epub 2013 Apr 30.
21. Guptill JT, Sanders DB, Evoli A. Anti-MuSK antibody myasthenia gravis: clinical findings and response to treatment in two large cohorts. *Muscle Nerve.* 2011;44(1):36–40. doi:10.1002/mus.22006.
22. Robeson K, Keung B, DiCapua D, et al. Is the rituximab response in acetylcholine receptor autoantibody myasthenia gravis durable? *Neurology.* 2014;84(10):Suppl S36.009.

23. Sanders DB, Rosenfeld J, Dimachkie MM, et al. A double-blinded, randomized, placebo-controlled trial to evaluate efficacy, safety, and tolerability of single doses of tirasemtiv in patients with acetylcholine receptor-binding antibody-positive myasthenia gravis. *Neurotherapeutics.* 2015;12(2):455–460. doi:10.1007/s13311-015-0345-y.
24. http://www.ninds.nih.gov/disorders/myasthenia_gravis/detail_myasthenia_gravis.htm#268403153. Updated November 2014.

11

A Fury in the Blood—Antiphospholipid Syndrome, Immune Thrombocytopenia, and Vasculitis

It took me almost 10 years to get a diagnosis. I had a history of headaches and started having blood clots in my legs in 1986. The vascular surgeon I was seeing found that my platelets were sky high, and I was told I had essential thrombocytosis. He put me on Coumadin to thin my blood. Almost immediately, my headaches went away, and after a while I stopped having the leg clots. My platelet count went back to normal, so they took me off the Coumadin, and right away I started having headaches again, and I had a mini-stroke. But when I told my primary care physician about it, he said that a stroke was unlikely for a woman my age with good blood pressure and cholesterol. He said it was probably an episode of low blood sugar, and didn't do any tests.

I was in my daughter's room when I had another stroke. I felt this stabbing pain in my head, like an ice pick. I thought I was speaking normally, my words sounded normal to me. But my daughter said, "Mom, your words are slurry and one side of your mouth is droopy. You're having a stroke," and she called 911. When we got to the ER the doctor on duty didn't think I had had a stroke (he also said I was too young, my blood pressure was too good, and so on) and sent me home. But the next day I couldn't get out of bed, and we went to another hospital closer by. They did an MRI and it showed that I had actually had five small strokes. They ordered a bunch of blood tests; one of them was a cardiolipin antibody test. The odd thing was that years before, my ophthalmologist had asked if I had had a cardiolipin workup. He said that anybody with unusual clotting under age 40 should have the test. . . . And in the hospital, after my stroke, the neurologist I saw suspected I had antiphospholipid syndrome. It took me months to get the results of the blood test they did after that stroke. By that time I had gone to a bigger hospital in the city to see a specialist, and he was the one who actually made the diagnosis of antiphospholipid syndrome.

Margaret, 56

Antiphospholipid Syndrome

Antiphospholipid syndrome (APS) is a disorder in which autoantibodies promote blood clots that can affect virtually any area of the body—causing seemingly unrelated problems like miscarriages and stroke.

First identified in the mid-1980s, antiphospholipid syndrome is an insidious disease that may not be diagnosed until after a woman has suffered several strokes, as in Margaret's case. In fact, APS is now thought to account for one-third of all strokes in people under age 50, as well as 20 percent of clots in the veins of the legs (*deep vein thrombosis, DVT*), and up to 15 percent of recurrent miscarriages. APS may have more widespread effects in the body than systemic lupus, since blood clots can block just about any blood vessel, from the tiniest capillaries in the eyes to the large vessels supplying the heart and brain.[1]

The formation of blood clots involves *platelets* (or *thrombocytes*), which originate in the bone marrow along with white and red blood cells, and proteins called *coagulation* or *clotting factors*. When you have a cut, platelets rush to the area to start plugging up the wound. First, each platelet adheres to the damaged blood vessel and becomes activated so they attach to each other (*aggregate*). Platelets are activated partly by chemicals secreted when a blood vessel is injured and by *thrombin*, a protein released during the clotting process itself (activated platelets also secrete chemicals needed for clotting). These chemicals stimulate coagulation factors in the blood and form a stringy protein called *fibrin,* creating long filaments that enmesh the platelets and other blood cells to form a semisolid plug in the wound that stops bleeding. Abnormal clot formation occurs when a blood vessel has not been punctured or cut, in other words, when there's no reason to clot.

This "coagulation cascade" is a complex process; anything that interferes with one step can cause either a tendency to abnormal bleeding or formation of blood clots (*thromboses*). In APS it is thought that autoantibodies react with proteins involved in the coagulation cascade and through still-unknown mechanisms disturb this process, leading to abnormal clot formation in veins or arteries.

APS can cause *venous thromboembolisms (VTEs)*, clots in leg veins called deep vein thromboses (DVTs) that can travel to the lungs (*pulmonary embolus*), or clots in major arteries leading the brain causing strokes or "mini-strokes" (*transient ischemic attacks, TIAs*), or heart attacks. In pregnant women, these autoantibodies can lead to clots in the placenta that block blood flow to the fetus, causing recurrent second trimester (or later) miscarriages.

Antiphospholipid syndrome is five times more common in women than in men, and sometimes runs in families. APS can occur with other autoimmune diseases—40 percent of people with the syndrome also have systemic lupus erythematosus (SLE), and 37 percent of SLE patients have *anti-beta2 glycoprotein I (anti-β2GPI) antibodies*[2] but it can also affect otherwise healthy women whose only outward sign may be repeated pregnancy loss.

Warning Signs of APS

- Repeated miscarriage (generally second trimester)
- Venous blood clots (including deep vein thrombosis and/or clots to the lungs)
- Atrial blood clots, transient ischemic attacks (TIAs), or mini-strokes
- Migraine headaches
- Thrombocytopenia
- Red, mottled rash on the legs (*livedo reticularis*)
- Heart valve disease

What Causes APS?

Antiphospholipid antibodies act against key proteins involved in clotting.

There are three main antiphospholipid antibodies (aPLs)—*anticardiolipin antibodies (aCLs)*, the *lupus anticoagulant (LAC)*, and *anti-beta2 glycoprotein I (anti-β2GPI)*.[3] Recent research has changed our understanding of the targets and actions of these antibodies, so the names originally given to them aren't really accurate descriptive terms.

For instance, the lupus anticoagulant doesn't have anticoagulant properties, but produces an increased risk of blood clotting. And, it turns out, aCLs don't actually bind to *cardiolipin* (a phospholipid found in high concentrations in heart and muscle tissue but present in all tissue). In other words, if you are found to have the LAC it does not mean you have a bleeding tendency. The reason for this paradox is that the autoantibodies react with proteins that in a test tube are needed to make the blood clot, but in the body these antibodies actually promote clots. β2GPI is a protein that binds to cell membranes and has natural anticoagulant properties, so binding to it and preventing its action can be a problem.

These aPLs are present in up to a third of women with lupus, and in women with rheumatoid arthritis, Sjögren's syndrome, and other autoimmune diseases, but they don't always cause clotting problems.

Other types of aPLs can be produced after infections (especially in older people) and do not seem to result in a clot. Infections linked to antiphospholipid antibodies include parvovirus (the respiratory virus that causes fifth disease), rubella, mumps, Lyme disease, HIV, and hepatitis A, B, and C. Additionally, aPLs are also found in women with immune thrombocytopenia (a condition in which there are low platelet counts, see pages 362 to 379).

There are a number of theories as to how these antibodies may come about. "Perhaps you get an infection, and there's inflammation and the cell phospholipids turn over and are exposed on the cell surface. But after the infection and inflammation go away, the normal antibody response doesn't die down, the antibodies start mutating, and sooner or later they start binding to an important blood clotting protein," suggests Joan T. Merrill, MD, an expert on APS and head of the department of clinical pharmacology at the Oklahoma Medical Research Foundation (OMRF) in Oklahoma City.

An infection may also set off another process that leaves clotting-related proteins exposed to an immune system attack. "When there is inflammation, these proteins bind to the surface of the cells of the bloodstream, and may fold in such a way that exposes little pieces of the protein that aren't normally seen by the immune system. Antiphospholipid antibodies may be binding to parts of these proteins that normally stay hidden until they are needed to stop blood clotting. So when the protein unfolds and exposes certain areas, instead of stopping blood clotting, the protein is attacked by antibodies," says Dr. Merrill, an OMRF professor of medicine who also heads up the Registry for the Antiphospholipid Syndrome.

Oxidative stress, the process by which cells react to and are damaged by oxygen, may also be involved.[2] Young women who have the LAC have an increased risk of stroke, but when there's also oxidative stress (from smoking, for example) and other physiological disruptions, the odds of a clot-induced stroke skyrocket.[4]

There may be something about the placenta itself that attracts anticardiolipin antibodies, which cause cell death and other adverse effects that can lead to fetal loss.

Perhaps molecular mimicry might be involved, where invading microbes have a similar structure to clotting proteins, so the immune system attacks both. While the bacteria are eventually eliminated, in vulnerable women immune cells may continue to target the normal proteins. Recent studies suggest that *Haemophilus influenzae* and other common bacteria may trigger production of certain antiphospholipid antibodies in genetically susceptible women.[3]

Several genes are probably involved in APS, and it may run in families. Some of the genes associated with rheumatoid arthritis and other autoimmune diseases (like the DR4 gene) are also found in women with APS, which may explain its coexistence with those diseases. Your genes may also determine the amount of aPLs you make. For example, women with higher levels of aCLs have more clotting events.[5]

I can tell you exactly when this all started. It was in February of 1989. I woke up in the middle of the night with a severe headache and joint pain.

I had had a little fever all week, I developed a kind of rash on my arm, and I was extremely tired. I went to bed that Friday night, and must have awakened around two in the morning in such pain that I couldn't bear to have the sheets on me. It was that bad and that fast. It was like I went to bed and woke up someone else. And the fatigue the next day was just crushing. Not like when you've cleaned your whole house and you're very tired. More like you've been turned inside out. But we thought it was the flu, because that's how flu hits. I had also had periods of confusion before that; I'd be at the grocery store and just stop and wonder what I was doing there with these coupons and this list. I went to my family doctor and he tested me for lupus, for Lyme disease, for mono, everything. But the tests all came up negative . . . and if you're a woman, they say, "Are you premenstrual, are you premenopausal, are you depressed?" Well, I wasn't depressed. I was very happy. I had just met a wonderful man. We don't live far from Yale (where it turns out they were studying this disease). I went there, and tested positive for antiphospholipid antibodies. They also did an MRI and saw evidence that I had had multiple small strokes. They counted a dozen lesions in the midbrain; they looked like little grains of rice on the MRI. This explained the confusion. And that was a relief, because after they run all those tests and find nothing, you begin to feel as if you really are going crazy.

Elaine, 58

Symptoms of APS

Elaine's and Margaret's stories are not that unusual. "Women with APS tend to have dramatic case histories," remarks Robert A. S. Roubey, MD, an associate professor of medicine at the University of North Carolina at Chapel Hill. "A woman comes into the office and says 'I have been pregnant five times and lost all the babies, and I have never been able to carry a pregnancy to term.' Or a young woman has a stroke out of the blue. Or a young woman has recurrent DVTs. Those are the three key symptoms of APS, and they are striking," says Dr. Roubey.

Recurrent miscarriages occur at specific points in a pregnancy in APS. "The most typical fetal loss associated with antiphospholipid antibodies occurs in the second trimester or later, which is a very unusual time to have a miscarriage. Perhaps 10 to 15 percent of these losses are associated with antiphospholipid antibodies," says Dr. Roubey. "While some women experience very early losses, before 10 weeks, they are not characteristic of APS and they can have many other causes, so it's difficult to make an association with these antibodies."

Repeated episodes of blood clots in leg veins (especially in the deep veins) and strokes (major and mini) are the other major symptoms of APS. Deep vein thromboses are dangerous because a piece of the clot can break off and travel to the lungs. Around 40 percent of women with APS experience DVTs, more often in primary APS.[6]

A third of women with APS also have reduced platelet counts (*thrombocytopenia*), often detected during routine bloodwork.[5] Although these women have longer than usual clotting times, they typically don't have bleeding episodes, Dr. Roubey points out.

Other complications of APS include heart attacks (often before age 45), likely due to blood clots in arteries that may be already narrowed by atherosclerosis, epileptic-type seizures, headaches (often migraines), vision problems caused by blockages (*infarcts*) in the tiny blood vessels of the eye, memory problems or dementia caused by mini-strokes (*multi-infarct dementia*), blood clots in the lungs (*pulmonary embolism*), and heart valve disease.[2]

"With heart valve disease in APS, you have fibrin deposits on the valves, most often the mitral valve, which thickens the valve so it doesn't close properly—this allows some blood to flow backward, which we call regurgitation," explains Dr. Roubey. "These fibrin deposits can break off and cause occlusions, and clots can also form on the valve. This also occurs in lupus, and is associated with anticardiolipin antibodies."

APS can cause skin problems, including a red or bluish rash on the legs (*livedo reticularis*), which looks like a "mesh network of veins underneath the skin," says Dr. Roubey.

These problems can appear sporadically, separated by months or years, and seem unrelated.

In some women, a series of clotting-related events affecting multiple organs (especially the kidneys and the heart) suddenly occurs over a period of days or weeks, sometimes after infections, surgery, or giving birth. This is called *catastrophic APS (CAPS)*, and it can be life threatening because clots can quickly affect multiple organs.[7]

When APS occurs by itself it is sometimes called *primary antiphospholipid syndrome (PAPS)* and is more common in younger women with recurrent, unexplained miscarriages. *Secondary APS* is associated with underlying autoimmune diseases, notably SLE and Sjögren's syndrome, and can even be drug induced. More recently they are being referred to as APS with or without associated rheumatic diseases.[1]

Patients are generally categorized by age, sex, and the complications they have, since symptoms may be caused by an underlying problem rather than by APS itself. Finding out whether other family members have APS may help some women to recognize symptoms and be treated earlier.

Around 20 percent of women with aPLs who suffer recurrent miscarriages may go on to develop leg clots.

Diagnosing APS

Any kind of abnormal blood clotting, whether in an artery or vein, and pregnancy losses that occur between the end of the first trimester to the middle of the second trimester should make a physician think of testing for antiphospholipid syndrome.

The presence of the *lupus anticoagulant (LAC)*, *anticardiolipin (aCL)*, and *β2GPI antibodies*, together with clinical signs and symptoms, are the gold standard for diagnosing APS.[1]

Under the most recent diagnostic criteria, you need a history of a clot, and the presence of an antiphospholipid antibody (seen in two lab tests at least 12 weeks apart) to be diagnosed with APS.[1] However, if you have antibodies but have never had a clot, your risk seems to increase along with the level of the antibody. So specific testing for one of these three antibodies (one of which includes a test to measure clotting times) is needed for a definitive diagnosis. Positive tests may help to predict which women are at risk for problems as well as for management of their treatment.

Antibodies are also called *immunoglobulins*. There are several categories of immunoglobulins—including *immunoglobulin G (IgG)*, *immunoglobulin M (IgM)*, and *immunoglobulin A (IgA)*. It's important to know the subcategory (or *isotype*) that the antiphospholipid antibody belongs to (in the case of aCL and aβ2GPI) if you're suspected of having APS, since the IgG isotype is associated with a greater risk of blood clotting. So your blood tests will not only report the level of antibodies, but also their isotype.

According to revised diagnostic criteria for APS,[1] you need to have one or more of the following clinical signs, along with any of the three antiphospholipid antibodies (for aCL and aβ2GPI it can be either the IgG or IgM subtype):

- Recurrent second trimester miscarriage
- Unexplained fetal loss after 10 weeks
- One or more premature births due to severe preeclampsia or placental insufficiency
- A venous blood clot (leg, lung)
- An arterial blood clot (heart, brain)

In addition, these clinical signs may factor into a diagnosis:

- Leg ulcers
- Thrombocytopenia
- Livedo reticularis

Tests You May Need and What They Mean

According to the latest guidelines, APS is defined by the presence of one or more *antiphospholipid antibodies (aPLs)* detected at least 12 weeks apart, plus a history of thrombosis (arterial or venous) and/or pregnancy complications.[1] The rationale for repeated testing is that some harmless aPLs may be produced after an infection or as a reaction to medication and these would be expected to be only transient.[8] There are three important blood tests:

Anticardiolipin antibodies (aCLs) are measured using a test called an *ELISA* (*enzyme-linked immunoabsorbent assay*), in which the clear part of the blood (*plasma*, devoid of cells such as white cells, red cells, or platelets) is analyzed for the presence of antibodies. An ELISA test is very sensitive and can detect even low levels (*titers*) of aCLs and other antibodies. The tests are reported as high titers (over 80 units), medium titers (20 to 80 units), or low titers (10 to 20 units); they also indicate whether the aCLs belong to the IgG subgroup. Generally, titers below 40 are not regarded as worrisome.

The **aCL antibodies** react with a specific type of phospholipid (called *cofactors*) in order to promote blood clots. A conventional ELISA test can detect whether aCLs react to *beta2 glycoprotein I.* Why have this additional test? For one thing, it can be more specific for APS than measuring the titer of aCLs. Studies have also shown that aCLs produced by infections don't react with beta2 glycoprotein I and are less likely to cause clotting. Finding aCLs that react with this cofactor is considered to be a good predictor of clotting (thrombotic) events.[8]

Beta2 glycoprotein I antibodies (anti-β2GPI) can also be detected using an ELISA test. Finding specific antibodies to β2GPI may be a better predictor than ACL of a woman's risk for clotting problems.

Lupus anticoagulant antibodies (LAC). This test is an important marker for a high risk of blood clots and fetal loss. Tests to measure the presence of a so-called lupus anticoagulant include an *activated partial thromboplastin time (aPTT)* test, in which clot-promoting factors are added to a sample of blood plasma from a patient with suspected APS and to normal plasma, and the time both samples take to coagulate is compared. Remember, the name of this test is very misleading because a positive result doesn't mean you are at risk for poor clotting—actually the opposite.

Recent research suggests that the type of aPL may indicate the risk for a vein or artery clot. One study found that the lupus anticoagulant and aCLs were associated with both venous and arterial thromboses, while β2GPI was strongly linked to arterial clots.[9]

Laboratory tests may also include assays for other, less common antiphospholipid antibodies (such as *phosphatidyl serine*); tests for deficiencies in *antithrombin* and in the clotting cofactors *protein C* and *protein S* (these protect against excessive clotting), and for *homocysteine* (a naturally occurring amino acid in the body that is harmful to blood vessels in high amounts and is also a risk factor for clots); and genetic tests for clotting disorders. A complete blood count (CBC) measures white and red blood cells, as well as platelets. The normal range for platelets is 150,000 to 450,000 per microliter (μL) of blood. A platelet count of less than 150,000 is considered to be thrombocytopenia (see pages 363 to 364) and may be present in patients with aPLs.

Magnetic resonance imaging (MRI) may be done if it's suspected that a woman has had strokes or mini-strokes. The damage from TIAs may be seen as small white spots scattered around the brain. You may also need Doppler ultrasound of your legs to look for VTEs, and perhaps pulmonary scans.

The Female Factor

Do female hormones play a role in APS? The answer is unclear.

"It probably has something to do with hormones, but it's not as simple as 'female hormones are bad, and male hormones are good.' There's a very complicated system of checks and balances in which hormones play an important role, and it looks as if people who get autoimmune diseases have a slightly different balance of hormones. But we don't really understand these issues very well," says Dr. Merrill.

Naturally occurring estrogens in the body help to keep blood vessels more supple and seem to prevent clogging and hardening of the arteries before menopause. On the other hand, it's important to know that estrogen increases production of clotting factors in the liver; therefore, adding estrogen (whether in oral contraceptives or postmenopausal hormone therapy) can increase the risk of blood clots. Estrogen can also lower levels of *protein S*, an anticoagulant protein that may be abnormally low in APS.

"So it's a question of balance, what other hormones are present or not present. We do not know that women with antiphospholipid antibodies should not take estrogen. The relationship of hormones to APS requires further study," adds Dr. Merrill.

Elaine's story continues:

You really need to take a careful family history. You can't just ask about one disease—you throw out a name and people may not know what it is. Or someone would say, "What's my thyroid got to do with anything? You have arthritis." People don't make the connections. I know I didn't. And until I was diagnosed and had my daughter tested, because she kept having miscarriages, I never would have connected the dots. But it turns out that my mother had arthritis, colitis, thyroid disease, and terrible migraines and died of a stroke when she was 48. Her father and two of my uncles died of strokes. My eldest daughter has had several miscarriages, she has headaches, and she has Crohn's disease. My other daughter has tested positive for aPLs. So autoimmunity runs in my family, but it never had a name.

APS Clusters

Antiphospholipid antibodies are found in women with a number of autoimmune diseases (including lupus, Sjögren's syndrome, scleroderma, polymyositis, and vasculitis), but they're not always associated with clotting problems. The autoimmune diseases that can cluster with APS include the following:

- Lupus
- Immune thrombocytopenia
- Raynaud's phenomenon
- Inflammatory bowel disease

Treating APS

Treatment for antiphospholipid syndrome usually involves measures to prevent blood clotting. This can include aspirin (which prevents platelets from clumping together) or anticoagulants like *heparin* or *warfarin*. The dose and length of treatment depends on whether you've had recurrent miscarriages and/or clots.

Corticosteroids and other drugs that dampen inflammation and immune system activity are not generally used in women with APS, since it's not considered an inflammatory disease. *Immune thrombocytopenia* (see page 369) can occur in APS, and although it responds to steroids, it may be absolutely necessary to prevent bleeding when there is an extremely low platelet count; the coexisting tendency for bleeding due to low platelet counts and the tendency for abnormal clotting poses a major problem for women receiving anticoagulants. So treatment for women with both disorders can be a delicate balancing act.

Anticoagulant therapy with *warfarin (Coumadin)* is prescribed if you have aPLs and have had any kind of clotting episode (including deep vein thromboses and transient ischemic attacks). If you haven't had a clot and are asymptomatic, aspirin may be prescribed.[10] A newer anticlotting drug, *Xarelto* (Rivaroxaban), is used for prevention of venous thromboembolism (DVT and PE).[11]

Treatment is usually prolonged, often lifelong, because the risk of recurrent vascular thromboses is so high. However, your level of anticoagulation will need to be monitored carefully with regular blood tests to make sure that you're not at risk for bleeding because your blood has been overtreated and does not clot at all.

Monitoring the level of anticoagulation is based on a numerical system called the *international normalized ratio (INR)*. In the past, coagulation standards were set at each lab; the INR is a means of standardizing the coagulation assay. The INR measures the balance of bleeding to coagulation by measuring your actual clotting time against an expected or control time.

Your INR will be measured with daily blood tests when you're first prescribed warfarin, until your doctor is sure clotting time is within a safe range. Blood tests will then be gradually reduced in frequency if your clotting time is stable.

The goal for APS patients with vascular thromboses is an INR between 2.0 and 3.0. At this range there's a higher risk of bleeding complications, so careful monitoring is needed. (A slightly lower level of anticoagulation may be needed in women with both APS and thrombocytopenia.) In addition, other risk factors for thromboembolic events—including high blood pressure and high cholesterol—must be aggressively controlled.[12]

Aspirin and heparin may be prescribed together or separately to prevent miscarriages in women with APS who have had recurrent pregnancy losses.[13]

Women who have had recurrent early miscarriages, regardless of whether they have had a history of clotting episodes when not pregnant, are usually given injections of *low-molecular-weight heparin* twice a day, along with low-dose aspirin (81 mg).

Low-molecular-weight heparin is *fractionated* to include only smaller heparin molecules. Low-molecular weight heparin (*Lovenox, Fragmin*) is generally longer acting and carries less risk of bleeding than regular (or *unfractionated* heparin). This is given by injection.

Prophylactic (preventive) therapy may be needed if you have antiphospholipid antibodies but no other clinical signs of APS, or if you do have APS and have experienced miscarriages but not thromboses, since there's a risk for developing clots later on in life. The first step may be low-dose (81 mg) aspirin.

APS patients at high risk of clots should avoid sitting for long periods during lengthy air travel; this increases the risk of deep vein thromboses (dubbed "economy-class syndrome").

Women with APS should avoid certain drugs that may increase their risk of clotting, including oral contraceptives and postmenopausal estrogen therapy (which increase production of clotting factors by the liver). *COX-2 inhibitors* (like *celecoxib*, see pages 36 to 37) prescribed for pain relief may have less anticlotting effects than aspirin, but there's a possibility that they can also increase the risk of clots.

Careful planning for any surgical procedure in women with APS is essential because of bleeding concerns with anticoagulants. Surgery may also trigger *catastrophic antiphospholipid syndrome (CAPS)* and damage multiple organs.[14]

Since CAPS can be fatal, it is treated aggressively with anticoagulants, corticosteroids, intravenous immunoglobulin, and/or plasmapheresis.[14]

How APS Can Affect You Over Your Lifetime

Fertility and Pregnancy

If you have antiphospholipid syndrome and aPLs, you will probably not have a problem getting pregnant, but you can lose the pregnancy—most commonly during the second trimester, but even in the first trimester.

The negative effects of APS on pregnancy may be due to abnormal function of the placenta. In normal pregnancies, the end portions of the spiral-shaped arteries that supply the placenta are open, and there's no smooth muscle layer, so blood flows freely to the fetus. In women with APS, some researchers have found narrowing of these small arteries, with a thickened inner lining and deposits not unlike those in cardiovascular disease, so blood flow to the fetus can be impeded (*placental insufficiency*).[15]

In addition, can be blood clots and even placental tissue death. Investigators are looking into the possible role of complement in damage to the placenta. Right now, the exact mechanism that causes poor functioning of the placenta in APS is not fully understood, so therapy to prevent pregnancy loss remains aimed at avoiding blood clots.[13]

An estimated 10 to 15 percent of women who suffer recurrent miscarriages may actually have antiphospholipid syndrome.[2]

"In women with clearly established APS, if the last pregnancy resulted in early loss, the chances of the next pregnancy also resulting in a loss are something around 70 to 80 percent, if you don't treat with anticoagulants," says Dr. Roubey. The treatment is generally a low dose of heparin and baby aspirin (see page 359). "There's some evidence that if you just take the baby aspirin, you can get the success rate up to 40 percent or so. But with low-molecular weight heparin, you usually can maintain the pregnancy 70 or 80 percent of the time."

If pregnancy loss occurs despite treatment with heparin, infusions of *intravenous gamma globulin (IVIG)* over a four- or five-day period may be a safe (but costly) alternative.[13]

Menopause and Beyond

If you have APS you should not use estrogen therapy to treat menopausal symptoms because of the risk of blood clots. "Antiphospholipid antibodies give you one risk factor for clotting, and you don't want to add another," remarks Dr. Roubey.

Nonhormonal menopausal remedies might be helpful as long as they don't promote clotting (as does evening primrose oil) or interfere with blood thinners and aspirin (as red clover/Promensil do).

Wild yams, which contain *diosgenin* (a precursor to natural progesterone (used by some drug companies to make prescription progestins), may also relieve hot flashes and other menopausal symptoms without promoting clotting. You should discuss any herbal or vitamin regimens with your doctor. (For details on nonhormonal menopausal remedies, see page 54.)

It's also important to note that the risk of recurrent thromboses may increase with age, so anticoagulant therapy must be continued with careful monitoring.

In 1992, I noticed I was getting these fried-egg-sized bruises on my forearm. If I bit my tongue it would bleed for a long time. . . . I would also have very heavy periods. At the time, I was a systems analyst for a pharmaceutical company. My tongue kept bleeding, and I didn't feel well. I went to a doctor, who eventually ran blood tests. My platelet count was around 6,000—there were virtually none in my blood. He told me I had a platelet disorder. He wrote down the name of the disease. At the time, I didn't even know what platelets were.

Joan Young, founder and former president,
Platelet Disorders Support Association

Immune Thrombocytopenia (ITP)

Immune thrombocytopenia (ITP) is a disorder in which the immune system attacks and destroys platelets in the blood, interfering with normal blood clotting. The disorder was formerly called *idiopathic thrombocytopenic purpura* (*purpura* refers to bruising or bleeding under the skin). It is sometimes referred to as autoimmune thrombocytopenic purpura. In this chapter, we'll use the term *immune thrombocytopenia.*

As discussed previously, when you get a cut, platelets gather in the area and almost immediately start to form a clot to seal off the area and limit bleeding. It's kind of like plugging up a leaky pipe. But if you don't have the materials to create that plug, the pipe keeps leaking. In ITP there's a shortage of platelets to form the plug because the immune system has targeted them for destruction in the spleen. As a result, blood clots don't form properly, allowing bleeding to continue for longer periods.

The spleen is a kidney bean–shaped organ located in the upper left abdomen, just behind your ribs, that produces some of the antibodies and immune cells that help fight off infections and removes worn-out red blood cells and antibody-coated particles like bacteria. Normally, platelets circulate in the blood for 10 days before being cleared by the spleen and replaced by others produced in the bone marrow. In women with ITP, this process of platelet clearance is sped up by autoantibodies at the same time as fewer platelets are made. These antibodies bind to platelets and cause the spleen and other organs to remove them from the blood prematurely. So platelets remain in the blood for only a short time, depending on how severe the disease is. The platelets are destroyed faster than they can be replaced.

A *thrombocyte* is a clotting cell, *penia* means low blood levels; thus *thrombocytopenia* means low platelets.

Since platelets are essential for stopping leakage of blood from damaged blood vessels, severe thrombocytopenia can cause bleeding, especially from smaller blood vessels in the skin and other parts of the body.

Low platelets can lead to prolonged and heavy menstrual periods, and bleeding from tiny blood vessels in mucosal surfaces such as the nose or gums. Bleeding can occur even with a minor injury that doesn't break the surface of the skin, so you bruise easily. Small bleeds can arise from blood vessels beneath the surface of the skin or mucosa, producing small red spots called *petechiae* inside of the mouth and on the legs. When the platelet count gets too low, bleeding can occur without provocation in the intestines or even the brain.

Normally you have 150,000 to 450,000 platelets per microliter of blood (usually written with Greek symbol μL). In severe cases of ITP, platelets are so depleted that the count can be close to zero; in milder cases, your platelet count may hover around 100,000 μL. However, bleeding (beyond bruising) usually does not occur until platelet counts fall below 30,000 to 50,000.[16]

Platelets have another function that has nothing to do with clotting. They store the mood-elevating brain chemical *serotonin*, which has effects not only in the brain but also in the body. Serotonin is involved in mood regulation, appetite, biological rhythms, and our sleep-wake cycle. So another consequence of having too few platelets can be a low level of serotonin, which may cause depression and fatigue. Whether this is the cause of the fatigue that is common in patients with ITP is not known.

ITP can occur at any age, but in adults it most often occurs between ages 20 and 40, affecting three times as many women as men. It can also occur in the elderly. In some cases, ITP occurs along with other autoimmune diseases

---

Warning Signs of Immune Thrombocytopenia

- Tiny spots of bleeding inside the mouth
- Easy or spontaneous bruising (purpura)
- Petechiae on the lower legs and ankles
- Bleeding gums
- Nosebleeds
- Fatigue
- Depression
- Muscle aches
- Heavy and/or continuous periods

---

such as lupus, antiphospholipid syndrome, rheumatoid arthritis, inflammatory bowel disease, and thyroid disease (see page 374).

While ITP can develop slowly in adults, in children it can come on suddenly (usually between ages two and four)—sometimes a couple of weeks after a viral illness—and may resolve on its own after a few weeks or months.

What Causes ITP?

The destruction of platelets and inhibition of platelet production are caused by autoantibodies called *antiplatelet antibodies*. But this autoantibody doesn't directly attack the platelet cell; it binds to the cell membrane and makes the cell a target for destruction by macrophages in the spleen.

You'll recall that macrophages (the "big eaters") are programmed to recognize foreign antigens like bacteria, ingest them, and take them out of circulation. While some macrophages patrol the bloodstream, some are produced by the spleen to help fight infectious agents there. When a receptor called the Fc receptor on those macrophages targets the antiplatelet antibody (which has an Fc part capable of being bound by the Fc receptor) on the surface of a platelet, the macrophage thinks it's a foreign cell and gobbles up the platelet, explains hematologist S. Gerald Sandler, MD, professor of medicine and pathology at MedStar Georgetown University Hospital in Washington, D.C.

Antiplatelet antibodies are produced by B cells in the sponge-like outer layer (*capsule*) of the spleen, lymph nodes, and bone marrow. Even after the spleen is removed, people with ITP may have elevated antiplatelet antibodies. So those B cells must also be present in other organs, like the liver and bone marrow, and in the circulation. The number of antibody-producing B cells may be increased in women with ITP, says Dr. Sandler, who's also director of transfusion medicine in the hospital's Department of Laboratory Medicine.

Numbers are also increased of "helper" T cells, which signal B cells to produce autoantibodies, perhaps telling other B cells to secrete antiplatelet antibodies. Platelet destruction can also occur in the liver (another organ that helps cleanse the blood).

What prompts the formation of these autoantibodies is not known. When the body is invaded by viruses or bacteria, production of antibodies called immunoglobulins may be stimulated. These antibodies may also act against proteins on platelets and function as antiplatelet antibodies. Most of the platelets destroyed in the spleen in this situation have been coated with these antiplatelet antibodies. The amount of platelet surface antiplatelet antibody correlates with the degree of thrombocytopenia.[17]

The structure of the platelets is thought to be totally normal in ITP; it's the antiplatelet coating that's not. "The macrophage is really looking for bacteria coated with the antibacteria immunoglobulin, the body's normal defense. And it will take bacteria and eat it up, get it out of the circulation, if it's got the antibody on it as part of the defense. In this case, we've also got a platelet that's cruising through with an abnormal antiplatelet antibody on it, so that's what's going to get picked up by the Fc receptor on the macrophage," says Dr. Sandler. "So what you have is a disorder where normal-looking platelets get taken out of the circulation by a cell in the spleen because they are coated with an antibody that shouldn't be on their surface."

At the same time, animal studies suggest ITP may in part be due to a problem with the development of platelets from stem cells, the cells in bone marrow that also develop into red and white blood cells.[16] A growth factor produced in the liver called *thrombopoietin (TPO)* acts on stem cells to transform (or *differentiate*) them into cells called *megakaryocytes*, which mature into platelets and are released into the bloodstream. TPO levels are not increased sufficiently to compensate for low platelets. This compounds the situation and may be one reason platelets are destroyed faster than new ones are made.

Infections and medications can also cause formation of antibodies. Since some cases of ITP are caused by drugs, occur after a virus, or worsen after a viral infection may mean that there are environmental triggers. ITP has been associated with Lyme disease, *cytomegalovirus*, *Epstein-Barr virus (EBV)*, *mycoplasmal* pneumonia, hepatitis C, and the ulcer-causing bacteria *Helicobacter pylori (H. pylori)*. Urea breath tests for *H. pylori* can determine if you'll need to be treated for that infection.

"There are infections that you don't completely clear that are associated with ITP. When you suppress them, it makes the thrombocytopenia better. For example, antiviral therapy boosts platelet counts in people with ITP with HIV-related thrombocytopenia or in hepatitis C," says hematologist James B. Bussel, MD, professor of pediatrics and director of the Platelet Disorders Center at the Weill Medical College of Cornell University.

There may be genes involved that increase the risk of developing ITP, but they have not been isolated yet. Potential genetic variations could include a gene that affects the Fc receptor, TPO, or other components of the immune system. "If we could find such genes it would then allow us to do tests in people and determine the optimal treatment for that individual," comments Dr. Bussel.

Joan's story continues:
If I had four hours a day when I could actually do something, that was a good day. I was incredibly fatigued; I couldn't walk out to get my mail. . . . I was obsessed with the marks on my body. I had red spots on my legs, and I would get enormous bruises. I had blood blisters in my mouth that looked like grapes. I went to my doctor to get a platelet count twice a week. Once it was zero; it was very frightening. I tried to keep my brain active with crosswords. I changed my diet, I adopted a macrobiotic diet, and that seemed to help a little bit. Then I got the flu, and my platelets fell to 10. . . . I had a number of treatments, but nothing seemed to work for me. Finally, I agreed to have a splenectomy . . . but two weeks after that, my platelets were as low as they were before. I tried herbs, I went on a macrobiotic diet, I did many other things to improve my health and tried a new regimen of drugs . . . and finally my platelets came back to a normal level.

Symptoms of ITP

ITP typically develops over months or years in adults, and there's typically no spontaneous bleeding until platelets fall below a certain level, usually around 30,000 to 50,000.

Your first symptoms may be heavy periods that last longer than usual. You may have nosebleeds (*epistaxis*), and your gums may bleed during normal brushing or routine dental work. Bleeding can occur even with a minor injury that doesn't break the surface of the skin, so you bruise easily (*purpura* is the Latin word for purple and refers to discoloration from bleeding under the skin). Sometimes this bruising (*thrombocytopenic purpura*) can occur on the arms or legs with no provocation at all, as it did with Joan.

Skin lesions develop as the tiny blood vessels beneath the surface of the skin or mucous membranes bleed, forming small red or purple spots (*petechiae*) inside the mouth and on the ankles and legs. The petechiae don't itch, and they're not raised (in contrast to those in *vasculitis*). Petechiae can merge together and form large bruise-like areas (*purpura*), which may occasionally develop into hemorrhagic blisters (*bullae*).

As your platelet count falls, there may be blood in the urine (*hematuria*), gastrointestinal bleeding, and, in rare cases, bleeding in the brain (*cerebral hemorrhage*).

Some women may become alarmed at the frequency of bruising and seek medical care. In an estimated in 50 percent of cases, ITP is diagnosed during routine blood tests that happen to include a platelet count that show abnormally low numbers. In most of these cases when an abnormally low platelet count is detected incidentally by a routine blood test, the platelet count is not in the very low range and returns to normal in a few weeks of "watchful waiting."

Diagnosing Immune Thrombocytopenia

A diagnosis of thrombocytopenia is made when an abnormally low platelet count cannot be attributed to another cause such as a coincidental infection, a drug, or disease known to be associated with thrombocytopenia. What *isn't* so simple is excluding other diseases that may be responsible for the low platelet count. But keep in mind that levels of platelets between 100,000 and 150,000 do not carry any risk of bleeding. With regard to lupus, the platelet count has to be below 100,000 to be considered one of the criteria for lupus. A number of diseases can cause low platelet counts, including lupus, antiphospholipid syndrome, Crohn's disease, Graves' disease, and *primary biliary cirrhosis*. Other diseases that can cause low platelet counts include *chronic lymphocytic leukemia*, *B-cell lymphoma*, and *Hodgkin's disease*. In some cases, a low platelet count occurs without apparent cause or other diseases (which is where the term *idiopathic* comes from, but it's often used interchangeably) or *nonimmune* thrombocytopenic purpura.

Secondary immune thrombocytopenia occurs in a number of multisystemic autoimmune and other diseases. At least 30 percent of women with systemic lupus erythematosus also have ITP and, in certain cases, it may be the first symptom that presents itself, says Dr. Bussel. Low platelet counts can also occur in rheumatoid arthritis and scleroderma.

However, unlike diseases where antibody testing can help make a diagnosis, testing for antiplatelet antibodies isn't useful in diagnosing ITP. "The diagnosis is based on a platelet count under 150,000, large platelets seen on a blood smear, and an otherwise normal blood count and physical exam, except for signs of bleeding, such as petechiae," explains Dr. Bussel.

Tests You May Need and What They Mean

Complete blood count (CBC) is the most important test for diagnosing thrombocytopenia. But you need the CBC, not just a platelet count, stresses Dr. Bussel. "You need to know the white cell count, the level of hemoglobin, the size of the red blood cells, the mean cell volume, all the red cell indices, to see if there are abnormal cells circulating," he explains.

In some people with thrombocytopenia, either red blood cells may be cleared faster by the spleen because of antibodies directed against them or there's bleeding from heavy menses, so a red blood cell count may be lower than normal.

Hematocrit (percent of red cells per volume of blood) and level of *hemoglobin* (the oxygen-carrying component of red cells) also indicates the amount of red blood cells.

A **peripheral blood smear** can reveal enlarged platelets (*megathrombocytes*), which are frequently seen with ITP and may be a sign that platelets are being destroyed and new large ones rushed out of the blood marrow to compensate. In the test, a blood sample is smeared onto a slide, stained, and viewed under a microscope.

A **direct Coombs test** may be done to see whether red cells have an antibody or complement on their surface (which is important in treatment with a drug called *WinRho*, pages 371 to 373). "You can have the same problem with red blood cells as you do with platelets, where there's an antibody that causes them to be broken down faster by the spleen," explains Dr. Bussel. "We might do this test to determine which patients could receive a treatment that places an immunoglobulin antibody on the red cells to make them a target instead of platelets. But if the red cells already have antibody on their surface, the drug would cause more red cell breakdown, or aggravated hemolysis."

Bone marrow aspiration may be needed in some cases to determine whether the number of *megakaryocytes*, the precursor cells to platelets, is normal. If megakaryocytes are increased, it can indicate that platelets are being destroyed by the spleen. *Myelodysplasia* (abnormal growth of bone marrow), a preleukemic syndrome found more often in people over age 60, can lead to abnormal megakaryocytes and low platelet counts and can be picked up with a bone marrow test. Bone marrow aspiration can also detect leukemia or marrow failure. However, bone marrow tests are not done routinely when tests look entirely like ITP.

Lupus autoantibody testing is highly advisable even if symptoms of arthritis do not exist with thrombocytopenia. Moreover, in some cases other autoantibodies are present (such as antiphospholipid antibodies), such as in lupus. "If other organ systems appear to be involved, it may be appropriate to see whether a woman has lupus. In this case, the thrombocytopenia would be the tip of the iceberg," says Dr. Bussel. Key autoantibodies in lupus include *antinuclear antibodies*, *anti-DNA antibodies*, and *antiphospholipid antibodies* (see pages 72 to 73.)

Thyroid stimulating hormone (TSH) tests may also be done, since there's as much as a 10 percent overlap with hypothyroidism in ITP, Dr. Bussel adds (see page 374).

Treating Immune Thrombocytopenia

ITP is an unpredictable disease. Some women simply have lowered platelet counts, but never progress to bleeding or other symptoms, and no treatment is needed. Other women may have platelet counts so perilously low that they are in danger of cerebral hemorrhage or other life-threatening bleeds, and immediate intervention is needed.

"There are really no hard-and-fast numbers. But in general, if your platelets are greater than 30,000, we don't start treatment unless you have symptoms, bleeding, need to undergo surgery, or are participating in at-risk activities like sports, or are fatigued without another explanation," says Dr. Bussel. "For newly diagnosed women whose platelets are under 10,000 or with bleeding symptoms, we would give IVIG in combination with prednisone. In some cases the platelet count will return to normal levels and retreatment may not be needed. Unfortunately, there's no way to predict which women will respond and which will need more therapy."

The most effective treatment to rapidly increase platelet counts—*intravenous immunoglobulin (IVIG), intravenous Rh (D) immune globulin (IV RhIG, WinRho),* and steroids—interfere with the destruction of platelets. Removing the spleen (*splenectomy*), and in certain cases rituximab, are the only curative treatments for ITP; splenectomy eliminates the main site of platelet destruction.

However, after the surgery, the destruction of platelets can resume in other organs, like the liver, even after many years of normal platelet counts. For this reason, it is generally accepted that there may be long-term remissions, but there is no "cure" for ITP, explains Dr. Sandler. Oral corticosteroids are the most commonly used nonsurgical treatment to maintain the platelet count.

Because of the serious side effects, women cannot continually take high doses and, in some patients, a short course of steroids followed by IVIG or WinRho will bring about a long-term remission.

Corticosteroids, most often prednisone, suppress overall immune function, decreasing the destruction of platelets and possibly increasing platelet production. The usual dose is 1 milligram of prednisone per kilogram of body weight (2.20 pounds) a day for up to two weeks until platelet counts come up to a "safe" level (over 30,000). The drug is then tapered off.

"No medication that can be taken orally has been shown to get the count up higher and quicker than prednisone. For this reason, it is usually part of all initial treatments for ITP," remarks Dr. Sandler. "Steroids are more useful for acute treatment, which we call induction, than they are for keeping platelet counts up over the long term, which we call maintenance."

Because of the side effects of high-dose steroids, they are not optimally continued for more than four weeks at a time. However, some women may need repeated cycles or prolonged use of steroids, increasing the risk of hypertension, diabetes, cataracts, and bone loss.

Intravenous immunoglobulin (IVIG) is prepared from human plasma and contains immunoglobulins for IgG, or gamma globulin. IVIG may work by blocking the receptors on macrophages that look for platelets coated with the

IgG antiplatelet antibody. "On these receptors there's a lock-and-key mechanism. If we flood the circulation with these other IgG molecules, then they're going to fit into the lock on that receptor and let the platelets go free," explains Dr. Sandler. "We call it a medical splenectomy. The spleen can't do two things at once, and if you occupy it with some other molecule, it won't eat platelets. You're really taking the spleen out of action." Recent research suggests that IVIG actually turns on inhibitory receptors and in that way prevents platelets from getting destroyed. IVIG may also increase the rate at which antibodies to platelets remain in the circulation. Thus, there are many possible mechanisms to explain the efficacy of IVIG.

Although IVIG can raise platelet counts within a day or so, large doses are required, which take three or more hours to be infused into the body. IVIG is also expensive—around $5,000 or more per infusion. Adverse side effects can include sudden headaches, backaches, flushing, chills, and (rarely) irritation of the membranes around the brain (*aseptic meningitis*) or kidney dysfunction and failure. The platelet count starts going down within days of an infusion as receptors become cleared of the IgG, so by the end of two to four weeks another infusion may be needed. However, the side effects are not as toxic as those of high-dose steroids (and IVIG doesn't cause bone loss).

Intravenous Rh (D) immune globulin *(IV RhIG, WinRho)* is also prepared from human immunoglobulins in plasma, but contains a specific antibody to a marker on red blood cells called D, making them a target instead of platelets. The drug is dubbed *anti-D.*

RhD is a protein (called an *antigen*) on the surface of the blood cells of 85 percent of people; they are considered Rh-positive. If you don't have it, you're Rh-negative.

Rh is used in blood typing, along with blood grouping (whether or not there are specific antigen markers on blood cells that make your blood type A, B, O, or AB as well as Rh positive or negative), to match donor blood with a recipient. Blood antibodies react to the antigens of the *same* type, causing blood cells to clump together and clog blood vessels. Type A blood has the A antigen, and type B has the B antigen. So if you have type A blood you can only accept a transfusion of type A blood; type B can only receive type B.[18]

There are two exceptions. Someone with type O Rh-negative blood is considered a "universal donor" because Type O has *no* antigens for type A or B blood and *no* antigens to Rh. Type AB positive blood is the "universal recipient" because that blood type has *both* A and B antigens, as well as Rh antigens. So "cross-matching" between blood types is vital.

(Rh becomes important in pregnancy. If an Rh-negative mother is pregnant with an Rh-positive fetus, the mother's blood develops antibodies to the fetus' Rh antigens. It's usually not a problem in the first pregnancy, but in subsequent pregnancies, the anti-Rh antibodies will clump the fetal blood. So the mother will need treatment with another special immune globulin preparation to destroy any Rh-positive cells of fetal blood that may get into her circulation, so the mother's immune system will not produce antibodies to Rh.)

When the "anti-D" drug is given to Rh (D)-positive women with ITP who haven't had a splenectomy, it prompts the immune system to order macrophages to target the D protein marker on red blood cells. "Anti-D goes onto normal red blood cells much as the IgG antibody attaches to platelets. Red cells are larger than platelets, and since these people have a normal red count, there are more coated red cells than platelets. So the red cells go in and literally stuff the mouth of the macrophage and the platelets are spared," explains Dr. Sandler.

The normal life of a red cell is around 120 days; WinRho accelerates the process of removal and keeps the macrophages in the spleen busy gobbling red cells. Platelet counts begin to rise within one to two days after an infusion of WinRho, and peak within a week or two. The response can last up to 30 days before another infusion is needed.

Studies of anti-D have shown a response rate of over 70 percent, bringing platelet counts to over 100,000 in many people, depending on the dose. It also contains special "detergents" and solvents that destroy viruses (such as hepatitis B and C) and remove other viruses, ensuring the drug's safety (since it's made from human plasma). WinRho takes around five minutes to infuse (a quick infusion is called a *push*), has fewer side effects, and is less costly than IVIG. But again, it works only in Rh (D)-positive women and those who have not had a splenectomy. In rare cases, WinRho may also cause excessive red cell breakdown. When red cells are broken up too quickly, hemoglobin is released in the bloodstream and excreted in urine, turning it pink.

The direct Coombs test may be able to identify patients at risk for excess hemolysis. A dose of prednisone before an infusion will help prevent fever and chills.

Anti-D may be used in adults as maintenance therapy. Studies show around 75 percent of patients respond, and continued treatments as needed will lead to resolution within six months in one-third to one-half of people, who will then need no further treatment, says Dr. Bussel.

WinRho is as effective as IVIG for maintaining remissions and is less toxic. However, only 85 percent of patients are Rh (D)-positive. For the remaining 15 percent of women who are Rh (D)-negative, infusions of IVIG may be used as maintenance therapy. However recent information suggests that IVIG may have mild curative effects.

If IVIG or WinRho infusions every three or four weeks maintain a safe platelet count, there's no reason to consider immediate splenectomy in most cases, remarks Dr. Sandler.

Splenectomy is 80 percent effective in bringing up platelet counts within days, and up to 65 percent of patients will have a lasting and substantial increase in platelets. Despite its function as a blood filter and fighter of infections, the spleen is actually not an essential organ. Once it's removed, many of its jobs are taken over by other parts of the lymphatic system; the liver filters the blood, and antibodies can be produced elsewhere. And the destruction of platelets will also take place elsewhere in the body, notably in the liver. You may also have small "accessory" spleens, which must be removed with the primary spleen. Splenectomy also carries a very small risk of serious infections.

The surgery can now be done laparoscopically, using small incisions, rather than as major abdominal surgery; you remain in the hospital for one to three days and can resume most normal routines in a week. Splenectomy may be riskier in older people and is done less frequently after age 65.

Unfortunately, some women's platelet counts do not go back up after treatment with prednisone, IVIG or WinRho, and splenectomy. "These are the most difficult people to treat, so we use a combination of drugs, which is more effective than single agents but can be more toxic," says Dr. Bussel. These can include a male hormone, *danazol (Danocrine)*; immune-suppressing agents such as *azathioprine (Imuran)*, *mycophenolate mofetil (CellCept)*; and chemotherapy drugs *vincristine (Oncovin)* or *vinblastine (Velban)*, *cyclophosphamide (Cytoxan)*, and *rituximab (Mabthera)*.

Romiplostim (Nplate)[19] **and eltrombopag (Promacta)**[20] are *thrombopoietin receptor agonists*, synthetic proteins that act similarly to thrombopoietin in the body to increase platelet production. They mimic the effects of natural thrombopoietin.

Nplate is given as a weekly injection under the skin.[21] Promacta comes in tablet form and needs to be taken on an empty stomach (two hours after a meal) and four hours before or after calcium intake, including any dairy products.[22] Both medications can cause increased blood clotting and must be monitored. They are not used in pregnant women, since they would be expected to cross the placenta into the fetus.

Other drugs that can raise platelet counts in severe unresponsive ITP include *colchicine* and *cyclosporine* (which may be more toxic).

Danazol is a weakened version of testosterone and causes a temporary menopause as well as androgenic side effects like acne, growth of facial hair, and a rise in LDL cholesterol. It may cause liver problems, so liver function tests must be normal before danazol is used and women on this drug must be monitored. For most people, it's very well tolerated and can help in weaning them off steroids.

If you have any neurological problems, vincristine can't be given, since it causes nerve damage. If you've been in remission and platelets start to fall again, corticosteroids and, in some cases, a combination of vincristine, IVIG, Solu-Medrol, danazol, and/or azathioprine are given.

Rituximab (Rituxan), which rapidly depletes peripheral B cells, is also effective in treating ITP, especially when used in combination with high doses of the corticosteroid *dexamethasone*.[23] Rituximab reduces cells that are the precursors of the antibody secreting type of B cells that produce both antibodies and autoantibodies, including antibodies that attach to platelets.[24]

ITP Clusters

ITP is seen in as many as 30 percent of women with lupus and in other autoimmune diseases. In some cases, your doctor will monitor platelet counts as part of your regular bloodwork. However, you should be alert for symptoms of ITP if you have any of the following autoimmune diseases:

- Antiphospholipid syndrome
- Rheumatoid arthritis
- Scleroderma
- Graves' disease, Hashimoto's thyroiditis
- Inflammatory bowel disease (Crohn's disease, ulcerative colitis)
- Primary biliary cirrhosis

I was diagnosed when I was 22. I was in my senior year in college in California, and I was feeling extremely fatigued. At first I chalked it up to staying up half the night to study; I wanted to graduate with highest honors. But after I had the flu that winter, I never really recovered. And I started to notice these little blood blister things in my mouth and had a couple of bad nosebleeds. I went to the university's medical center—we had a major medical school there—and the blood tests came back showing that my platelets were extremely low, around 1,900 . . . a hematologist explained that I had thrombocytopenia, that my platelets were disappearing from my body, and that the flu virus had probably made it worse. I figured they would be giving me a blood transfusion or something (that's how little I knew then), but they put me on steroids, 60 milligrams of prednisone, which they said would bring my platelet count up. It did, but the side effects were awful. My face ballooned, I gained 30 pounds, and I had mood swings. They finally tapered me off it when my counts went up to 230,000. I was thrilled to be off that drug!

I went to our medical library and started reading all I could about this disease, and what I read really scared me to death. I had always had very heavy periods, which seemed to go on forever; I figured that was just me. But I must have had ITP since my teens. The disease changed a lot of my habits; I stopped shaving my legs and used a cream hair remover. I bought an electric toothbrush so I wouldn't brush my teeth too hard (once I ended up with a mouthful of blood after I accidentally bit my tongue). I stopped playing handball (which I used to love), because I was afraid of the bruising. After I got off the prednisone, I worked hard at losing the weight and my face started to look normal. My fiancé and I had planned to be married at Christmastime and I wanted to look nice. I made it through the wedding, and then my platelets dropped again and I was right back on prednisone. I went through three cycles of the stuff and my platelets finally seemed to stabilize, and I thought I was out of the woods.

When I was 27 I became pregnant. Fortunately, my hematologist referred me to an OB who had handled a number of ITP pregnancies. My platelets stayed in the 90s during my first and second trimester, but when they started falling again, I was back on prednisone. My OB assured me that prednisone would not harm my baby, but there was an outside chance that my baby would be born with ITP. When Callie was born they found she had a platelet count of 28,000, so they took her to the neonatal intensive care unit, and she stayed there for a few days. She was put on a liquid form of prednisone for four weeks, and her platelet count went up to 250,000 and has stayed normal ever since, thank God. After that, I decided to have a splenectomy—I was tired of the way this disease seemed to dominate my life. My platelets have been normal ever since the surgery, and we hope to have a second child. The only catch is that my ITP could come back during pregnancy. But it's a chance I guess I'll take.

Audrey, 32

How ITP Can Affect You Over Your Lifetime

Having low platelets can affect menstrual periods and can complicate pregnancy; some cases of ITP may even be caused by pregnancy.

Menstruation and Fertility

Low platelet counts that delay clotting can cause very heavy menstrual periods that last longer than a week. For some women who have had ITP for years with no other symptoms, heavy periods may simply seem "normal." Iron replacement may be important.

Some women who experience heavy menstrual bleeding take oral contraceptives (OCs) to regulate their cycles and lessen bleeding. While this is generally safe for most women with ITP, a few will have the estrogen component of the oral contraceptives worsen their ITP. Therefore when possible we use OCs low in estrogen and high in progesterone, says Dr. Bussel.

But a note of caution. Some women with low platelets have antiphospholipid antibodies as described earlier in this chapter. For those women who test positive for these antibodies, birth control pills containing estrogens may be dangerous in that they increase the risk of blood clotting. So it is wise to have aPL checked before going on birth control pills if you have a history of ITP. It may seem paradoxical that low platelets that cause bleeding can be associated with aPL that can cause blood clotting; however this is a situation that can happen.

Pregnancy and Postpartum

Many cases of ITP are first diagnosed during pregnancy, and, in fact, the disease can be triggered by pregnancy. (There is a separate, nonautoimmune problem called gestational thrombocytopenia that often occurs during the third trimester, where platelet counts may drop slightly to around 80,000 but return to normal after delivery.)

It was previously thought that pregnant women with ITP might experience some worsening of their disease. But this may not always be the case, says Daniel W. Skupski, MD, professor of OB/GYN at the Weill Medical College of Cornell University.

Dr. Skupski and colleagues studied 96 pregnancies in 53 women over a 16-year period to look at the severity of ITP in pregnancy, recording how often women had bleeding episodes (especially around the time of delivery), and kept track of whether the disease worsened or improved over time. "Major bleeding complications were limited to one case of early placental separation and four cases of postpartum hemorrhage, which is no different from the rate of these types of problems in women without ITP," says Dr. Skupski. "It appeared that, as a general rule, ITP improved in the early part of pregnancy, returned to baseline later in pregnancy, was not different in severity during pregnancy as opposed to when not pregnant, and did not appear to worsen in subsequent pregnancies."

During pregnancy your platelet counts will be monitored, and if need be, you'll be put on oral corticosteroids if they drop too low. IVIG is used only when clearly indicated. "Our experience with IVIG is that it doesn't produce problems for the pregnancy or for the fetus," says Dr. Skupski. When platelet counts were below 50,000 around the thirty-eighth week of pregnancy, treatment with IVIG produced an increased count such that labor could be induced and epidural anesthesia could safely be used. Premature births do not seem to be associated with ITP.

Marked neonatal thrombocytopenia can occur in up to 15 percent of infants born to women with ITP, because of maternal antibodies crossing the placenta. Having a previous baby born with thrombocytopenia increases the chance another child will be affected. Your platelet count does not have any bearing on your baby's.[25] That's because autoantibodies against the platelets may be present in the mother but not necessarily result in low counts. However when crossing the placenta, which all IgG isotypes do, they can attack the fetal platelets.

In neonatal thrombocytopenia, a baby may be born with a low platelet count or platelets may begin to drop in the first week after delivery. Oral corticosteroids and intravenous immunoglobulin can help bring platelet counts up. However, the baby's platelet count usually stabilizes and starts to rise within three to four weeks, as maternal antibodies gradually decrease (interestingly maternal antibodies may not fully clear until about six months).

While ITP itself doesn't appear to worsen because of pregnancy, in some women platelet counts may settle at a lower level after giving birth and dip further with each subsequent pregnancy, says Dr. Skupski. This may be because the disease tends to worsen over time, rather than any effect of pregnancy. And it does not necessarily cause bleeding or other symptoms.

Menopause and Beyond

Estrogen therapy (ET) for menopausal symptoms may lower platelet counts in some women with ITP, says Dr. Bussel. Preliminary studies suggest that taking a higher dose of progestin for 10 days every month together with estrogen may counter those effects. Progestin also prevents overgrowth of cells in the uterus that can lead to cancer, and women who have not had a hysterectomy are generally advised to take combined hormone replacement therapy.

"However, because it can lower platelet counts, I generally do not advise women to take estrogen for osteoporosis prevention. There are other drugs that are more effective for this purpose," he adds. "If a woman feels that she needs estrogen for menopausal symptoms, I would advise her to do so in conjunction with measuring platelet counts regularly, to make sure it is not having any adverse effects on her ITP."

Nonhormonal menopausal remedies may be helpful for some women. However, red clover (sold under the brand name of *Promensil*) can promote bleeding and should not be used by women with bleeding disorders like thrombocytopenia.

If you've ever taken prednisone or other corticosteroids, you have an increased risk of osteoporosis, so you should have regular bone mineral density testing, especially after menopause. You also need to take supplemental calcium and vitamin D, and possibly drugs, to prevent or treat osteoporosis. (See page 57.)

As you get older, you're more likely to be taking one or more medications for other health problems, such as high blood pressure or high cholesterol. There are prescription drugs (as well as over-the-counter drugs and supplements) that can lower platelet counts. For example, the cholesterol-lowering drug *atorvastatin (Lipitor)* binds to plasma proteins and may infrequently cause severe thrombocytopenia. Tylenol can also reduce platelet counts, as can the heartburn medicine *cimetidine (Tagamet).*

Women with cardiovascular disease may need low-dose aspirin (81 mg a day), but it needs to be monitored carefully. "I advise women to take aspirin if their platelet counts are 50,000 to 60,000 and they are stable. They will get the same benefits from aspirin just as other people with cardiovascular disease do," says Dr. Bussel. "If you don't take prophylactic aspirin because you have ITP, and your platelet counts improve, you can run the risk of strokes and heart attacks. So it is something that must be used cautiously."

Other drugs for heart-related conditions can affect platelet counts, including diuretics like *chlorothiazide* and *chlorthalidone*; *digoxin* (any digitalis preparation); calcium channel blockers like *diltiazem* (*Cardizem*), and antiarrhythmics such as *procainamide (Pronestyl-SR).*

Many commonly used antibiotics like *ampicillin*, *cephalosporin*, and *sulfamethoxazole* can also affect platelet counts. So alert your hematologist to all medications you're taking.

Vasculitis

Vasculitis means inflammation of blood vessels, and the different disorders that result (*vasculitides*) can affect every type of blood vessel from the major arteries to the tiny capillaries, from small venules to large veins.

Inflammation from vasculitis causes two types of damage. It can weaken a section of the blood vessel wall, causing it to stretch and bulge out like a tiny balloon (an *aneurysm*). In rare cases, the bulging vessel wall can become so weak that it ruptures and bleeds. In other cases, the inflamed blood vessel wall becomes narrowed, restricting blood flow (*ischemia*). A blood vessel may even close off (*occlusion*), blocking blood flow altogether. Sometimes the body compensates for hampered blood supply by rerouting blood to other blood vessels (*collateral blood supply*), but sometimes there simply isn't enough collateral flow and the affected tissue dies (*infarction*).

Vasculitis can affect one organ, such as the kidneys, or it can affect several organ systems at once (*systemic vasculitis*); symptoms can vary depending on the parts of the body affected. Vasculitis is often called the "great mimicker" because its symptoms can mimic those of other diseases.

Women are at particular risk for two types of systemic vasculitis: *Takayasu's arteritis*, which affects the aorta and its branches, and *giant cell arteritis* (*GCA*, also called *temporal arteritis*), an inflammation of the arteries that primarily supply the head.

Other types of systemic vasculitis include *polyarteritis nodosa*, *eosinophilic granulomatosis with polyangiitis (EGPA)*, formerly termed *Churg-Strauss syndrome*, and *granulomatosis with polyangiitis (GPA)*, formerly called *Wegener's granulomatosis*.[26]

Different forms of vasculitis are now classified in terms of the size of the blood vessels that are affected. GCA and Takayasu's are both considered **large vessel vasculitis** under this new nomenclature.[27] Vasculitides that affect **medium-sized** vessels are polyarteritis nodosa and Kawasaki disease. **Small vessel vasculitis** is associated with *antineutrophil cytoplasmic antibodies (ANCA)*. ANCA-associated vasculitis includes GPA and EGPA (a rare disease).

Takayasu's is nine times more common in women and typically occurs before age 40; GCA affects two to three times more women than men, usually later in life.

GPA affects men and women equally at any age and can be life threatening. It most often affects the upper respiratory tract (the sinuses, nose, and trachea) but can also cause problems in the ears, eyes, skin, lungs, heart, kidneys, and the nervous system.

What Causes Vasculitis?

Some forms of vasculitis are thought to be separate from autoimmune diseases, while others are a consequence of systemic inflammatory disease that can inflame and damage blood vessels, such as scleroderma or lupus.

There are autoantibodies that act against components of blood vessel walls, including the cells lining the inside of the vessel (*endothelial cells*) and the thin cell membrane that separates the vessel lining from the smooth muscle (*basement membrane*). When autoantibodies attack the vessel wall, it causes immune complexes to form inside the wall and attract inflammatory cells. (Immune complexes are latticelike structures created when antibodies bind to antigens.) Immune complexes that form in the blood of lupus patients may also attach themselves to the endothelial cells, damaging the blood vessel lining. Some evidence suggests that this may also occur in rheumatoid arthritis and in Sjögren's syndrome. Autoantibodies in diseases like lupus may also cause blood vessel damage.

The vasculitides that occur independently such as *giant cell arteritis* or *Takayasu's arteritis*, are believed to be caused by damage from autoreactive T cells, which provokes an inflammatory reaction in the blood vessel wall. Overexpression of the inflammatory cytokine *tumor necrosis factor alpha (TNFα)*, involved in diseases like rheumatoid arthritis and Crohn's disease, is also thought to contribute to vasculitis.

Much of the pathophysiology of vasculitic diseases has not been worked out. Different immune cell types are in each, and different layers of the vessel wall are affected.

Vasculitis can also be triggered by a past or present infection (including hepatitis) that leads to formation of immune complexes, by certain cancers, or by an allergic reaction to medication (such as sulfa drugs, *sulfonamides*). In most cases the trigger is not known.

Genes also play a role. Some forms of vasculitis cluster in families and may affect certain racial groups more often. Caucasians (especially those of Scandinavian descent) are more prone to temporal arteritis and polymyalgia rheumatica (PMR); Asian women are more susceptible to Takayasu's arteritis.

Symptoms of Vasculitis

The symptoms of vasculitis can be nonspecific; inflammation can often provoke body-wide symptoms such as fever, fatigue, aches, and a general feeling of just being ill. There may be appetite loss, weight loss, and an absence of energy.

Other symptoms depend on the area of the body or even the type of blood vessel that's affected, says Hal J. Mitnick, MD, a clinical professor of medicine at the New York University School of Medicine with a special expertise in vasculitis. "Vasculitis affects the venous system more often than the arterial system, probably because veins are 'leakier' than arteries." explains Dr. Mitnick. The damage caused by vasculitis in the smallest veins (venules) may allow leakage of both plasma and red blood cells. "The most common syndrome is leukocytoclastic vasculitis, predominantly an inflammation of the venules," he adds.

When red blood cells leak from the venules, it usually produces a rash you can feel that has some bruising associated with it, called *palpable purpura.* When the rash appears as flesh-colored hives that don't go away in less than 24 hours, it's due to inflammation that doesn't usually involve red cell leakage. This is called *urticarial vasculitis.*

Vasculitis in the blood vessels of the eyes can cause vision loss, or if the kidneys are affected it can lead to progressive kidney failure and/or high blood pressure. Some forms of vasculitis have specific symptoms:

Giant cell arteritis (GCA) causes inflammation that damages large- and medium-sized arteries, often the temporal arteries along the sides of the head at the temples, just in front of the ears (hence the disorder's other name, temporal arteritis). It usually occurs after age 50 (the average age of a GCA patient is 70).[28]

Eighty percent of people with GCA have severe, throbbing headaches, usually in the temples or forehead on one or both sides of the head. The scalp over the affected blood vessels may feel tender and sore (it may even hurt to brush or comb your hair). Many women with GCA have facial or jaw soreness (especially with chewing), says Dr. Mitnick. Depression is also common. If the ophthalmic artery is blocked, it can cause vision loss. If larger arteries leading to the arms or legs are affected, women may have fatigue or aching in the limbs or intermittent claudication, muscle aching during exercise.

Muscle aches or pain can also be due to coexisting *polymyalgia rheumatica (PMR)*. PMR occurs in about 30 percent of women with giant cell arteritis. It is often characterized by the rapid onset of muscle pain or aching in the large muscle groups, especially those around the shoulders and hips. Symptoms of PMR can be somewhat vague, and it's not uncommon for it to be initially misdiagnosed as an infection, rheumatoid arthritis, or other illness that affects muscles (or even cancer).

Takayasu's arteritis, chronic inflammation of the aorta and its branches, has two phases: The systemic phase causes body-wide symptoms of inflammation as well as joint pains and nonspecific aches and pains. In the occlusive phase, women develop symptoms because of the closing off of the affected blood vessels, usually during repetitive activities (*claudication*). Most commonly, sharp pains occur in the arms while cutting meat, or in the calves of the legs while walking. A woman may also experience dizziness when abruptly standing up after sitting or lying down, headaches, and visual problems.

Takayasu's is often called the "pulseless disease" because it can result in a pulse that's barely felt. This occurs because blood vessels are narrowed to such an extent that the normal push of blood being pumped through the aorta from the heart cannot be felt in the wrist, neck, elbow, or lower extremities. When a stethoscope is placed over an affected blood vessel, a whooshing sound called a bruit (pronounced *broo-ee*) can be heard as blood pushes through narrowed blood vessels.

Although high blood pressure is common in Takayasu's (from narrowing of arteries in the kidneys), restricted blood flow in the arms or ankles can make it difficult to get an accurate blood pressure reading. Unfortunately, the disease can be present for some time before symptoms appear, and some women are not diagnosed until they suffer a stroke or other complication of the occlusive phase.

Granulomatosis with polyangiitis (**GPA**, formerly **Wegener's granulomatosis**), results from inflammation in blood vessels in a variety of tissues and can produce the same body-wide inflammatory symptoms as other forms of vasculitis. This can cause inflammation of the nose or sinuses, with a persistent runny nose (*rhinorrhea*), nasal crusts and sores, nosebleeds, nasal discharge, and facial pain. When GPA affects the middle ear, it can cause middle ear inflammation (*otitis media*), pain, and hearing loss. Respiratory tract symptoms include a cough, bloody phlegm, and chest pain. You may also experience hoarseness, vocal changes, wheezing, or shortness of breath, caused by inflammation of the trachea. GPA can also affect the kidneys.

Diagnosing Vasculitis

Because many vasculitis symptoms are nonspecific, diagnosis can be difficult. Often a biopsy of the skin or other affected areas may help in confirming a diagnosis. For example, a skin biopsy can reveal inflamed blood vessels beneath the second layer of skin (the *dermis*).

Erythrocyte sedimentation rate (ESR) is one of the blood tests that measure inflammation. As you'll recall, the ESR measures the speed at which red blood cells settle in a vertical glass tube. When inflammation is present, the cells settle to the bottom faster than in people who don't have inflammatory conditions. Women with vasculitis may also have a slight anemia, which can be detected with a red blood cell count.

The diagnosis of giant cell arteritis is based on the symptoms noted on page 382 and a finding of abnormal blood flow in the arms, legs, or aorta. Your physician will look for tenderness of the scalp or temples and visual abnormalities; your SED rate will be high (greater than 50). A temporal artery biopsy involves taking a small tissue sample from a part of the temporal artery located in the hairline in front of the ear. When viewed under a microscope, the tissue from the temporal arteries reveals inflammation and unusually large macrophages, or "giant cells." A biopsy can be helpful in most cases, but the disease can "skip" areas of the artery, so a biopsy on both sides of the head may be done, says Dr. Mitnick. The use of color Doppler ultrasound to image the temporal arteries has been proposed as a useful diagnostic test, but is not always accurate.

Polymyalgia rheumatica (PMR) can mimic many illnesses, and it can only be diagnosed after these other illnesses are excluded. During your physical exam, your doctor will look for pain, aching, and stiffness in the shoulder, pelvic, and hip regions. A high ESR is common among patients with PMR. Sometimes a short course of low-dose corticosteroids is given; if symptoms disappear fairly quickly, then it's likely to be PMR.

C-reactive Protein (CRP) is also elevated in giant cell arteritis and polymyalgia rheumatica, but there are no established biomarkers for these or other forms of vasculitis.[23]

The primary diagnostic test for Takayasu's arteritis is **magnetic resonance angiography (MRA)**. Thickening of the aortic wall can be seen on MRA. In some cases, damage to the aorta, the aortic valve, or other large blood vessel is found and surgery is needed to repair it. In angiography, a special dye (which appears opaque on x-ray) is injected into an artery and x-rays are taken of key blood vessels. In many cases, the aorta will show long areas of narrowing (*stenosis*). But these narrowed areas can also be found in many or all of the large blood vessels.

GPA is diagnosed by the results of a physical exam, together with symptoms, lab tests, x-rays, and sometimes a biopsy of affected tissue (skin, nose, lung, or kidney). These factors are also used to judge whether the disease is active or in remission. Other tests include a blood test for *antineutrophil cytoplasmic antibodies (ANCAs)*, antibodies to enzymes located in the cytoplasm of white blood cells called *neutrophils*, a red blood cell count to test for anemia, an ESR (or SED rate), and urinalysis to detect protein in the urine (proteinuria), and x-rays of the sinuses or chest may also be done. Tests for ANCA in GCA and PMR can rule out other autoimmune diseases.

Lupus manifestations may represent vasculitis. "To a greater or lesser extent, lupus is a vasculitic illness," remarks Dr. Mitnick. "There are frequent skin manifestations, but there may also be vasculitis affecting internal organs, such as the kidneys, lungs, or brain. When a patient with lupus nephritis becomes hypertensive, we worry the renal arteries are affected with vasculitis. Likewise, if a lupus patient has a stroke, we wonder about vasculitis in the brain, cerebral vasculitis."

Treating Vasculitis

Vasculitis is treated according to the stage of disease, the level of disease activity, and whether there's vessel damage. The initial treatment goal of ANCA-associated vasculitis is remission, and then the maintenance of remission, with maintenance treatments continuing for 18 to 24 months.[29]

Corticosteroids, most commonly prednisone, are the usual treatment for the most common types of vasculitis. Corticosteroids relieve symptoms of both giant cell arteritis and polymyalgia rheumatica within days and slow or stop the progression of the disease.[25] While low doses of corticosteroids are effective in treating PMR, higher doses (40 to 60 mg of oral prednisone a day) are often required initially to control temporal arteritis and Takayasu's arteritis. Unfortunately, the blindness that can occur in rare cases of temporal arteritis may not be reversible with treatment. (This is why it is so important to diagnose the disease before permanent damage takes place.)

Steroid sparing agents, such as low doses of *methotrexate, cyclophosphamide (Cytoxan)*, or *azathioprine (Imuran)* may be used so that lower doses of prednisone can be used. Cyclophosphamide can cause bladder irritation, bleeding, and cancer.

Angioplasty may also be used to trast Takayasu's and GCA. In angioplasty, a balloon-tipped catheter is threaded into blood vessels to widen narrowed arteries, such as in the kidneys. In some cases, damage from severe inflammation can require bypass procedures or aortic valve replacement, but the surgery must be done when the disease is inactive. Active GCA may last only a year or two, but continued low-dose treatment may be needed after remission.

Because GPA can be life threatening, it is treated with high doses of prednisone and azathioprine and methotrexate.[30] Extended treatment with corticosteroids may be needed, so eventually the dose of prednisone is slowly decreased. Some women may have a remission, but it's difficult to predict how long it will last. Methotrexate and azathioprine can be effective in maintaining remission.[31] However, half of all GPA patients may have a relapse, so close monitoring is vital.

In clinical trials, infusions of the B-cell-depleting drug rituximab (Rituxan) every six months were shown to be more effective than azathioprine in maintaining remission in ANCA-associated vasculitis, especially GPA.[32] Rituxan may also be effective in a rare form of ANCA-associated vasculitis, EGPA.[33]

Biologic drugs, including those that block the inflammatory cytokine *tumor necrosis factor alpha (TNFα)*, are also being used to treat different forms of vasculitis.[34] These include *etanercept (Enbrel)* and *infliximab (Remicade)*.[35] However, anti-TNF drugs are apparently not effective in Wegener's.

Intravenous immune globulin (IVIG) may have benefit as an adjunctive therapy in ANCA-associated vasculitides, particularly in particularly in relapsing disease, recent studies suggest. One preliminary study from France found that just one course of IVIG in combination with corticosteroids or other immunosuppressants produced remission in over half of patients with GPA, EGPA, and another rare ANCA vasculitis called *microscopic polyangiitis (MPA)*.[36]

How Vasculitis Can Affect You Over Your Lifetime

Vasculitis in women of reproductive age does not affect pregnancy and fertility, but the medications use to treat it can.

Menstruation and Fertility

As mentioned in previous chapters, prednisone can cause menstrual irregularities but can safely be used during pregnancy and breast-feeding. Because prednisone (and similar drugs) can lead to osteoporosis, women may need bone-building drugs and bone scans to monitor bone mineral density regardless of their age. However, the effects of vasculitis on pregnancy and fertility have not been studied.

Menopause and Beyond

Because vasculitis often arises in later life, when the risk of heart disease also increases, researchers are investigating connections between the two conditions. Blood vessel inflammation is known to be a component of cardiovascular disease, and people with vasculitis also have an increased risk of arteriosclerosis, or narrowing of blood vessels by fatty plaques. Blood clots can form at the site of active inflammation, and vasculitis itself can also cause heart attacks and strokes. For now, women with vasculitis would do well to take steps to reduce any of the accepted risk factors for coronary disease, such as obesity, high blood pressure, high cholesterol, and a sedentary lifestyle. And stop smoking!

Notes

1. Miyakis S, Lockshin MD, Atsumi D, et al. International consensus statement on an update of the preliminary classification criteria or antiphospholipid syndrome (APS). *J Thromb Haemost.* 2006;4:295–306.
2. Giannakopoulo B, Steven A, Krilis SA. The pathogenesis of the antiphospholipid syndrome. *N Engl J Med.* 2013;368:1033–1044. doi:10.1056/NEJMra1112830.
3. Chaturvedi S, McCrae KR. Recent advances in the antiphospholipid antibody syndrome. *Curr Opin Hematol.* 2014;21(5):371–379. doi:10.1097/MOH.0000000000000067.
4. Urbanus RT, Siegerink B, Roest M, et al. Antiphospholipid antibodies and risk of myocardial infarction and ischaemic stroke in young women in the RATIO study: a case-control study. *Lancet Neurol.* 2009;8:998–1005.
5. Haemostasis and Thrombosis Task Force, British Committee for Standards in Haematology. Investigation and management of heritable thrombophilia. *Br J Haematol.* 2001; 114:512–528.
6. Cervera R, Serrano R, Pons-Estel GJ, et al. Morbidity and mortality in the antiphospholipid syndrome during a 10-year period: a multicentre prospective study of

1000 patients. *Ann Rheum Dis.* 2015;74:1011–1018. doi:10.1136/annrheumdis-2013-204838.

7. Asherson RA, Cervera R, de Groot PG, et al. Catastrophic antiphospholipid syndrome: international consensus statement on classification criteria and treatment guidelines. *Lupus.* 2003;12(7):530–534.
8. Tripodi A, deGroot PG, Pengo V. Antiphospholipid syndrome: laboratory detection, mechanisms of action and treatment. *J Intern Med.* 2011;270:110–122. doi:10.1111/j.1365-2796.2011.02362.x.
9. Reynaud Q, Lega JC, Mismetti P, et al. Risk of venous and arterial thrombosis according to type of antiphospholipid antibodies in adults without systemic lupus erythematosus: a systematic review and meta-analysis. *Autoimmun Rev.* 2014;13(6):595–608. doi:10.1016/j.autrev.2013.11.004.
10. Arnaud L, Mathian A, Ruffatti A, et al. Efficacy of aspirin for the primary prevention of thrombosis in patients with antiphospholipid antibodies: an international and collaborative meta-analysis. *Autoimmun Rev.* 2014;13:281–291.
11. https://www.xarelto-us.com/.
12. Erkan D, Yazici Y, Peterson MG, Sammaritano L, Lockshin MD. A cross-sectional study of clinical thrombotic risk factors and preventive treatments in antiphospholipid syndrome. *Rheumatology (Oxford).* 2002;41(8):924–929.
13. de Jesus GR, Agmon-Levin N, Andrade CA, et al. 14th International Congress on Antiphospholipid Antibodies Task Force. Report on obstetric antiphospholipid syndrome. *Autoimmun Rev.* 2014;13:795–813. http://dx.doi.org/10.1016/j.autrev.2014.02.003.
14. Erkan D, Leibowitz E, Berman J, Lockshin MD. Perioperative medical management of antiphospholipid syndrome: hospital for special surgery experience, review of literature, and recommendations. *J Rheumatol.* 2002;29(4):843–849.
15. Sebire NJ, Backos M, El Gaddal S, et al. Placental pathology, antiphospholipid antibodies, and pregnancy outcome in recurrent miscarriage patients. *Obstet Gynecol.* 2003;101:258–263.
16. Neunert C, Lim W, Crowther M, et al. The American Society of Hematology. 2011 evidence-based practice guideline for immune thrombocytopenia. *Blood.* 2011;117(16):4190–4207. doi:10.1182/blood-2010-08-302984.
17. Ballem PJ, Segal GM, Stratton JR, et al. Mechanisms of thrombocytopenia in chronic autoimmune thrombocytopenic purpura. Evidence of both impaired platelet production and increased platelet clearance. *J Clin Invest.* 1987;80:33–40.
18. Moini J. *Phlebotomy Principles and Practice*. Burlington, MA: Jones & Bartlett; 2013.
19. Rodeghiero F, Ruggeri M. Treatment of immune thrombocytopenia in adults: the role of thrombopoietin-receptor agonists. *Semin Hematol.* 2015;52(1):16–24. http://dx.doi.org/10.1053/j.seminhematol.2014.10.006.
20. Kim YK, Lee SS, Jeong SH, et al. Efficacy and safety of eltrombopag in adult refractory immune thrombocytopenia. *Blood Res.* 2015;50(1):19–25.

21. How Nplate works. http://www.nplate.com/patient/how-nplate-may-help/how-nplate-works.html. http://pi.amgen.com/united_states/nplate/nplate_pi_hcp_english.pdf.
22. https://www.gsksource.com/gskprm/htdocs/documents/PROMACTA.PDF.
23. Patel VL, Mahe'vas M, Lee SY, et al. Outcomes 5 years after response to rituximab therapy in children and adults with immune thrombocytopenia. *Blood.* 2012;119(25): 5989–5996.
24. Platelet Disorder Support Association. B-cell depletion (anti-CD 20). http://www.pdsa.org/treatments/conventional/b-cell-depletion.html.
25. Bussel JB, Skupski DW, MacFarland JG. Fetal alloimmune thrombocytopenia: consensus and controversy. *J Maternal-Fetal Med.* 1996;5(5):281–292. [Article first published online January 6, 1999]. doi:10.1002/(SICI)1520-6661(199609/10)5:5<281::AID-MFM6>3.0.CO;2-D.
26. Falk RJ, Gross WL, Guillevin L, et al. Granulomatosis with polyangiitis (Wegener's): an alternative name for Wegener's granulomatosis. *Arthritis Rheum.* 2011;63:863.
27. Jennette, JC, Falk RJ, Bacon PA, et al. 2012 Revised international Chapel Hill Consensus Conference nomenclature of vasculitides. *Arthritis Rheum.* 2013;65(1):1–11. doi:10.1002/art.37715.
28. Weyand CM, Goronzy JJ. Giant-cell arteritis and polymyalgia rheumatica. *N Engl J Med.* 2014;371:50–57. doi:10.1056/NEJMcp1214825.
29. Kallenberg, CGM. Key advances in the clinical approach to ANCA-associated vasculitis. *Nat Rev Rheumatol.* 2014;10:484–493. Published online July 1, 2014. doi:10.1038/nrrheum.2014.104.
30. Pagnoux C, Mahr A, Hamidou MA, et al. Azathioprine or methotrexate maintenance for ANCA-associated vasculitis. *N Engl J Med.* 2008;359(26):2790–2803.
31. Hoffman GS. Therapeutic interventions for systemic vasculitis. *JAMA.* 2010;304(21): 2413–2414. doi:10.1001/jama.2010.1676.
32. Guillevin L, Pagnoux C, Karras A, et al for the French Vasculitis Study Group. Rituximab versus azathioprine for maintenance in ANCA-associated vasculitis. *N Engl J Med.* 2014;371(19):1771–1780. doi:10.1056/NEJMoa1404231.
33. Fanouriakis A, Kougkas N, Vassilopoulos D, et al. Rituximab for eosinophilic granulomatosis with polyangiitis with severe vasculitic neuropathy: case report and review of current clinical evidence. *Sem Arthritis Rheum.* 2015. doi:10.1016/j.semarthrit.2015.03.004.
34. Henderson CF, Seo P. Biologic agents in systemic vasculitis. *Int J Clin Rheumatol.* 2011;6(4):453–462.
35. Jarrot PA, Kaplanski G. Anti-TNF-alpha therapy and systemic vasculitis. *Mediat Inflamm.* 2014. http://dx.doi.org/10.1155/2014/493593.
36. Crickx E, Machelart I, Lazaro E, et al. Intravenous immunoglobulin as immunomodulating agent in ANCA associated vasculitides: a French nationwide study of 92 patients. *Arthritis Rheumatol.* 2015 Oct 16. doi:10.1002/art.39472. [Epub ahead of print].

12

Assault on the Liver—Autoimmune Hepatitis and Primary Biliary Cirrhosis

I turned yellow when I was a senior in college. Having jaundice was the first sign that there was something really wrong with me. I had been under a lot of stress, was feeling tired and lethargic, and had no appetite. But I hadn't been sleeping or eating that well, and I had just gotten over the flu. So nothing really rang alarm bells until a friend of mine said to me, "You don't look so well—you look yellow." I looked in the mirror, and sure enough, I was. I went to the college health center and they tested me for everything possible: mono, hepatitis A, hepatitis C, Epstein-Barr virus. My tests did show I'd been exposed to Epstein- Barr virus, but there were no viruses in my blood. The only thing they found was that my liver enzymes were off the charts. But I tested negative for primary biliary cirrhosis and gallstones. So no one knew what was wrong with me. The college sent me to a couple of local doctors; one of them was even a liver doctor. And he said it was probably mono, that 4 percent of people with mono had jaundice. He told me I'd been working too hard, and to take it easy. It took two and a half months and four doctors to find out what I really had.

Hannah, 27

The liver is the body's main chemical processing plant. Autoimmune diseases can cause it to seriously malfunction, spilling chemicals into areas where they shouldn't be and damaging the processing equipment.

The liver's amazing processing system makes bile to help digest food; stores iron (along with vitamins and minerals); and stockpiles carbohydrates, glucose, and fat until the body needs them for energy. The liver manufactures components of blood, including clotting factors to stop bleeding and help wound healing, and detoxifies the various chemicals we ingest, including alcohol and drugs (both legal and illegal). In fact, much of what we eat, drink, breathe, and even absorb through the skin passes through the liver to be detoxified and excreted in bile. The liver also makes cholesterol, a fat needed by all the cells in our body, and proteins that help carry fats in the bloodstream (having too much of certain types of cholesterol and other blood fats contributes to heart disease). It also produces complement, which plays a role in many autoimmune diseases.

Autoimmune hepatitis (AIH) and *primary biliary cirrhosis (PBC)* affect the small bile ducts in the liver. *Sclerosing cholangitis* affects the larger bile ducts and is primarily seen in men. These diseases are caused by an immune attack on specific cells in the liver and bile ducts, producing inflammation and scarring (*cirrhosis*), eventually compromising the liver's ability to function. Autoimmune hepatitis occurs four times more often in women than men; PBC strikes women 6 to 10 times more often than men, mostly in middle age and later life.

"I often use an analogy to describe the liver as a tree. The *hepatocytes*, the cells of the liver, are the leaves; the bile ductules are the twigs and small branches, and the bile duct is the trunk. In autoimmune hepatitis, the immune system attacks the hepatocytes, the leaves of the tree; in PBC, it attacks the bile ductules, the twigs. And in sclerosing cholangitis, it attacks the bile duct, the trunk of the tree and the major branches," explains hepatologist Henry C. Bodenheimer, Jr., MD, professor of medicine at the Hofstra North Shore-LIJ School of Medicine.

"Think of these diseases as arthritis of the liver or bile ducts. Just as in arthritis, where there's inflammation in the joints and destruction of the joints, there is inflammation and scarring in the liver," says Dr. Bodenheimer, who also serves as medical director of the Medicine Service Line for the North Shore Health System in Manhasset, New York.

In some women, the scarring becomes so extensive that the liver begins to fail and a transplant is needed. Although some women can experience a remission, autoimmune hepatitis is a disease that may require lifelong treatment.

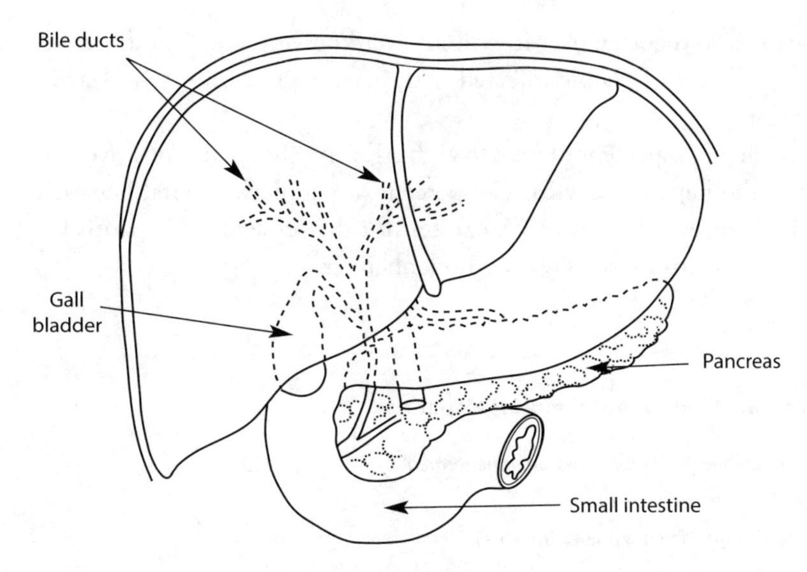

The Liver and Bile Ducts

Autoimmune Hepatitis

When you think of hepatitis, you probably think about the infectious kind—hepatitis A, B, or C—but autoimmune hepatitis is not like infectious hepatitis. It's a distinct condition, caused by an immune system assault on the liver. Why this happens is still unknown; a number of genes have been linked to vulnerability to the disease, and there are some suspect environmental factors. AIH typically hits women during their twenties, and there's another peak during the sixties. Between 10 and 20 percent of cases of chronic hepatitis are due to AIH.

The disease does not often make its presence known early. The most pronounced outward sign, yellowing of the whites of the eyes and the skin (*jaundice*), appears only after the liver has sustained severe damage. Only in 25 percent of cases does AIH begin with an acute episode of hepatitis.[1]

What Causes Autoimmune Hepatitis?

While there's no link between autoimmune hepatitis and any of the infectious hepatitis viruses, some women with AIH may have had a past infection with hepatitis C and gotten over it without ever knowing they had it. Between 15 and 40 percent of people infected with hepatitis C completely clear it from their system.[1]

As many as 5 percent of people with AIH may have false-positive antibody tests to the hepatitis C virus (10 percent of people with viral hepatitis may also have autoantibodies). "We can test for the presence of hepatitis C virus, and do a sensitive test," says Dr. Bodenheimer.

Warning Signs of Autoimmune Hepatitis

- Cessation of menstruation (*amenorrhea*)
- Decreased fertility
- Fatigue, feeling unwell (*malaise*)
- Poor appetite
- Joint pain (*arthralgias*)
- Upper abdominal discomfort
- Swelling of the abdomen and legs
- Yellowing of the skin and whites of the eyes (*jaundice*)
- Abnormal liver tests
- Elevated bilirubin
- Dilated capillaries under the skin (*spider angiomas*)

Instead of a viral attack on liver cells, in autoimmune hepatitis the damage is done by T cells and liver-specific autoantibodies, including *antinuclear antibodies (ANAs), smooth muscle cell antibodies (SMA)*, and *anti-liver microsomal antibody type 1 (anti-LKM-1)* also known as *liver kidney microsomal type 1 antibodies*.[1] But the trigger of this attack is not known.

A liver biopsy will reveal T cells and plasma cells (activated B cells), which manufacture autoantibodies (see pages 4 to 5). As inflammation and damage progress, liver tissues become hardened (*fibrotic*) and scarred. Progressive scarring called *fibrosis* spreads throughout the liver, leading to extensive damage termed *cirrhosis*. Eventually liver blood flow is impaired, choking off vital nutrients, and cells begin to die (*necrosis*). As more and more liver cells die, the liver begins to fail. Although immunosuppressant drugs can slow this process, some women eventually require a liver transplant.

Among the genes associated with autoimmune hepatitis are genes linked to rheumatoid arthritis, in particular genes called *DR3 and DR4*.[1] Patients with DR3 often have a faster progression of the disease and fewer remissions, and require a transplant more often. Women may also have other immune abnormalities or a family history of autoimmune diseases, such as thyroid disease or ulcerative colitis.

Autoimmune hepatitis may be triggered by environmental factors, such as a virus, bacteria, chemicals, or drugs.[2]

Drugs linked to AIH include the antibiotic *minocycline*, cholesterol-lowering drugs called *statins*, and, possibly, the tumor necrosis factor-alpha (TNFα) blockers *adalimumab (Humira)* and *infliximab (Remicade)*.[1] Drug-induced autoimmune hepatitis can be reversed when the medication is stopped.[2]

Some studies have suggested—but not proven—that AIH can develop after infection with hepatitis A, B, or C. Other suspect viruses include Epstein-Barr virus (EBV), measles virus, and herpes simplex type 1 (HSV-1).

Molecular mimicry, in which liver cells resemble invading pathogens, may be another mechanism involved in AIH.[1]

However, no single trigger has yet been linked to AIH. Other cofactors may be needed, such as genes, female hormones, alcohol, and nicotine that upregulate or downregulate the immune system or liver enzymes that metabolize drugs, which, by being unusually elevated, may provoke an immune reaction.

Hannah's story continues:

I was getting ready to go home for Christmas when I saw the first liver doctor, who had said I had mono. I even asked him if it was OK to drink alcohol. He told me it was fine to have a beer or two. That amazes me now. By then, the jaundice had gone away, I started feeling better. I got my appetite back. I figured he must be right; it was mono. But while I was visiting my mother that January, the jaundice came back. I lost my appetite, and had this gurgling in my stomach, which I realized later were other symptoms of autoimmune hepatitis. My stools had also been white and my urine bright yellow, but I hadn't paid it much attention the first time. My mother said my eyes were the color of electric daffodils—that's how yellow I was when the jaundice came back. My mother made me promise I'd see a doctor.

When I got back to college, I did go back to the local hepatologist, who realized it wasn't mono. He tested me for antinuclear antibodies and smooth muscle antibodies and said, "You have this rare disease, autoimmune hepatitis." I had a liver biopsy, and fortunately my liver wasn't damaged—there was no cirrhosis. The most uncomfortable thing about the biopsy is that even though the needle goes into your right side, you feel a pain in your left shoulder. But I was very lucky. Some people only have symptoms when their liver is so damaged that their only hope is a liver transplant.

Diagnosing Autoimmune Hepatitis

AIH can be present for some time before producing any symptoms at all. Typically, the disease has been present for at least six months (or longer) before a woman is diagnosed.

"Often a woman will come in after having abnormal liver test results. She may be taking medications that require liver monitoring, or maybe she's just not feeling well. Fatigue is a very common symptom," remarks Dr. Bodenheimer.

Up to 40 percent of people with AIH present with apparent acute liver injury, but others can have a subclinical disease with very small elevations of liver enzymes.

There can be ethnic and racial differences in the way AIH presents, as well. For example, African Americans have cirrhosis more frequently than do white women. Asian Americans may have milder, later onset AIH, while Native American women may have more advanced disease and other immune disorders.[3]

Tests You May Need and What They Mean

Liver Enzyme Tests are often part of routine blood work and include *bilirubin*, various liver proteins, biliary associated *liver enzymes* like *alkaline phosphatase* (indicating inflammation or blockage of bile ducts), and *aminotransferases*, which are elevated when there's inflammation or injury to liver cells. These enzymes can be elevated in a number of conditions, viral hepatitis, alcoholic liver disease, medication-induced liver disease, nonalcoholic "fatty" liver (excess fat deposits), and liver tumors. So when liver enzymes are elevated, these other problems must be ruled out.[4]

Gamma globulins/immunoglobulins components of blood plasma that respond to bacteria or viruses, especially *immunoglobulin G (IgG)*, are considered a hallmark of the disease.

Liver biopsy is the usual way of diagnosing AIH to see whether there is inflammation and/or scarring.

Your liver is located on the right side of your body underneath the diaphragm. Under local anesthesia and ultrasound guidance, a hollow needle is gently inserted between the right lower ribs to take a small tissue sample the size of a pencil lead that's analyzed by a pathologist. If autoimmune hepatitis is present, the tissue sample will show an infiltration of T cells and plasma cells, as well as scarring and tissue death. Even though the tissue sample is small, a liver biopsy usually indicates what's going on in the rest of the liver, as well as how severe the disease is, says Dr. Bodenheimer.

Autoantibody Tests. Almost all AIH patients have autoantibodies. In North America, an estimated 96 percent have *antinuclear antibodies (ANAs)* or *anti-smooth muscle antibodies (SMAs)* or both. These are detected in liver cells by using a staining process that makes them fluorescent when seen under a special microscope (a technique called *immunofluorescence*).

There are two subcategories of AIH, depending on which antibodies are found.

The most common is type 1, or classic AIH, in which there are elevated ANAs and SMAs. In the less common type 2 AIH, levels of *LKM-1 antibodies* and/or *anti-liver cytosol type 1 antibody (anti-LC-1)* are elevated and the disease seems to have a more rapidly progressing course.[3] However, the subcategory of AIH you have will *not* determine your treatment. LKM-1 is mostly found in young women and children.[1]

Around 80 percent of AIH patients have type 1, with the majority women ages 16 to 30.[3]

The International Autoimmune Hepatitis Group (IAIHG) has a 17-point scoring system to help diagnose AIH.[5] In the scoring system, being a woman is two points; having elevated aminotransferases is another two points.

Included in the list: levels (*titers*) of autoantibodies (ANAs, SMAs) are one to three points each, depending on the level detected; increased gamma globulin (two times the normal level is three points); and having another autoimmune disease is one point. If your score is 10 to 15 points, the diagnosis is "probable" AIH; a total score of 15 or greater is "definite AIH."[5]

This scoring system can also be used to determine if asymptomatic patients need treatment. The IAIHG is studying a simpler system for routine clinical use.[6]

Autoimmune Hepatitis Clusters

Women who have autoimmune hepatitis often have previously had or may develop other autoimmune diseases within several years. These diseases are varied and may affect any part of the body, from the joints to the skin.

- Thyroid disease
- Ulcerative colitis
- Rheumatoid arthritis
- Type 1 diabetes
- Celiac sprue
- Lupus
- Myasthenia gravis
- Sjögren's syndrome
- Vitiligo

The Female Factor

Seventy to eighty percent of autoimmune hepatitis occurs in women, usually before age 30 and less often after age 50 (in older age, it's more common in men), says Melissa Palmer, MD, clinical professor of medicine at New York University School of Medicine and Global Head of Clinical Development in Hepatology at Shire Pharmaceuticals. But research into possible hormonal aspects is scant.

It is known that processing (*metabolism*) of male and female hormones by the liver can be abnormal in people who have cirrhosis. "Both testosterone and estrogen can be altered in some people with cirrhosis. In women, estrogen metabolism may be inhibited in some way, and that could be a contributing factor in why some women with cirrhosis have abnormal menstrual cycles or, in severe cases, stop menstruating," explains Dr. Palmer. "In men, it seems to go the opposite way. Men with cirrhosis often get feminization—*gynecomastia*, enlarged breasts—and a change in hair distribution."

Primary biliary cirrhosis (PBC) is a disease predominantly of middle age and older women, but there's no indication of any link to low estrogen in menopause. "Women may be diagnosed later in life, but they may have had the disease for years. If you biopsy the liver years before the disease was diagnosed, it will usually show some microscopic changes," she remarks.

Hannah's story continues:

I started on the prednisone and Imuran a week after my diagnosis. At first I didn't want to take them; I knew they were really powerful drugs and I was afraid of what they might do to my body. But I also knew that they would help get rid of the inflammation and calm down my immune system.

I was put on a big dose of prednisone, 60 milligrams a day, which acted like caffeine for me—it gave me lots of energy. I didn't gain a lot of weight, but I did get the steroid moon face. On the advice of a naturopathic physician I had been seeing since before I was diagnosed, I also started taking calcium and magnesium to prevent osteoporosis from the steroids. Thanks to her, I was doing that from the beginning.

Treating Autoimmune Hepatitis

Treatment for autoimmune hepatitis is generally indicated if you have:

- Any AIH symptoms
- Significantly elevated liver enzymes
- A liver biopsy showing active inflammation

Immunosuppressive drugs are the standard treatment for autoimmune hepatitis. You may be given "monotherapy" with prednisone or prednisolone, or a combination therapy with *azathioprine (Imuran)*, with either prednisone or another steroid called *budesonide (Entocort EC)*. Adding azathioprine helps keep the needed dose of corticosteroids low. Budesonide is more rapidly taken up by the liver, so it has fewer systemic side effects than prednisone.

Even with combination therapy, as many as 80 percent of women will have some side effects with corticosteroids, such as bone loss, weight gain, and mood swings (see pages 42 to 43).[7]

Prednisone is usually started out at a high dose (60 mg a day), tapered over three months to a lower dose (30 mg), and then reduced to a maintenance dose (20 mg or less).[7] Prednisone starts to improve aminotransferase values and IgG within three to four weeks. However, it can take six to eight weeks for the benefits of azathioprine (50 mg to 150 mg a day) to kick in. So if azathioprine is prescribed, it's usually started as soon as possible after a diagnosis is made.

Remission is currently defined as the complete normalization of aminotransferase liver enzymes and IgG in lab tests, along with no symptoms or *histological signs (cellular evidence)*, such as inflammation, of hepatitis in a liver biopsy. Be aware that histological improvement may lag behind biochemical remission by three to eight months. However, rates of histological remission actually increase the longer therapy is continued, up to approximately 80 percent after 36 months.[7]

Up to 65 percent of women with AIH will experience complete remission. After at least two years in remission, some patients can be weaned off immunosuppressant therapy.

"If they have a flare, they go back on medication, usually permanently. There are no clear-cut triggers for a relapse, but factors like viruses or stress may be important," explains Dr. Palmer. "Infection with one of the hepatitis viruses may cause a flare, or they may have a worse course of hepatitis A or B. So we recommend that all patients be vaccinated against hepatitis A and B."

There are risks to long-term maintenance therapy. In younger women, who may require lifelong treatment, there's a slightly increased risk of cancer with long-term, higher-dose azathioprine. Symptoms of steroid withdrawal, such as body and joint aches, can also occur if corticosteroid doses are reduced too abruptly. Plus, there's the risk of corticosteroid-induced osteoporosis.

Most women with autoimmune hepatitis will need lifelong treatment. However, 10 to 30 percent of women will stay in remission without medications after a minimum of four years of maintenance therapy.

A liver biopsy is performed to make sure there is no inflammation before maintenance medications are stopped. Relapses occur most often during the first year after stopping medications, but can also arise many years later, so close follow-up is needed.

Also needing surveillance are women diagnosed with AIH before age 18, those with histological cirrhosis when first diagnosed, and soluble liver antigen/liver pancreas antigen (SLA/LP) antibodies, all of which may be risk factors for poorer outcomes.[8]

Immunosuppressive drugs used in transplantation medicine, including *cyclosporine*—either regular (*Sandimmune*) or modified (*Neoral*)—*tacrolimus (Prograf)*, and *mycophenolate mofetil, MMF (CellCept)*,[9] offer alternatives for difficult-to-treat AIH patients. MMF seems especially beneficial for women who are azathioprine-intolerant or those who have haven't responded to treatment, and it has very rapid steroid-sparing effects.[7]

Note that regular and modified cyclosporine are absorbed differently and cannot be substituted for each other. It's important to make sure you received the same cyclosporine drug each time you get a new prescription refill.[10]

The B-cell-depletion drug *rituximab* (*Rituxan*, see pages 79 to 80)[11] and the tumor necrosis factor-alpha blocker *infliximab* (Remicade),[12] both used in other autoimmune conditions, have met with some success in treating refractory AIH.

Liver transplants can replace a damaged liver, but do not correct the underlying problem in autoimmune hepatitis. "If you start out with a liver that's badly damaged and you put in a new one, it 'resets' the clock. You do have the potential for the return of the disease. But you are starting over and recurrence may take years. Immunosuppressants may also slow the process down," says Dr. Bodenheimer. "It can be a pretty aggressive disease with or without a transplant, however. What we're doing is fixing the results of the disease, but not the immune system problem that caused it."

How Autoimmune Hepatitis Can Affect You Over Your Lifetime

Menstruation and Fertility

The first sign of AIH in young women is often a stoppage of menstruation, *amenorrhea*.

"Because of menstrual cycle irregularities, it's hard for some women to become pregnant," remarks Dr. Palmer. However, treatment with prednisone and azathioprine can normalize menstrual cycles and ovulation, so women can have successful pregnancies and deliveries. Women without cirrhosis have normal fertility.

Oral contraceptives containing estrogen may cause the growth of benign tumors (*hemangiomas, hepatic adenoma*, and *focal nodular hyperplasia*), so women with AIH are usually advised to take all-progestin birth control pills (or a long-acting injection of *medroxyprogesterone*, *Depo-Provera*). Women who have fluid in the abdomen (*ascites*) are advised to avoid progesterone because it can cause sodium and fluid retention.

Oral contraceptives do not protect against sexually transmitted diseases, including hepatitis B (and in rare cases, hepatitis C). Again, AIH is *not* infectious.

Pregnancy

Women may have a remission of AIH during pregnancy. "That's because of the immunosuppressive effects of pregnancy, and perhaps higher estrogen levels," says Dr. Palmer. "Some women may have a disease flare during pregnancy, but that's rare."

Although prednisone is considered safe, azathioprine is usually discontinued as soon as a woman becomes pregnant. Guidelines from the American Association for the Study of Liver Disease (AASLD) advise that "patients must be counseled regarding the uncertain risk of azathioprine in pregnancy, and azathioprine should be discontinued, if possible, in patients during pregnancy."[13]

Women with AIH planning to become pregnant are advised to discontinue azathioprine approximately six months before conceiving, says Dr. Palmer.

If a woman's steroid dose was reduced because she was also taking azathioprine, she may need an increased dose. If a woman has had a flare of AIH or liver-related complications (such as bleeding from varices), pregnancy should be postponed for at least a year, she adds.

[Author's note from Dr. Buyon: "Azathioprine has been used safely during pregnancy without evident side effects in the baby in lupus, and recent data in other diseases support its use when needed. As always, a balance between the benefits on maternal health and potential fetal effects should be discussed with patients."]

Potential harm to a fetus can't be ruled out with oral budesonide, and it has been found in breast milk.[14] MMF carries the risk of first trimester pregnancy loss and certain congenital abnormalities, such as cleft lip.[15] It's not known whether rituximab will harm an unborn baby, and it can also be excreted in breast milk.[16] Cyclosporine and tacrolimus also pose risks. So use of these medications is generally not recommended during pregnancy, unless the potential benefits of treatment outweigh the risks.

Hannah's story continues:

The problem with our medical system is that you see specialists. So I have a doctor that focuses on my liver. And I have a gynecologist who focuses on that. And I have an internist I see for everything else. The gynecologist knows that I have autoimmune hepatitis, but he hasn't discussed any of the gynecologic or reproductive issues with me. My hepatologist knows I'm taking birth control pills, but he never asked which one or what dose. You have to find out so much for yourself. For instance, I noticed that in the three years I've been taking the pill, the symptoms of the prednisone have been minimal. I had bad acne when I first started prednisone, and that cleared up. They're both good doctors, but neither really looks at the whole person. I found out on my own about the other diseases that people can have with autoimmune hepatitis. The first liver doctor I saw didn't tell me much about the effects of prednisone on bones, maybe because of my age. This year I had a bone density scan that showed that I had lost a lot of bone despite taking calcium. So now I'm taking Fosamax once a week. I was a bit scared of it at first; you can't lie down for a half hour after taking it or it can harm the esophagus, and you can't eat anything for two hours after taking it. Really, you do need a doctor who will give you all the information.

Menopause and Beyond

Oral estrogens for menopausal symptoms are not recommended for women with AIH.

"I usually shy away from oral estrogens in women with liver disease, since estrogens may elevate liver enzymes. Women experiencing severe hot flashes or other symptoms who wish to use estrogen can use the estrogen patch or estrogen cream with an oral progestin. Transdermal estrogen enters the bloodstream directly, bypassing the liver on the first pass, so it has lesser effects on the liver," says Dr. Palmer.

There are several types of estrogen patches, which look like large, clear bandages. They are worn on the lower abdomen, upper thigh, or buttocks and are changed once a week (*Climara*, *FemPatch*) or twice a week (*Alora*, *Vivelle*, or *Estraderm*). Estrogen creams (like *Premarin*) are inserted into the vagina with an applicator to prevent atrophy and drying of tissues. Very little is absorbed into the bloodstream.

There's no physical reason for sexual dysfunction in women with AIH, but, as in any chronic disease, depression and fatigue can affect libido. Note that androgen therapy may be dangerous. "Some androgens, like anabolic steroids, have been shown to lead to liver cancer. They really have not done the studies to see what kinds of effects androgens will have on someone with liver disease," remarks Dr. Palmer.

As with other autoimmune diseases, chronic use of corticosteroids causes bone loss. "I give alendronate or one of the other antiresorptive drugs, and I usually follow women with bone density tests," says Dr. Palmer. "I also tell patients they need to do weight-bearing exercises to protect their bones, as well as take calcium and vitamin D."

Women with AIH (and primary biliary cirrhosis) are advised to avoid iron, vitamin A, and niacin, which can be toxic to the liver in high doses, unless they are found to be deficient in these vitamins.

"Women may not realize they are getting so much iron, for example, if they take a multivitamin. Also, some herbs may be coated with iron, and this information may not be listed on the label. But too much iron can speed any kind of liver disease," cautions Dr. Palmer. "I advise women to buy a multivitamin without iron, and not to take any over-the-counter products that contain vitamin A or iron. The best thing is to take vitamins separately.

The only supplements I find helpful are calcium and vitamin D." However, women in advanced stages of PBC may actually have a deficiency in vitamin A, so get vitamin A levels checked, adds Dr. Palmer. "Supplementation is recommended only if a deficiency is found and a woman experiences night blindness, a side effect of vitamin A deficiency."

Cases of autoimmune hepatitis that arise in later life can also pose a problem. Women may already have osteoporosis or other medical problems, and steroid drugs may make them worse. So the decision to treat aggressively is highly individualized in older age.

Primary Biliary Cirrhosis (PBC)

Primary biliary cirrhosis is another autoimmune disease that damages the liver, but it results from an autoimmune attack on the *bile ducts* rather than on liver cells.

Bile, which helps break down fat during digestion, is stored in the gallbladder and released through the bile ducts into the *duodenum*, where fat enters the small intestine.

In PBC, the immune system attacks the smaller bile ducts and *ductules*, causing damage and leakage of bile acids into nearby tissues. Bile acids are toxic and injure liver cells, attracting T cells and causing small, granular inflammatory lesions (*granulomas*) to form as the liver attempts to contain bile seepage. Copper, normally excreted in bile, also accumulates in liver cells, as does *bilirubin*, the orange-yellow pigment that gives bile its color (bilirubin is normally excreted in stool). In PBC, cells in the small bile ducts overgrow, eventually replacing the ducts with hardened scar tissue.[17] Bile flow is reduced (*cholestasis)* and may eventually be blocked.

Warning Signs of PBC

- Fatigue
- Itching
- Dry eyes (Sjögren's syndrome)
- Jaundice

- Gastrointestinal bleeding
- Problems with taste or swallowing
- Clubbing of nails; whitening of nails

Immune damage is concentrated around blood vessels of the liver and causes increased blood pressure (*portal hypertension*) in the network of veins that carry blood to the liver from the stomach and other organs of the digestive system. The increased pressure causes bulging of the veins (*varices*) and bleeding in the stomach and esophagus.

As tissue injury progresses in the liver, inflammation and scarring spread and liver function becomes impaired. PBC is slow, chronic, and progressive, eventually causing liver failure, and is a common reason for a liver transplant.[17]

What Causes Primary Biliary Cirrhosis?

The cause of PBC is not known. Some research suggests that the immune system may mistake liver cells for bacteria, such as *Escherichia coli (E. coli)*, especially associated with recurrent urinary tract infections. In addition, *Epstein-Barr virus (EBV)* and *cytomegalovirus* are among the infectious agents associated with bile duct injury. Some drugs and environmental toxins have also been associated with PBC, but there's little evidence of any direct cause and effect. Progression of the disease may be hastened by changes in bile composition, making the bile ductules more susceptible to injury.

Autoantibodies seen in PBC are not specific to the bile ducts, but attack the tiny energy-producing components within cells called mitochondria, *antimitochondrial antibodies (AMAs)*. Ninety percent of people with PBC have circulating AMAs.

A variant of the disease, *PBC-AIH overlap syndrome*, is characterized by damage from cholangitis and bile duct destruction, along with elevated serum *alanine aminotransferase*, elevated IgG, and *smooth muscle antibodies (SMA)*. A liver biopsy will also show patches of cell death (*necrosis*) around the bile ducts.[18]

PBC is 10 times more common in women and mostly affects those ages 35 to 65. But PBC can also occur in young women and in the elderly, adds

Dr. Bodenheimer. There's a genetic component, with a higher prevalence among first-degree relatives with the disease and among women with family members who have other autoimmune diseases. Notably, sisters of women with PBC may have as much as a fourteen fold greater risk of the disease.[17] Smoking may also increase the risk of PBC.

A majority of women with PBC also have another autoimmune disease, which may be present years before PBC is diagnosed. Between 50 and 75 percent of women with PBC may have *Sjögren's syndrome. Scleroderma* is also common. About 6 percent of women with PBC also have rheumatoid arthritis, and another 6 percent have thyroid disease. Some experts recommend testing women with thyroid disorders for AMAs.[18] Other autoimmune diseases seen in women with PBC include *pernicious anemia, autoimmune thrombocytopenia, celiac disease,* and *polymyositis.* Women with PBC may also be at higher risk for liver and other cancers, including lymphoma and cancers of the breasts, ovaries, and thyroid.[17]

Symptoms of PBC

As with AIH, fatigue may be one of the earliest symptoms of primary biliary cirrhosis, occurring in as many as 78 percent of patients. You may find that you're unable to exert yourself physically, especially with exercise.

Another common symptom is intense itching (seen in over 60 percent of women), which may worsen at bedtime. The dry mouth of Sjögren's syndrome can alter taste and hamper swallowing and even vocal cord function. Dry eyes are also common, and there may be enlargement of the parotid glands in women who also have Sjögren's.[17]

Women may also complain of upper abdominal pain on the right side. There may be weight loss and diarrhea with pale, bulky stools. Some women may have brownish hyperpigmentation of the skin. Signs of later disease and liver failure include fluid in the abdomen, gastric bleeding, and jaundice (caused by accumulation of bilirubin in the skin and other tissues).

Advanced PBC is also associated with bone loss (see page 411); in some cases, poor absorption of vitamin D (a fat-soluble vitamin) may contribute.[17] The degree of osteoporosis can be severe, with spinal fractures and compression that result in back pain and muscle spasms. Older women may experience spontaneous (nontraumatic) fractures of the ribs and bone pain.

Up to 60 percent of people with PBC have no symptoms at all (some may even have normal aminotransferase levels). As with AIH, routine blood work may reveal abnormalities in liver test results that alert a woman's doctor to a problem. In PBC, the red flag is an elevation in the enzyme *alkaline phosphatase* (an enzyme that increases in bile with cholestasis) over normal levels (20 to 70 units per liter, U/L). Cholesterol may also be mildly elevated, due to backflow of bile fats into the blood and increased cholesterol production by liver cells. However, some women may have normal liver enzymes and even in advanced disease may show no outward signs.

However, two physical signs are the hallmarks of PBC: One is yellow, fatty nodules in the skin, caused by abnormal cholesterol metabolism. When these nodules appear around the eyes, they are called *xanthelasmas*, and when they arise in folds or creases of the skin (such as on the hands, elbows, or knees) they are termed *xanthomas*. People with PBC may also display abrasions and breaks in the skin caused by scratching to relieve intense itching (*excoriations*); these scratch marks can often bleed.[17]

Diagnosing PBC

It's often difficult to tell PBC from autoimmune hepatitis, because both cause the death of liver cells (necrosis). Blood tests and liver biopsy can help distinguish PBC from other *cholestatic* liver disorders and reveal the extent of damage to bile ducts, granulomas, and fibrosis, along with infiltration of inflammatory cells.

Diagnostic criteria include AMA titers, levels of *alkaline phosphatase* one and a half times the upper limit of normal over a six-month period, and liver histology showing *nonsuppurative destructive cholangitis (CNDC, or syndrome of primary biliary cirrhosis)* and destruction of the *interlobular bile ducts (Canals of Hering).*[19] A liver biopsy also helps to "stage" PBC to evaluate the progression and extent of liver and bile duct damage, and whether there's liver cirrhosis. In early disease, with diagnostic blood test results, a liver biopsy may not be needed to diagnose or manage PBC.

AMAs are detected in blood or liver cells using *immunofluorescence*. The amount of AMA does not indicate how severe PBC is or predict how rapidly it will progress. Unlike *antinuclear antibodies (ANAs)*, which often decline after treatment for other autoimmune diseases, AMAs do not respond to treatment.

Cholesterol can also be elevated in PBC; it can top 1,000 mg per deciliter of blood (mg/dl) in late-stage disease.

PBC Clusters

Autoimmune thyroid disease occurs in around 20 percent of women with primary biliary cirrhosis.[17] Many of the same diseases that cluster with autoimmune hepatitis also occur with PBC. They include:

- Thyroid disease
- Sjögren's syndrome
- Rheumatoid arthritis
- Scleroderma
- Raynaud's phenomenon
- Lupus
- Celiac disease
- Pernicious anemia
- Vitiligo

A majority of women with PBC have other autoimmune disorders (see list), which must be treated separately. Because of the overlap with autoimmune hepatitis, some patients are given a trial of prednisone to help distinguish between the two; PBC does not respond to corticosteroids, but AIH does.

Treating PBC

Ursodeoxycholic acid (UDCA), or *ursodiol (Actigall, URSO 250, URSO Forte)* is the most common treatment for PBC. Taken orally, it improves symptoms, prolongs survival, and postpones the need for a liver transplant.

Ursodiol lowers levels of alkaline phosphatase, bilirubin, and other liver enzymes and is also prescribed to dissolve certain kinds of gallstones. Side effects may include abdominal pain, indigestion, nausea, chest pain, and itching.[20] Ursodiol can interact with cholesterol-lowering medications, aluminum-based antacids (such as *Rolaids*), and estrogens.

Ursodiol may also be given in combination with corticosteroids, especially budesonide (which is highly absorbed into the liver). PBC-AIH overlap syndrome is treated with corticosteroids or azathioprine.

Newer treatments for PBC are being tested, including *obeticholic acid*, which reduces bile acid synthesis and aids excretion of bile.

"The therapies we have do not cure the disease, and patients not adequately controlled by medication may progress to needing a liver transplant," says Dr. Bodenheimer.

A liver transplant is the only definitive treatment for end-stage PBC, improving the course of the disease as well as survival. However, it doesn't eradicate the underlying problem. PBC can also recur after a transplant. One-year survival after transplant is 85 to 90 percent and five-year survival is about 75 percent, with many patients going on to live 20 and more years.

The itching associated with PBC is treated with *cholestyramine resin (Questran, Questran Light)* taken three times a day. Questran is a bile-acid binder that comes in powder form and must be mixed with water or other liquids. The main side effect is constipation. It can also interact with estrogens and progestins, as well as thyroid medications such as *Synthroid*. Questran can also interfere with the normal digestion and absorption of fats and fat-soluble vitamins. The effects of Questran during pregnancy have not been well studied, so women need to take it under a doctor's supervision.

How PBC Can Affect You Over Your Lifetime

Ursodiol can interfere with the estrogens in oral contraceptives, so women may need to use a second form of birth control or another method of contraception.

An estimated 25 percent of women with PBC are of childbearing age, and most available evidence indicates they have uneventful pregnancies.[21]

In one retrospective study, researchers at a liver center in Toronto assessed outcomes in women who were pregnant at the time of PBC diagnosis or became pregnant after being diagnosed. In 80 percent of patients, liver biochemistry remained normal during pregnancy, and 72 percent had a postpartum biochemical flare. However, no adverse events were seen during pregnancy and postpartum, and risks to the baby don't seem to be influenced by biochemical disease activity.[21] Biochemical disease activity and severe itching can increase during or after pregnancy.

While there's no evidence to indicate that ursodiol can harm an unborn baby, it's not recommended during pregnancy unless clearly needed. It's not known whether the drug passes into breast milk, so caution is advised for those women who are breast-feeding.

Menopause and Beyond

Ursodiol can also interfere with the effectiveness of oral estrogen in hormone therapy, so women are advised to use estrogen patches or cream (see pages 53 to 54).

Osteoporosis is a serious concern for postmenopausal women in general, but women with PBC may have a greatly accelerated course. Older women with PBC can have vertebral fractures, spinal compression, loss of height, and sudden rib fractures. Women with PBC may need to be put on drugs such as alendronate to slow bone loss.

The Risk of Cancer

Liver cancer can develop in anyone with cirrhosis, but the incidence is low in both PBC and autoimmune hepatitis. "The risk of liver cancer in women with autoimmune liver disease is increased compared to the general population, but not as much as in people with the viral hepatitis," remarks Dr. Palmer. "We really don't know why. In hepatitis C there's a 25 percent chance of developing liver cancer, but in autoimmune hepatitis and PBC it's much, much lower, perhaps around 2 to 6 percent in PBC. Preventing the development of cirrhosis will also prevent liver cancer."

Notes

1. Manns MP, Lohse AW, Vergani D. Autoimmune hepatitis—update 2015. *J Hepatol.* 2015;62:S100–S111.
2. Bjornsson E, Talwalkar J, Treeprasertsuk S, et al. Drug-induced autoimmune hepatitis: clinical characteristics and prognosis. *Hepatology.* 2010;51:2040–2048.
3. Manns MP, Czaja AJ, Gorham JD, et al. AASLD Practice guidelines: diagnosis and management of autoimmune hepatitis. *Hepatology.* 2010;51(6):2193–2213. doi:10.1002/hep.23584.
4. Liberal R, Grant CR, Longhi MS. Diagnostic criteria of autoimmune hepatitis. *Autoimmunity Rev.* 2014;13:435–440. http://dx.doi.org/10.1016/j.autrev.2013.11.009.
5. Alvarez F, Berg PA, Bianchi FB, et al. International Autoimmune Hepatitis Group report: review of criteria for diagnosis of autoimmune hepatitis. *J Hepatol.* 1999;31:929–938.
6. Czaja AJ, Manns MP. Advances in the diagnosis, pathogenesis, and management of autoimmune hepatitis. *Gastroenterology.* 2010;139:58–72. doi:10.1053/j.gastro.2010.04.053.
7. Manns MP, Taubert R. Treatment of autoimmune hepatitis. *Clin Liver Dis.* 2014;3(1):15–17. doi:10.1002/cld.306.
8. Kirstein MM, Metzler F, Geiger E, et al. Prediction of short- and long-term outcome in patients with autoimmune hepatitis. *Hepatology.* July 14, 2015. doi:10.1002/hep.27983. [Epub ahead of print].
9. Gatselis N, Georgia Papadamou G, et al. Mycophenolate for the treatment of autoimmune hepatitis: prospective assessment of its efficacy and safety for induction and maintenance of remission in a large cohort of treatment-naïve patients. *J Hepatol.* 2011;55(3):636–646.
10. Medline Plus. Cyclosporine information. http://www.nlm.nih.gov/medlineplus/druginfo/meds/a601207.html.
11. Burak KW, Swain MG, Santodomingo-Garzon T, et al. Rituximab for the treatment of patients with autoimmune hepatitis who are refractory or intolerant to standard therapy. *Can J Gastroenterol.* 2013;27:273–280.
12. Weiler-Normann C, Quaas A, Weigard C, et al. Infliximab as a rescue treatment in difficult-to-treat autoimmune hepatitis. *J Hepatol.* 2013;58(3):529–534. doi:http://dx.doi.org/10.1016/j.jhep.2012.11.010.
13. Manns MP, Czaja AJ, Gorham JD, et al. Diagnosis and management of autoimmune hepatitis. *Hepatology.* 2010;51(6). doi:10.1002/hep.23584.
14. Prescribing information about budesonide. http://www.nlm.nih.gov/medlineplus/druginfo/meds/a608007.html.
15. Information about mycophenolate mofetil. http://www.rxlist.com/cellcept-drug.htm.
16. Rituximab prescribing guide. http://www.gene.com/download/pdf/rituxan_prescribing.pdf.
17. Purohit T, Cappell MS. Primary biliary cirrhosis: pathophysiology, clinical presentation and therapy. *World J Hepatol.* 2015;7(7):926–941. doi:10.4254/wjh.v7.i7.926.

18. Reshetnyak VI. Primary biliary cirrhosis: clinical and laboratory criteria for its diagnosis. *World J Gastroenterol.* 2015;21(25):7683–7708. doi:10.3748/wjg.v21.i25.7683.
19. Bowlus CL, Gershwin EM. The diagnosis of primary biliary cirrhosis. *Autoimmunity Rev.* 2014;13:441–444. http://dx.doi.org/10.1016/j.autrev.2014.01.041.
20. URSO 250®/URSO Forte®, Urosiol. Package insert. http://www.accessdata.fda.gov/drugsatfda_docs/label/2008/020675s013lbl.pdf.
21. Efe C, Kahramanoğlu-Aksoy E, Yılmaz B, et al. Pregnancy in women with primary biliary cirrhosis. *Autoimmun Rev.* 2014;13:931–935. http://dx.doi.org/10.1016/j.autrev.2014.05.008.

13

Fellow Travelers—Fibromyalgia, Chronic Fatigue, Endometriosis, and Interstitial Cystitis

I was diagnosed with juvenile rheumatoid arthritis when I was in eighth grade. But I've been fortunate in that I only seem to get bad flares every few years. I was always able to stay active in some way; I've even run marathons. When I have a flare, the pain and fatigue are very bad . . . it's hard to do my job . . . I can't write or type, I can't open a car door, or even turn the key in the ignition . . . but I would take different drugs and it would get better. Even with those problems, I had started to think of my RA as kind of predictable. But then I started to develop pain in other areas of my body. Not in the joints, but in the muscles around them . . . and at very specific points like my shoulders, elbow, or knees. And I got this overwhelming aching fatigue, like I had the flu . . . I couldn't seem to think straight . . . I just wanted to sleep all the time, but I never really felt rested. This was unlike any of the RA flares I'd ever had, and none of the drugs I normally took seemed to help it. My rheumatologist kept saying it was my RA getting worse, but the blood tests did not show any signs of a flare and my joints were not affected. My doctor finally diagnosed me with fibromyalgia.

Cate, 30

Fibromyalgia

Fibromyalgia is *not* an autoimmune disease. However, it occurs so often with autoimmune diseases, particularly rheumatoid arthritis (RA), Sjögren's syndrome, and systemic lupus erythematosus (SLE), and has such a major impact on so many women's lives, that we felt it should be included in this book.

Symptoms of fibromyalgia can overlap with autoimmune connective tissue diseases, and it's often difficult to tell whether it's an RA or SLE flare or not. Additionally, new insights have been gained into the nature of this disorder—its characteristic signs, its possible causes, and its effects on women with autoimmune diseases.

Fibromyalgia isn't a new problem by any means. In the 1880s it was called *neurasthenia*,[1] a vague ailment attributed to "weakness or exhaustion of the nervous system" that sent women to their beds with aches and pains, unexplained fatigue, and depression (and maybe a swig of "Lydia Pinkham's Vegetable Compound," a popular cure-all containing 20 percent alcohol). But it wasn't until 1975 that two Canadian researchers studying rheumatoid arthritis patients described the distinct symptoms—including sleep disorders, diffuse musculoskeletal pain, and tenderness at specific points around the body—that characterize fibromyalgia.[2]

It was first called *fibrositis*, meaning "muscle inflammation," but studies later showed there was no inflammation in the muscles of patients with the disorder.

Today, the constellation of symptoms known as *fibromyalgia syndrome (FMS)* is recognized as a distinct medical disorder involving pain amplification or hypersensitivity, with myriad dimensions.

The American College of Rheumatology (ACR) first established formal diagnostic criteria for FMS in 1990,[3] updating those criteria in 2010,[4] making further tweaks in 2011.[5] The newer ACR criteria include high levels of fatigue, unrefreshing sleep, and cognitive problems (trouble thinking or remembering things) plus chronic pain in multiple areas.

The biggest change is the way fibromyalgia is diagnosed. The 1990 criteria called for examination of 18 "tender points" (see illustration), specific points of the body sensitive and painful to the touch. This has been replaced by findings of persistent musculoskeletal pain in areas *correlating* to those tender points. There's also a severity scale (SS) score for other symptoms (see page 422), which requires more careful attention to how patients

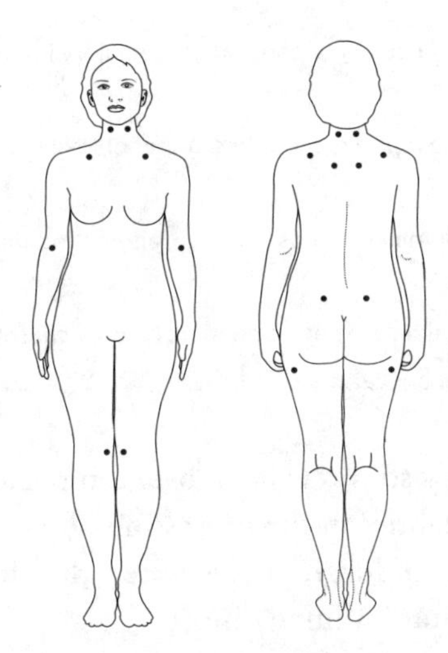

2011 ACR guidelines for FMS correlate the 1990 'tender points' with localized areas where there is pain and sensitivity.

Source: American College of Rheumatology

experience the disorder. Mood, which can vary and is very difficult to quantify, is not considered in the criteria.

The ACR says the old system missed 25 percent of fibromyalgia patients, while the newer criteria accurately identify more than 90 percent of patients. A simple six-item self-report FMS questionnaire is also being studied.[6]

While it's not 100 percent accurate, experts say the updated ACR criteria can help distinguish symptoms of RA, SLE, and other autoimmune diseases from fibromyalgia and may improve treatments for both.

The list of FMS-associated symptoms is long and very general—so it's quite easy to *self-diagnose*. In addition, there are no clinical or laboratory tests that can confirm the diagnosis. This is why fibromyalgia has been, and remains, a controversial and difficult diagnosis.

Some Warning Signs of Fibromyalgia

The symptoms must be present for three months or more with no other likely cause.

- Fatigue
- Unrefreshing sleep

- Cognitive problems (inability to concentrate, memory impairment)
- Depression
- Persistent pain in the hip, jaw, shoulders, upper or lower arms, and legs.
- Chronic headaches
- Irritable bowel (abdominal cramps, bloating, alternating diarrhea and constipation)
- Depression
- Irritable bladder (frequent, painful urination, bladder spasms)

Fibromyalgia typically strikes women between the ages of 20 and 40, possibly caused by abnormalities in the processing of pain signals by the central nervous system. Some studies have suggested that it may be triggered by injuries, infections, or autoimmune diseases.

Between 2 and 4 percent of women in the general population may be affected, two to seven times more women than men[7] depending on which set of criteria is used.

Up to 25 percent of women with autoimmune diseases, including rheumatoid arthritis, lupus, and Crohn's disease, may meet updated ACR criteria for fibromyalgia.

Fibromyalgia symptoms also overlap with other autoimmune "fellow travelers" such as *chronic fatigue syndrome*, *irritable bowel syndrome (IBS)*, and *interstitial cystitis (IC)*.

What Causes Fibromyalgia?

The underlying causes of fibromyalgia are still unknown. Some experts believe that some stressor or trauma—be it a physical injury, immune overstimulation (as in autoimmune disease), hormonal alterations (such as being hypothyroid), infections, extreme emotional stress, or a combination of factors—triggers disturbances in the central nervous system of susceptible women, leading to oversensitivity to even low levels of pain. It's been likened to having the "volume turned up" to pain and other stimuli.

Fibromyalgia can run in families, primarily among women, mostly affected by pain amplification. "We don't have a single candidate gene, and it's probably a combination of genetic factors, but the evidence is that there's a predisposition to this disorder," remarks Laurence A. Bradley, PhD, professor of medicine in the division of Clinical Immunology and Rheumatology at the University of Alabama at Birmingham. "There may be multiple disruptions in the function of structures in the central nervous system involved in pain transmission and modulation, along with dysregulation of neurotransmitters involved in pain processing and stress hormones."

However, without genetic factors or biomarkers that may signal enhanced risk, there's no way to make reliable predictions at this time as to who is especially vulnerable to FMS, with or without a family history, Dr. Bradley stresses.

Brain activity in processing pain seems to be different in people with FMS. "We identified resting state abnormalities in cerebral blood flow in two brain structures involved in processing pain in patients with fibromyalgia, compared to healthy people. And in non-patients who report pain, we also saw low levels of blood flow in one of those structures," says Dr. Bradley. Many people with fibromyalgia appear to have abnormalities in the *autonomic nervous system* (which governs breathing, heart rate, and blood pressure, among other things), causing symptoms like *orthostatic hypotension* (dizziness when going from a sitting to standing position).

Brain chemicals that may be affected in FMS include *serotonin* (which helps regulate mood, sleep, and appetite) and *norepinephrine* (a stress hormone). Studies have also found levels of *substance P*, a chemical that helps transmit pain signals, to be up to three times higher in the spinal fluid of fibromyalgia patients than levels in healthy individuals.[8]

A small study at the Cedars-Sinai Medical Center in Los Angeles also found increased levels of inflammatory cytokines stimulated by substance P in blood samples from 56 people with fibromyalgia, compared to 36 healthy people.[9] One cytokine, *interleukin-8 (IL-8)* promotes pain, and another, *interleukin-6 (IL-6)*, induces hypersensitivity to painful stimuli, fatigue, and depression. (IL-6 is also elevated in people with lupus and rheumatoid arthritis.) Researchers believe that these inflammatory cytokines may play a role in increased pain sensitivity.

"The evidence is not very consistent, but there is some question as to whether there may be abnormalities in some of the cytokines that promote inflammation in people with fibromyalgia. However, there is no reliable evidence so far that there is an immune system problem in fibromyalgia, and certainly not an autoimmune problem," says Dr. Bradley, who has studied the disorder for years.

"Nevertheless, there are individuals with autoimmune diseases such as rheumatoid arthritis who develop fibromyalgia as a secondary condition," he adds.

Psychological factors also come into play. The lifetime incidence of mood disorders like depression and anxiety in people with fibromyalgia ranges from 40 to 70 percent, but that may be an overestimate. "When we compare people being treated for fibromyalgia with non-patients, nonpatients tend to have lower scores on questionnaires that measure depression or other kinds of psychological distress, and they often feel they're more able to use their internal resources to cope with their pain than the people who are treated in the clinic," comments Dr. Bradley.

Symptoms of Fibromyalgia

The main symptoms of fibromyalgia—fatigue, unrefreshing sleep, cognitive problems (dubbed "fibro fog"), and chronic pain in multiple areas of the body—are frustratingly nonspecific.

While many women with fibromyalgia also have painful connective tissue diseases like lupus or rheumatoid arthritis, in many cases no physical joint, bone, or tissue damage or inflammation can be found.

Fibromyalgia pain often waxes and wanes, shifts from one area of the body to another, and is often accompanied by numbness or tingling. Some women complain that they "ache all over," while others report pain only in certain regions of the body, like the lower back and hip. In fact, many women may initially be diagnosed with lower back problems or an overuse injury like tennis elbow (*lateral epicondylitis*) or heel pain (*plantar fasciitis*).

Other problems common in fibromyalgia include headaches, dry eyes, jaw pain (*temporomandibular joint syndrome, TMJ*), noncardiac chest pain, heartburn, painful periods, urinary frequency and urgency (*irritable bladder*), and pelvic pain. Women with FMS may also have other, more regional pain-related syndromes, such as *irritable bowel syndrome*, interstitial cystitis, endometriosis, and vulvar pain syndromes (*vulvodynia* and *vulvar vestibulitis*, a chronic irritation, rawness and pain in the vulva. labia, or the *vulvar vestible*, a crescent shaped opening around the vaginal opening).

"Many of these symptoms and syndromes cluster together. For example, it's much more likely for someone with chronic pain to have irritable bowel syndrome or TMJ syndrome than someone who doesn't have chronic pain," observes noted FMS authority Daniel J. Clauw, MD, a professor of medicine in the division of rheumatology and director of the Center for the Advancement of Clinical Research at the University of Michigan, Ann Arbor.

A majority of women with fibromyalgia report severe fatigue; at least half of those who meet the criteria for FMS will also meet diagnostic criteria for chronic fatigue syndrome (CFS), says Dr. Clauw. "While the defining symptom of CFS is fatigue, you also have to have pain-based symptoms."

In FMS, fatigue and pain are worse after physical activity, and women may also experience major problems with concentration and memory. Other symptoms can include weight gain (or loss); intolerance to heat, cold, and loud noises; and problems with vision or hearing. Women may also complain of "allergic" symptoms, ranging from drug reactions and multiple chemical sensitivities to respiratory symptoms like runny nose and nasal congestion.

Symptoms of fibromyalgia may come on after viral infections, such as *Epstein-Barr virus* (infectious mononucleosis), *Lyme disease, parvovirus*, or *Q fever*, all of which have a pain component. "Two to 3 percent of people who develop these infections will never completely recover and end up with fibromyalgia or chronic fatigue syndrome," says Dr. Clauw. There's also a subset of people who develop hypothyroidism and have chronic widespread pain. And even after their thyroid hormone is replaced and they are made euthyroid, they never regain their baseline state of health and have something indistinguishable from fibromyalgia."

Certain medications, like the cholesterol-lowering drugs called *statins*, can provoke chronic widespread muscle pain, which persists even after the drug is stopped. Symptoms mimicking fibromyalgia can also occur when women are being tapered off high-dose corticosteroids. However, regular pain medicines (like aspirin, ibuprofen, or acetaminophen) don't help the pain of fibromyalgia, and that's often what brings a woman to her doctor's office.

The symptoms of fibromyalgia and autoimmune disorders overlap, including joint and muscle pain, fatigue, and morning stiffness, as well as a feeling that the hands or feet are swollen. Some women may have symptoms similar to *Raynaud's phenomenon* (see page 131), but their entire hand turns pale or red, instead of just the fingers. Facial flushing and a mottled red rash on the legs (*livedo reticularis*) are also common in fibromyalgia, and women may initially be misdiagnosed with lupus. FMS often coexists with autoimmune diseases.

Diagnosing FMS

The 2010–2011 ACR classification criteria for fibromyalgia include three major symptoms—**fatigue, unrefreshing sleep, and cognitive problems** (trouble thinking or remembering things)—plus a variety of other nonspecific symptoms (see page 417) and persistent pain in at least seven areas of the body:[5]

- Shoulder girdle (shoulder blades and collar bone)
- Left or right hip (buttock and area where the hip joint meets the upper thigh bone)
- Left or right jaw
- Upper back/lower back (right or left)
- Upper arm/lower arm (right or left)
- Upper leg/lower leg (right or left)

According to the ACR criteria, the number of painful areas adds up to a **widespread pain index (WPI)**. Symptoms are assessed with a severity score of 5 or above (on a scale of 1 to 12). Or, both the WPI and the SS must add up to 9 or above to meet the criteria.

The Fibromyalgia Network (www.fmnetnews.com) has adapted the ACR criteria into a self-assessment form, which may be valuable to bring to a doctor visit (see Appendix A).

If you, or your doctor, suspect you have fibromyalgia, you'll undergo a thorough physical examination to exclude neurological, orthopedic, and rheumatological causes for your symptoms.

More acute, short-term pain may be due to an injury or disease flare, and may need a more extensive workup. Physical signs of inflammation like swollen joints (*synovitis*) or muscle weakness are not signs of fibromyalgia. But inflammatory and noninflammatory mechanisms can both cause fibromyalgia symptoms, so having a response to anti-inflammatory medications doesn't automatically rule out FMS. Since one in three lupus patients also have fibromyalgia, often doctors attribute symptoms to SLE and try to treat them with prednisone. However, lupus patients don't usually have the overall pain sensitivity seen in fibromyalgia.

Tests You May Need and What They Mean

There are no diagnostic tests or blood markers for fibromyalgia.

Your doctor may order a complete blood count; blood tests for liver, kidney, and thyroid function, and a sedimentation rate or level of C-reactive protein to detect inflammation. Unless your pain has come on suddenly or there's evidence that you may have an autoimmune disease, testing for markers such as rheumatoid factor (RF) or antinuclear antibodies (ANAs) is usually not done.

If you have dizziness when going from a prone to standing position, your blood pressure will be measured as you do this to see if you have a sudden drop in pressure (*orthostatic hypotension*, or *orthostatic instability*), a common symptom in fibromyalgia. If you're having pain and stiffness in weight-bearing joints, x-rays or other imaging may be done to look for evidence of arthritis, either rheumatoid arthritis or *osteoarthritis* (the wear-and-tear kind that breaks down cartilage in the joints).

Cate's story continues:

My husband was fine through my RA flares, but he doesn't understand this.

It really has put a strain on our relationship. He keeps saying, "Why do you need to sleep so much? Why can't you do things? Why are you upset so easily? Can't you take something for the pain?" It's very frustrating. I know if my RA got bad, there are drugs I could take to help it. But nothing really seems to make fibromyalgia better . . . I've had antidepressants . . . I've taken bigger doses of pain medications. The only thing that really seems to help is exercise. So I just force myself to go out and walk or run. It's hard, and I can't exercise as much as I used to, and that gets me down sometimes, much more so than having RA. But I refuse to give in to this. Since I've had RA for so long I understand what's going on in my body. But fibromyalgia? This, I just don't understand.

Treating Fibromyalgia

Treatment for fibromyalgia usually involves a combination of medication and exercise, along with behavior modification techniques, cognitive behavioral therapy, and stress reduction.

"Regular analgesics don't work very well in pain amplification syndromes. Things like acetaminophen and nonsteroidal anti-inflammatory drugs have virtually no effect in pain amplification syndromes. Opioids (such as *tramadol*) also do not seem to work well," comments Dr. Clauw. "The best drugs for these syndromes are those that act on the central nervous system and the neurotransmitters serotonin and norepinephrine."

Three medications have been approved specifically for fibromyalgia: *duloxetine (Cymbalta),*[10] *milnacipran (Savella),*[11] and *pregabalin (Lyrica).*[12]

Cymbalta and Savella act like antidepressants that prevent excess reabsorption (*reuptake*) of the neurochemicals *serotonin* and *norepinephrine* in the brain, helping to dampen overactive pain signals from nerves (*neuropathic pain*). They can also aid sleep and improve fatigue.

It's unknown whether Cymbalta can harm an unborn baby, but it may cause problems in a newborn if taken during the third trimester of pregnancy. So you need to let your doctor know if you plan to (or want to) become pregnant.[9,10]

The most common side effect with Savella is nausea. Other side effects include headache, constipation, dizziness, insomnia, hot flushes, excessive sweating, dry mouth, and palpitations.[11]

A 2013 study of milnacipran led by Dr. Clauw showed it produced clinically meaningful improvements in FMS pain for up to three years.[13]

Lyrica also affects the brain chemicals *serotonin* and *norepinephrine*, helping to block overactive nerve signaling. It also targets *substance P* and another excitatory neurotransmitter, *glutamate*.[8] Lyrica's side effects can include dizziness, drowsiness, and weight gain.[12]

Other medications used in fibromyalgia include the tricyclic antidepressant *amitriptyline (Elavil)*, the muscle relaxant *cyclobenzaprine (Flexeril)*, the selective serotonin reuptake inhibitor (SSRI) antidepressants *paroxetine (Paxil)* and *fluoxetine (Prozac)*, and *tramadol*, a weak opioid and serotonin and norepinephrine reuptake inhibitor (available with and without acetaminophen).[14]

A review of drugs used in fibromyalgia concluded that there are few differences between the three newer medications; they provide an improvement in pain of 30 percent in half of patients who take them, and improvements in pain of 50 percent in a third of patients. Paroxetine, fluoxetine, and tramadol are considered second-line treatments, the review noted.[14]

Atypical antidepressants, such as *bupropion (Wellbutrin)* and *nefazodone (Serzone),* which affect the neurotransmitters norepinephrine and dopamine, have been shown to help FMS patients whose major complaints are fatigue or cognitive problems.

Women who have orthostatic hypotension or palpitations may benefit from increasing fluid intake, along with sodium and potassium; low doses of *beta-blockers* are also helpful in women with these signs of *autonomic nerve dysfunction.*

Nondrug Therapies

Moderate aerobic exercise and gentle stretching with Tai Chi or yoga may be the best prescription for fibromyalgia pain.

Exercise has been shown to relieve pain by boosting *endorphins* (the body's natural painkiller) as well as depression in patients with rheumatoid arthritis. Physical therapy and other techniques to ease pain include cortisone injections, injections of local anesthetic (such as *procaine*), massage, moist heat, *myofascial release therapy* (in which pressure is applied to trigger points to "release" tightened muscles), *chiropractic* (a technique of spinal manipulation), and *acupuncture* (the application of hair-thin needles to specific points along the body called *meridians*, triggering the release of endorphins and stimulating nerve endings). However, there have been only a few studies of these therapies in fibromyalgia.

Cognitive behavioral therapy (CBT) is well studied in pain syndromes and other chronic problems. CBT teaches coping skills and behavioral changes to help you manage negative thoughts that can make pain worse. "Every randomized, controlled trial of cognitive behavioral therapy in any chronic illness has been shown to be effective," remarks Dr. Clauw.

One recent study looked at CBT combined with a tailored exercise program in fibromyalgia. Researchers assigned newly diagnosed patients to 16 twice-weekly sessions of CBT followed by exercise tailored to their pain-related behaviors (including relaxation training, aerobic exercises, and strength and flexibility exercises) with a booster session after three months.[15] The program proved to be highly effective in improving both short- and long-term physical outcomes such as pain, fatigue, and functional disability, as well as psychological outcomes including negative mood and anxiety.

With CBT, you'll learn relaxation techniques (such as deep breathing and positive visual imagery), how to reframe negative thoughts and behaviors that intensify pain responses, how to effectively solve problems, and how to pace activities to accommodate whatever limitations you may have. The ultimate goal is to provide you with tools to take control over your fibromyalgia . . . and your life.

Chronic Fatigue Syndrome

Many autoimmune diseases can cause fatigue that is chronic. However, chronic fatigue syndrome (CFS) is *not* autoimmune.

CFS is believed to involve interactions between the immune and central nervous systems, but the cause is unknown. The Institute of Medicine (IOM) suggests it may be triggered by infection, physical trauma, and exposure to environmental pollutants, chemicals, and heavy metals.[16]

Symptoms of CFS often overlap with other illnesses. They can come on suddenly, often after a viral infection, with extreme fatigue and a cognitive "fog" that can last for months or even years. Infections that have been linked to CFS include colds, bronchitis, hepatitis, and infectious mononucleosis (*Epstein-Barr virus*).

CFS symptoms may linger or come and go frequently for more than six months. They include fatigue and weakness, muscle and joint aches, headaches, inability to concentrate, allergic symptoms, and tender lymph nodes.

For most people, CFS symptoms plateau early in the course of illness and later wax and wane, with some people completely recovering.

There are no clinical or blood tests, no brain scans, nor other imaging techniques to diagnose CFS—and it's often dismissed as "psychosomatic."

But CFS is very real. Patients with the syndrome are "typically unable to perform their normal activities, and as many as one-fourth are homebound or bedridden, sometimes for extended periods," a recent report comments.[17]

The IOM report estimates between 826,000 and 2.5 million people in the United States may be affected by CFS.

Under diagnostic criteria set by the Centers for Disease Control and Prevention (CDC), CFS can be diagnosed if a person has had six or more consecutive months of severe fatigue unrelieved by sufficient bed rest and four of these eight symptoms:[18] flu-like symptoms, memory impairment, tender lymph nodes, muscle pain, pain in multiple joints, new-onset headaches, unrefreshing sleep, or malaise lasting more than 24 hours after exertion.

The IOM says a more accurate—and less stigmatizing—name for this complex disorder may be *myalgic encephalomyelitis/chronic fatigue syndrome (ME/CFS)*.[16]

Under the IOM's criteria, a patient would have to have three key symptoms: a substantial reduction or impairment in the ability to engage in pre-illness levels of occupational, educational, social, or personal activities that persists for more than six months and is accompanied by fatigue, which is often profound, is of new or definite onset (not lifelong), is not the result of ongoing excessive exertion, and is not substantially alleviated by rest; "post-exertional malaise"; and unrefreshing sleep.[16]

In addition, patients would also need to have either cognitive impairment or *orthostatic intolerance* (dizziness and lightheadedness when standing up abruptly).[16]

Whichever criteria are eventually adopted, such vague, nonspecific symptoms make the syndrome a "diagnosis of exclusion," which often delays care. In multiple surveys, 67 to 77 percent of chronic fatigue patients say it took longer than a year to get a diagnosis and about a third say it took longer than five years. Due to competing criteria and symptoms often met with skepticism, "it is almost certainly the case that the majority of affected patients are never diagnosed," comments one researcher.[17]

There are no drugs approved to treat CFS or other specific treatments for the syndrome. Since it shares many symptoms with FMS, the same kinds of medications and therapies that help women with fibromyalgia may also work with CFS. These include cognitive behavioral therapy, graduated exercise programs, and low-dose tricyclic antidepressants to help with sleep and pain.

Nonsteroidal anti-inflammatory drugs (NSAIDs), such as ibuprofen, may help ease body aches or fever, and nonsedating antihistamines may help relieve allergic symptoms, such as runny nose. Learning how to manage fatigue and plan activities can help improve day-to-day functioning.

I've probably had endometriosis since I was 16, when I started having severe pain with my periods. It has taken a tremendous toll on me. I developed severe osteoporosis from treatments among other endometriosis-related factors, and over the years I've had five surgeries for endometriosis, including hysterectomy. After that, I took hormones for a few years because I had severe menopausal symptoms, but my endometriosis kicked in again, so I had to stop them temporarily. I was diagnosed with Hashimoto's thyroiditis in 1991, and I have also developed horrific joint pain. I also have terrible allergies.

Although we really can't say yet (in 2015) whether endometriosis is autoimmune, it is obviously an immune-mediated disease, and women with endometriosis have a greater risk for hypothyroidism, fibromyalgia, chronic fatigue syndrome, rheumatoid arthritis, lupus, Sjögren's syndrome, and multiple sclerosis, as shown in a study from our research registry published with the National Institutes of Health.

Mary Lou Ballweg, founder and president,
Endometriosis Association

Endometriosis

Endometriosis is a painful, chronic condition that affects an estimated 89 million women and girls worldwide, according to the Endometriosis Association, upwards of seven and a half million women just in the United States and Canada.

The problem arises when endometrial tissue, which normally lines the uterus, is found outside the uterus, where it grows in response to estrogen. These implants cause pain and inflammation, irritating the pelvic cavity, the reproductive organs, and/or the bowel. As the inflammation heals, scar tissue can form weblike growths called *adhesions*, which can also cause pain.

Like fibromyalgia, endometriosis often involves a heightened sensitivity to pain.[19] In fact, according to the American Society of Reproductive Medicine (ASRM), 70 to 90 percent of women who suffer with pelvic pain may have endometriosis.[20]

And, like FMS and CFS, it is *not* considered an autoimmune disease. However, over the years, some evidence has accumulated to suggest there may be an immune component. Experts note that endometrial implants are tolerated as self-antigens but act as irritants to promote inflammation, and levels of inflammatory cytokines found in many autoimmune diseases are also elevated in women with endometriosis.[21]

One study, presented back in 2002 at the World Congress on Endometriosis, found that 12 percent of women with endometriosis also had an autoimmune disorder, such as lupus or multiple sclerosis.[22] In contrast, only 2 percent of women in the general population have either disease.

In another study, researchers from the Endometriosis Association and the National Institutes of Health (NIH) polled 3,680 women aged 14 to 89 with surgically diagnosed endometriosis and asked whether they had ever been diagnosed with an autoimmune disorder, an endocrine disorder, fibromyalgia, chronic fatigue syndrome, and allergies or asthma. More than 20 percent reported having a coexisting condition; 35 percent had either FMS or chronic fatigue, more than 12 percent had asthma (20 percent of the women with autoimmune diseases reported having asthma), and 63 percent of the women suffered allergies.[23] "This suggests an *association* of endometriosis with autoimmune diseases," the researchers concluded.

Warning Signs of Endometriosis

- Unusually painful menstrual periods ("killer cramps")
- Chronic pelvic pain
- Painful sex
- Infertility
- Fatigue
- Diarrhea, painful bowel movements, and other gastrointestinal symptoms at the time of a menstrual period

---

What Causes Endometriosis?

Despite decades of research, the exact cause of endometriosis remains unclear. The earliest theory linked endometriosis to "retrograde menstruation," the purported backward flow of menstrual discharge through the fallopian tubes into the pelvic cavity.

What has become evident is that women with the disease have some type of immune dysregulation that fails to destroy the rogue tissue.

Normally, the scavenger cells of the immune system (*macrophages*) get rid of foreign cells and bacteria, but in endometriosis these "big eaters" don't clean up all the stray endometrial cells and cell fragments. The macrophages gobble the errant endometrial cells and present the remains of their dinner to T cells, which recognize the tissue as self and don't attack. There's also reduced activity of *natural killer (NK)* T cells, which don't need to be sensitized to react against viruses or tumors. So inflammation and irritation caused by the implants continue, possibly leading to production of cytokines that foster the growth of endometrial implants.

Studies also show the inflammatory cytokine *tumor necrosis factor-alpha (TNFα)*, elevated in autoimmune diseases, is also elevated in endometriosis, preventing normal programmed cell death and allowing endometrial implants to proliferate.[24] However, drugs that inhibit TNFα have no effect on endometriosis.[25]

Other research has found elevations of other inflammatory cytokines, including *interleukin-6 (IL-6)* and *interleuken-8 (IL-8)*.[26] "The theory has been that abnormal amounts of these cytokines and other chemicals produced by immune cells, along with retrograde flow, may overwhelm the immune system's ability to eliminate migratory endometrial cells," says David L. Olive, MD, director of the Wisconsin Fertility Institute in Madison. "There are subtle immunologic disorders that occur with endometriosis. Are they the primary disorder or are they the result of endometriosis? We simply don't know."

Endometriosis is considered a chronic pain syndrome. Cytokines produced in reaction to endometrial implants may cause malaise, fatigue, fever, and other inflammatory symptoms. Pain from implants may be caused by chemicals such as *prostaglandins* (which are also produced by the uterine lining and cause menstrual cramps). "It's unclear why endometriosis causes pain in some women, and not in others. It may be specific to the site of the implants, the amount of prostaglandins secreted by the implants, or the implants may secrete chemicals such as nerve growth factor, which can increase the local nerve density as well as increase inflammation," adds Dr. Olive.

Autoimmune diseases are characterized by the presence of autoantibodies, and researchers have looked for such antibodies in blood and secretions from women with endometriosis. Scientists have found *anti-endometrial antibodies*, which may be triggered by the presence of the endometrial implants and contribute to symptoms. *Antinuclear antibodies (ANAs)* found in lupus have been detected in women with endometriosis, but those antibodies are also found in women without autoimmune disease and in healthy women.

"Endometriosis may coexist with autoimmune disease, but this does not seem to be a common phenomenon. The presence of autoreactive antibodies in the serum of some patients with endometriosis may be a natural by-product of inflammation and local tissue destruction. The finding of antibodies to ovarian and endometrial nuclear antigens in patients with endometriosis supports the concept of endometriosis being a multiple antibody autoimmune condition. These autoreactive antibodies may play a role in pregnancy loss and infertility in patients with endometriosis, wrote the authors of a 2012 review.[23]

However, they conclude that endometriosis remains "enigmatic"—and its autoimmune connection still inconclusive.

Symptoms of Endometriosis

The most common symptom of endometriosis is severe pain before and during menstrual periods, caused in part by prostaglandins produced by the endometrial implants.

However, some women may have no symptoms at all and are diagnosed only when they're unable to become pregnant, sometimes due to scars or adhesions that block the release of eggs from the ovaries or their passage into the fallopian tubes, inflammation, or other factors.

Common sites for endometrial implants include the outer surface of the uterus and supporting ligaments, the space between the uterus and the rectum (called the *cul-de-sac*), the ovaries, and the membrane that lines the pelvic cavity. As the implanted tissue grows under the influence of estrogen, it can invade nearby organs, including the intestines and the bladder, causing painful bowel movements, irritable bowel symptoms, diarrhea and/or constipation, and intestinal upsets during menstruation.

A survey by the Endometriosis Association found that more than 87 percent of patients felt fatigued and exhausted; over a third were unable to carry out normal activities one to two days a month, and 57 percent had allergies. Sixty-four percent of the 4,000 women surveyed experienced painful intercourse. In addition, 43 percent of the women reported low resistance to infection, around 30 percent had low-grade fevers, and others reported severe problems with yeast infections (*candidiasis*) and yeast allergies. Up to 65 percent of women with endometriosis experience their first symptoms before the age of 20.

Diagnosing Endometriosis

While endometriosis can produce nodules or cysts on the ovary and cul-de-sac that can be felt during a pelvic exam, laparoscopy is the gold standard for a diagnosis.

Laparoscopy uses a thin, lighted telescope to look inside the pelvis and inspect the reproductive organs. It's done under general anesthesia, using small incisions in the abdomen to insert the fiber-optic scope to view the pelvic organs, and surgical instruments for a biopsy.

Implants can be vaporized (burned away), *excised* (cut out), or *ablated* (destroyed) during later laparoscopy using a laser or *electrocautery* instruments.

Treating Endometriosis

Medical treatment is aimed at suppressing the female hormones that fuel the growth of endometrial implants, using various hormones to prevent or lessen menstruation. It's not a cure; recurrence rates range from 30 to 60 percent. Surgery can eradicate endometrial implants and remove adhesions that cause pain, but cannot cure the disease.

Hormonal Therapy

Oral contraceptives are usually the initial treatment for endometriosis. Various formulations and strengths of estrogen and progesterone act together to prevent ovulation; the progestins in the pill suppress growth of endometrial tissue, reduce production of prostaglandins, and lessen pain. Oral contraceptives provide short-term relief in 50 to 80 percent of women and are considered the first-line treatment of endometriosis.[25]

Danazol (Danocrine, Cyclomen) is a derivative of testosterone, which reduces the amount of estrogen produced by your body to menopausal levels. A six-month regimen reduces the size and extent of endometrial implants by up to 50 percent; a majority of women experience pain relief, and as many as 70 to 100 percent of women go into remission. Danazol has androgenic side effects, including acne, growth of facial hair, water retention, and weight gain. It can also raise cholesterol. Danazol cannot be used during pregnancy.[27] In recent years newer drugs have largely replaced danazol.

GnRH agonists mimic the natural *gonadotropin releasing hormone* produced by the body that regulates estrogen production, but are much more potent. These drugs fool the body into thinking you're in menopause, reducing the symptoms of endometriosis. GnRH agonists approved by the FDA for endometriosis come in several forms, including *leuprolide (Lupron)*, given as injections; *nafarelin acetate (Synarel)* and *buserelin acetate (Suprefact)* in nasal spray form; or *goserelin acetate (Zoladex)*, an implant placed under the skin of the abdomen.[27]

These relieve pain in most women and produce up to a 90 percent regression of implants. The artificial menopause they create has all the symptoms of natural menopause: hot flashes, vaginal dryness, decreased sex drive, mood swings, and fatigue. GnRH agonists cannot be used during pregnancy.[27]

GnRH agonists also cause accelerated bone loss (around twice the normal rate of the first year of menopause) increasing the risk of osteoporosis. If prolonged treatment is needed, drugs are given to prevent bone resorption, including *alendronate (Fosamax)* and *risedronate (Actonel)*.

Other FDA-approved hormonal treatments for endometriosis are the progestogens *depot medroxyprogesterone acetate (Depo-Provera)* and *norethindrone acetate (Aygestin)*, which inhibit the growth of endometrial tissue.[27]

Surgery is usually done when hormonal therapy fails or if a woman doesn't wish to take hormones. Endometriosis surgery is usually done laparoscopically, making small incisions to admit tiny surgical instruments, lasers, or electrocautery devices that remove or destroy implants.

Laparoscopic surgery is done as a day surgery under general anesthesia. Laparoscopic surgery causes far less pain than open abdominal surgery, and recovery is faster; most women return to work within a week. For severe, invasive implants in and around the bowel or bladder, open abdominal surgery (*laparotomy*) may be needed.

Surgical procedures to eradicate implants should always be performed by a skilled endometriosis specialist.

How Endometriosis Can Affect You Over Your Lifetime

Endometriosis takes its biggest toll during a woman's reproductive years, sometimes causing pain during her teens.

Menstruation and Fertility

Endometriosis can cause extremely painful menstrual periods and, according to surveys by the Endometriosis Association, more than 40 percent of women with endometriosis report fertility problems. Surgery to remove adhesions or blockages that interfere with the release and uptake of an egg can improve fertility. But some women aren't helped by surgery and turn to in vitro fertilization. However, hormones needed for these procedures may stimulate endometrial implants, so experts urge women to proceed cautiously.

Women with endometriosis also have a high rate of tubal (*ectopic*) pregnancies and an increased risk of miscarriage. Some studies suggest that autoantibodies may interfere with the implantation of the fetus. Some studies have suggested that a combination of low-dose aspirin and prednisone improved pregnancy and implantation rates in women undergoing in vitro fertilization who were found to have autoantibodies, but experts say evidence to date does not support its use.[28]

Menopause and Beyond

For some women, pregnancy brings temporary relief from endometriosis, and menopause usually ends symptoms in women who have moderate disease. *Estrogen therapy (ET)* can occasionally reactivate endometriosis (even in women who have had a hysterectomy).

The course of endometriosis in later life has not been well studied. But studies suggest that women with endometriosis may have an increased risk of ovarian and breast cancer, as well as melanoma.

Interstitial Cystitis

Interstitial cystitis (IC) is another chronic pain condition that some scientists suspect may have an immune component.

IC (also called *painful bladder syndrome* or *bladder pain syndrome*) is a chronic disorder that causes nerve endings in the bladder to be irritated by elements in urine, resulting in bladder pain on filling, so it holds less urine. The cause is not known. It was once thought to be inflammatory, but bladder biopsies show very little inflammation.

One theory is that the cells lining the bladder are somehow "leaky" in women with IC, allowing substances in urine to penetrate the bladder wall, irritating muscle tissue and nerve endings, resulting in symptoms of urinary urgency and pain.

Other research has suggested that IC may be an autoimmune problem, with autoantibodies attacking bladder tissue.[29] Around 25 percent of women with IC are found to have increased levels of *antinuclear antibodies (ANAs)*, but, again, these are also found in healthy women. Autoantibodies to *mitochondria*, the energy-generating components of cells, found in women with scleroderma, have also been found in around 2.5 percent of IC patients. However, it's not known exactly what role these autoantibodies may play.

Mast cells, which play a role in allergies and in inflammation, have turned up in bladder biopsies of some women with IC, and 40 percent of IC patients also have allergies.

There's also a connection with chronic pain disorders. One study by Temple University found that 25 percent of women with IC have *irritable bowel syndrome*, almost 20 percent have migraines, 13 percent had endometriosis, and 10 percent had vulvodynia (see page 420).

The Temple study found that other IC patients have been diagnosed with (or have occasional symptoms of) fibromyalgia, ulcerative colitis, chronic fatigue, lupus, and asthma. However, experts say there are probably multiple causes for IC, which affects as many as 3.3 million U.S. women.[30]

The most common symptom is an urgent need to urinate, sometimes as many as 60 times over a 24-hour period. Women also experience a burning or cramping pain before and after urinating. Over half of women with IC have pain during or after intercourse, possibly due to spasms in pelvic muscles caused by irritation.

IC is diagnosed by *cystoscopy*.[31] The procedure is done under general anesthesia: the bladder is filled with water (*distended*) and drained, and then a flexible, lighted fiber-optic scope is inserted into the urethra to examine the lining of the bladder to look for tiny hemorrhages, ulcers (*Hunner's ulcers*), or cracks in the mucosa. Distention of the bladder with water (*hydrodistention*) may have therapeutic effects for some women.[30]

Bladder training and physical therapy, along with other self-care, noninvasive treatments, are recommended as first-line treatments by the American Urological Association (AUA).[32]

Dimethyl sulfoxide (DMSO) is an FDA-approved drug that is infused into the bladder by a catheter weekly (or every other week) for four to six weeks.[32] Because DMSO is absorbed into the bladder wall, it may directly lower inflammation and block pain, as well as prevent muscle contractions that cause urinary pain, frequency, and urgency.[32]

Lidocaine has also been used as a bladder infusion and has helped reduce pain for some women.[32]

Pentosan polysulfate sodium (Elmiron) is given orally. It seems to help coat the bladder lining, protecting it from irritants. Other treatments include the tricyclic antidepressant *amitriptyline (Elavil)*, which lessens nerve pain in some women, and seems to increase bladder capacity, and the antihistamine *hydroxyzine (Atarax)*. Since both can cause drowsiness, they're usually taken at bedtime.

Some women have found injections of *Botox (botulinum toxin)* into the bladder wall helpful. But it can be painful and may cause damage requiring periodic catheterization.[32]

Dietary changes—avoiding "bladder irritants" like alcohol, citrus fruits and juices, spicy foods, coffee, vinegar, and high-oxalate foods like spinach and rhubarb—may help some women.

There are no cures for interstitial cystitis. But, as with other chronic pain syndromes, women are urged to learn stress management techniques to help cope with the disorder.

Notes

1. Inanici FF, Yunus MB. History of fibromyalgia: past to present. *Curr Pain Headache Rep.* 2004;8(5):369–378. doi.10.1007/s11916-996-0010-6.
2. Moldofsky H, Scarisbrick P, England R, Smythe H. Musculoskeletal symptoms and non-REM sleep disturbance in patients with "fibrositis syndrome" and healthy subjects. *Psychosom Med.* 1975;37(4):341–351.

3. Wolfe F, Smythe HA, Yunus MB, et al. The American College of Rheumatology 1990 criteria for the classification of fibromyalgia. Report of the Multicenter Criteria Committee. *Arthritis Rheum.* 1990;33(2):160–172.
4. Wolfe F, Clauw DJ, Fitzcharles MA, et al. The American College of Rheumatology preliminary diagnostic criteria for fibromyalgia and measurement of symptom severity. *Arthritis Care Res.* 2010;62(5):600–610. doi:10.1002/acr.20140.
5. Wolfe F, Clauw DJ, Fitzcharles MA, et al. Fibromyalgia criteria and severity scales for clinical and epidemiological studies: a modification of the ACR preliminary diagnostic criteria for fibromyalgia. *J Rheumatol.* 2011;38(6):1113–1122. doi:10.3899/jrheum.100594.
6. Marcus DA, Bernstein C, Albrecht KL. Brief, self-report fibromyalgia screener evaluated in a sample of chronic pain patients. *Pain Med.* 2013;14(5):730–735. First published online April 11, 2013. doi:10.1111/pme.12114.
7. Lawrence RC, Felson DT, Helmick CG, et al. Estimates of the prevalence of arthritis and other rheumatic conditions in the United States, Part II. *Arthritis Rheum.* 2008;58(1):26–35. doi:10.1002/art.23176.
8. Becker S, Schweinhardt P. Dysfunctional neurotransmitter systems in fibromyalgia, their role in central stress circuitry and pharmacological actions on these systems. *Pain Res Treatment.* 2012. doi:10.1155/2012/741746.
9. Wallace J, Linker-Israeli M, Hallegua D, et al. Cytokines play an aetiopathogenetic role in fibromyalgia: a hypothesis and pilot study. *Rheumatology.* 2001;40(7):743–749. doi:10.1093/rheumatology/40.
10. U.S. Food and Drug Administration Medication Guide, Cymbalta. http://www.fda.gov/downloads/Drugs/DrugSafety/ucm088579.pdf.
11. U.S. Food and Drug Administration Medication Guide, Savella. http://www.fda.gov/downloads/Drugs/DrugSafety/ucm089121.pdf.
12. U.S. Food and Drug Administration Medication Guide, Lyrica. http://www.fda.gov/downloads/Drugs/DrugSafety/UCM152825.pdf.
13. Clauw DJ, Mease PJ, Palmer RH, Trugman JM, Wang Y. Continuing efficacy of milnacipran following long-term treatment in fibromyalgia: a randomized trial. *Arthritis Res Ther.* 2013;15:R88. doi:10.1186/ar4268.
14. Hauser W, Walitt B, Fitzcharles MA, Sommer C. Review of pharmacological therapies in fibromyalgia syndrome. *Arthritis Res Ther.* 2014;16(1):201. doi:10.1186/ar444116:201.
15. van Koulil S, van Lankveld W, Kraaimaat FW, et al. Tailored cognitive-behavioral therapy and exercise training for high-risk fibromyalgia patients. *Arthritis Care Res.* 2010; 62(10):1377–1385. doi:10.1002/acr.20268.
16. IOM (Institute of Medicine). *Beyond Myalgic Encephalomyelitis/Chronic Fatigue Syndrome: Redefining an Illness.* Washington, DC: The National Academies Press; 2015. http://www.iom.edu/mecfs.
17. Clayton EW. Viewpoint: beyond myalgic encephalomyelitis/chronic fatigue syndrome. An IOM report on redefining an illness. *JAMA.* 2015;313(11):1101–1102. doi:10.1001/jama.2015.1346. Published online February 10, 2015. doi:10.1001/jama.2015.1346.

18. Centers for Disease Control and Prevention (CDC). Chronic fatigue syndrome (CFS). http://www.cdc.gov/cfs/diagnosis/index.html.
19. Stratton P, Khachikyan I, Sinaii N, Ortiz R, Shah J. Association of chronic pelvic pain and endometriosis with signs of sensitization and myofascial pain. *Obstet Gynecol.* 2015;125(3):719–728.
20. American Society for Reproductive Medicine. Highlights from fertility and sterility: ASRM's practice committee issues new report on endometriosis and pelvic pain. *ASRM Bull.* 2014;16(15). http://www.asrm.org/news/article.aspx?id=12866#top.
21. Matarese G, De Placido G, Nikas Y, Alviggi C. Pathogenesis of endometriosis: natural immunity dysfunction or autoimmune disease? *Trends Mol Med.* 2003;9(5):223–228.
22. Schenken RS. Contributions from the VIII World Congress on Endometriosis. *Fertil Steril.* 2002;78(4):663–664. doi:http://dx.doi.org/10.1016/S0015-0282(02)03978-X.
23. Sinaii N, Cleary SD, Ballweg ML, Nieman LK, Stratton P. High rates of autoimmune and endocrine disorders, fibromyalgia, chronic fatigue syndrome and atopic diseases among women with endometriosis: a survey analysis. *Hum Reprod.* 2002;17(10):2715–2724.
24. Eisenberg VH, Zolti M, Soriano D. Is there an association between autoimmunity and endometriosis? *Autoimmun Rev.* 2012;11(11):806–814. doi: http://dx.doi.org/10.1016/j.ijgo.2006.03.005.
25. Johnson NP, Hummelshoj L, for the World Endometriosis Society Montpellier Consortium. Consensus on the current management of endometriosis. *Hum Reprod.* 2013;28(6):1552–1568. Advanced access publication March 25, 2013. doi:10.1093/humrep/det050.
26. Koga K, Osuga Y, Yoshino O, et al. Elevated interleukin-16 levels in the peritoneal fluid of women with endometriosis may be a mechanism for inflammatory reactions associated with endometriosis. *Fertil Steril.* 2005;83(4):878–882. doi:10.1016/j.fertnstert.2004.12.004.
27. Quaas AM, Weedlin EA, Hansen KR. On-label and off-label drug use in the treatment of endometriosis. *Fertil Steril.* 2015;103(30):612–625. http://dx.doi.org/10.1016/j.fertnstert.2015.01.006.
28. Gelbaya TA, Kyrgiou M, Li TC, et al. Low-dose aspirin for *in vitro* fertilization: a systematic review and meta-analysis. *Hum Reprod Update.* 2007;13(4):357–364. doi:10.1093/humupd/dmm00.
29. van de Merwe JP. Interstitial cystitis and systemic autoimmune diseases. *Nat Clin Pract Urol.* 2007;4(9):484–491.
30. Berry SH, Elliott MN, Suttorp M, et al. Prevalence of symptoms of bladder pain syndrome/interstitial cystitis among adult females in the United States. *J Urol.* 2011;186:540–544.
31. National Institute of Diabetes and Digestive and Kidney Diseases (NIDDK). Interstitial cystitis/painful bladder syndrome. 2013. http://kidney.niddk.nih.gov/kudiseases/pubs/interstitialcystitis/.
32. Hanno PM, Burks DA, Clemens JQ, et al. Diagnosis and treatment of interstitial cystitis/bladder pain syndrome. Revised 2014. https://www.auanet.org/common/pdf/education/clinical-guidance/IC-Bladder-Pain-Syndrome-Revised.pdf.

14

Navigating the New Medical Maze

I was incredibly lucky—it only took me a couple of months to get a diagnosis. I now have an excellent liver doctor. But his focus is on the liver, not on the fact that I have an autoimmune disease. He doesn't discuss my diseases with me in that context. He discusses my medications and my liver function tests, and he makes sure that I'm doing OK. I get my blood work done at my GP's office. And even then I don't see the doctor. Once I found the American Autoimmune Related Diseases Association, I was able to learn a lot about autoimmunity and my own disease. And I was able to connect with other women who have these diseases, and it's really wonderful. We exchange e-mails and we call each other. That support is really important. But I do wish there were doctors who specifically dealt with autoimmunity, so you could get a more complete picture of what's going on. You learn things bit by bit, and so much is left for you to figure out on your own.

HANNAH

Hannah is lucky. The typical woman with an autoimmune disease may spend an average of four years, see five different doctors, and shell out over $50,000 before she gets a correct diagnosis. Some women have a tough time just getting their symptoms taken seriously.[1] A 2013 survey by the American Autoimmune Related Diseases Association (AARDA) found that 51 percent of patients were labeled "chronic complainers" by their doctors in the early stages of their illness.[1] All too many women are told their symptoms are "all in their head" and are referred to a psychiatrist instead of a rheumatologist or endocrinologist, remarks Virginia Ladd, founder and president of AARDA.

Autoimmune diseases consume more than $100 billion annually in healthcare dollars and are the fourth leading cause of illness in American women, after heart disease, lung cancer, and breast cancer. Yet there are few centers that "triage" women to the proper care and help them form a care team, says Ladd. No specialty in *autoimmunology* exists, so it may not be easy to find the proper doctor to manage your care.

> *There needs to be an autoimmune specialty. We can have wacko symptoms that often make no sense. And each specialist is only looking at his one specialty. We need to have doctors who get the big picture. In my medical odyssey there were actually only two doctors who did not suspect what I had. The specialists, the ophthalmologist, the neurologist, the rheumatologist, and the hematologist, all suspected it was antiphospholipid syndrome. But my primary care physician and the first ER doctor I saw discounted it. I do think that part of it is that outside of big cities, in rural areas particularly, doctors may be insular and they are not comfortable with collaborative diagnoses in the way that doctors at major medical centers are. So I would tell women to get to a major medical center in a big city.*
>
> Margaret

Who Should Be Your Doctor?

If you think you have an autoimmune disease—or need better care for an existing problem (or problems)—you need to find the right specialist to obtain the proper diagnosis, treatment, and follow-up. As a starting point, AARDA suggests identifying the type of medical specialist who deals with your major symptom, then looking for physicians who have board certification in that particular area. They should be certified by one of the specialty boards of the American Board of Medical Specialties (http://www.abms.org/verify-certification/).

The following are some general guidelines for choosing a specialist:

Rheumatoid arthritis, lupus, Sjögren's syndrome, and other connective tissue diseases are usually managed by a **rheumatologist**. This is a specialty that encompasses diseases of the joints, bones, and muscles, and related diseases in which the immune system may be in imbalance resulting in inflammation. A rheumatologist may have dual board certifications in internal medicine and rheumatology from the American Board of Internal Medicine, and will often belong to the American College of Rheumatology (ACR).

As your treatment progresses, other professionals can often help, including nurses, physical or occupational therapists, orthopedic surgeons, psychologists, and social workers. Physical therapists are certified by the American Board of Physical Medicine and Rehabilitation. If you should need joint replacement, you'll need an orthopedic surgeon certified by the American Board of Orthopaedic Surgery; they can often be found through the American Association of Orthopaedic Surgeons (AAOS).

Endocrine disorders, including thyroid disease and type 1 diabetes, require the care of an **endocrinologist**. This specialist can also deal with issues of osteoporosis that arise from corticosteroid treatments.

Women with diabetes ideally should look for a physician who specializes in managing diabetes—an endocrinologist who's a **diabetologist**, says Mount Sinai diabetologist Dr. Carol Levy. Your care team might include a certified diabetes educator (who may be a registered nurse or registered dietitian) to help you learn to manage glucose self-testing and insulin injections and structure a healthy eating plan that fits your likes, dislikes, and lifestyle. "Many internists will not have access to these people, so I recommend looking for a hospital that has a diabetes program or clinic," Dr. Levy advises. "This is a lifelong condition that needs lifelong management, so it's important to have an endocrinologist who can follow you. Your condition can change over time; you can develop complications or other autoimmune endocrine diseases, or new treatments may come out that will benefit you. So, ideally, the best person to manage your care is an endocrinologist."

A diabetologist is an endocrinologist who specializes in diabetes and is board certified in Diabetes and Metabolism by the American Board of Internal Medicine; other board certifications include those with Special Qualifications in Endocrinology and/or Reproductive Endocrinology.

For neurological diseases, such as multiple sclerosis and myasthenia gravis, a **neurologist** is the best physician to diagnose and manage your condition. He or she should be board certified by the American Board of Neurological Surgery.

Gastrointestinal diseases, including Crohn's disease, ulcerative colitis, and celiac disease, should be managed by a **gastroenterologist**. Autoimmune hepatitis and primary biliary cirrhosis are managed by gastroenterologists who specialize in liver disease called **hepatologists**. Your gastroenterologist should be a Diplomate of the American Board of Gastroenterology. For surgery, you'll need a physician board certified in Colon and Rectal Surgery by the American Board of Colon and Rectal Surgery. The professional group is the American Society of Colon and Rectal Surgeons.

Specialists in blood disorders, called **hematologists**, can manage not only platelet disorders like immune thrombocytopenia, but also antiphospholipid syndrome. However, even if APS occurs without another autoimmune connective tissue disease, such as lupus, your rheumatologist can often manage APS. A hematologist is board certified in that specialty by the American Board of Internal Medicine and will usually be a member of the American Society of Hematology.

A **dermatologist** is best qualified to manage autoimmune skin disorders, including psoriasis, alopecia areata, and vitiligo. They can have general certification in Dermatology, with special qualifications in Dermatological Immunology/Diagnostic and Laboratory Immunology (for biopsies) from the American Academy of Dermatology.

A **reproductive endocrinologist** or **gynecologist** who specializes in infertility is ideally suited for diagnosing primary ovarian insufficiency and helping you get pregnant. The American Board of Obstetrics and Gynecology offers general certification in Obstetrics and Gynecology, with special Qualifications in Reproductive Endocrinology. A good OB/GYN will often be a fellow of the American College of Obstetricians and Gynecologists (ACOG). Infertility specialists are usually members of the American Society for Reproductive Medicine (ASRM).

Asthma and allergies can coexist with some autoimmune diseases. Specialists in this area are certified by the American Board of Allergy and Immunology. They typically belong to the American College of Asthma, Allergy and Immunology (ACAAI) or the American Association of Allergy, Asthma and Immunology (AAAAI).

In general, large teaching hospitals affiliated with medical schools are more likely to have an array of specialists to consult. You can also find an appropriate specialist by visiting the websites of the various professional organizations. Support groups for various disorders often keep lists of specialists and can be a valuable resource in finding the right doctor. (See Appendix A.)

Being followed by the right kind of specialist can make a difference to your care. For example, the American College of Rheumatology (ACR)[2] and the European League Against Rheumatism (EULAR) strongly recommend that women with RA be followed by a rheumatologist.[3] That's because rheumatologists are more likely to know about and follow current treatment guidelines. For example, one study that examined the treatment of patients with RA belonging to a large health insurance plan in Pittsburgh found 67 percent of those being followed by a rheumatologist were prescribed disease-modifying antirheumatic drugs (DMARDs), compared to only 27 percent of those seen by a non-rheumatologist. And RA patients seen by non-rheumatologists were more likely to be given narcotics for their pain, rather than drugs that also target inflammation to dampen pain.

The specialist you pick can depend on those within the "network" of your health insurance (see page 444). Once you've made a list of potential providers, interview them. Ask each doctor how many patients he or she has treated with your particular problem. The more patients the doctor sees with your disease, the more skilled he or she is likely to be in treating it.

However, personal "fit" is important too. Even if you have found "the" expert in the field, the personal empathy may not be there. You'll be revealing some of the most intimate details of your life to this person, so if you don't feel comfortable talking to him or her, keep looking until you find the right fit. Too many of us choose a doctor who will have a major impact on our quality of life based on just one visit. Even though he or she may be an expert on your disease, you're the expert on your own experiences with your illness.

Are You Covered?

The implementation and the impact of the 2010 *Affordable Care Act (ACA)* vary from state to state and with insurance providers, and the ACA itself may be undergoing changes as other provisions take effect. Two resources to help you keep abreast of changes as they occur are healthcare.gov and the Henry J. Kaiser Foundation, kff.org. The Kaiser Foundation in particular reports regularly on healthcare issues and costs that directly affect you. (See Appendix A.)

Under the ACA, several types of insurance plans are offered by health marketplaces in participating states, and they are tiered in five categories according to how much of your medical expenses they will cover. As this book goes to press, "Bronze" plans cover 60 percent of medical costs by in-network providers; mid-level "Silver" plans cover 70 percent, "**Gold**" plans pay 80 percent on average, and "**Platinum**" plans cover 90 percent of costs.[4] All of these plans can limit you to "network" physicians and some may cover "out-of-network" services. However, you may find some of the better doctors for your condition might be out of network and you'll have to find this out and figure what your costs may be and how to pay for care. "**Catastrophic coverage**" plans pay less than 60 percent and are available only to people who are under 30 and/or have a hardship exemption.[5]

If you enroll in a "silver plan" and you make $30,000 a year or less, you may be able to qualify for assistance to reduce your out-of-pocket costs for doctor's visits, hospital care, and prescription drugs.[4,6]

Types of plans may include:

- **Health Maintenance Organizations (HMO).** A network of healthcare providers who agree to provide services to the group, often at a set fee per patient. Specialists are covered by HMOs, but you must pick a primary care provider on the HMO list (PCP) to make a referral. You may also have to live or work in the HMO's area to obtain coverage.
- **Preferred Provider Organizations (PPO).** Specialists are included in a PPO network, and you can see the doctor of your choice, in most cases without a referral. You'll be charged a small co-pay for each specialist visit.
- **Exclusive Provider Organization (EPO).** A managed care plan that allows you to see any healthcare provider within the EPO network, including specialists. Anyone outside the EPO will not be covered.
- **Point of Service (POS).** In a POS plan you pick a PCP for routine care within the network and he or she will refer you to a specialist. If you're willing to pay more, you can see an out-of-network specialist.[5]
- **High Deductible Health Plan (HDHP).** You have to pay out a certain amount before coverage kicks in. Deductibles are typically around $1,250 for an individual and $2,500 for a family. These may be linked to a Health Savings Account (HSA).

With the advent of the ACA, some patients report changes in their access to care—and the cost of that care.

AARDA and the National Coalition of Autoimmune Groups (NCAPG) conducted a survey in 2013 among 357 people with one or more autoimmune diseases, and preliminary results found many were directly affected by the ACA. While 66 percent were able to keep seeing their specialist, 45 percent were concerned about their continued access to care.[7]

About a third of patients report that the services they receive were decreased or remained the same. Insurance premiums have increased for 42 percent. Some people have had to switch insurance plans.[5] In general, however, costs have risen only moderately since the ACA took effect.[8]

As this book went to press, you may qualify for tax subsidies to help pay premiums for plans purchased through federal insurance exchanges if you make between $12,000 and $47,000 a year (as an individual).[5]

The upshot: we will all have to stay on top of changes in the law (check www.healthcare.gov for updates) and in the marketplace (your co-pays and other out-of-pocket costs)—and become active advocates for our own medical care.

When I was diagnosed with autoimmune hepatitis and my family started talking about it, we realized there was a family history of autoimmune disease. My mother has Hashimoto's thyroiditis, and my grandfather was also hypothyroid. My grandmother had type 1 diabetes. So there was definitely a history, but we'd never talked about it as autoimmunity. It turns out my dad's brother also had hypothyroidism. So we have it on both sides of the family. But no one had liver disease, at least that I know of.

HANNAH

I never even asked questions until recent years, and found out we had an extensive family history of thyroid disease that stretched into my second and third cousins. I've persuaded my brother to be tested, since his daughter has a thyroid problem. And it wasn't just thyroid—my father had Crohn's disease and Hashimoto's, my second cousin had celiac disease, and another cousin has lupus. And honestly, I might never have known.

LYNNE

What You Can Do to Take Charge

Taking charge of your care means getting as much information as you can, keeping track of symptoms and medications, and coming prepared to every doctor visit.

Make a Family Tree

Ask questions about other family members and make a family medical tree. It's not simply an exercise in genealogy. In some cases, testing may be advised for close family members, especially in cases of type 1 diabetes and thyroid disease. You may need additional testing for autoimmune diseases that cluster with your particular problem.

Thyroid autoimmunity is somehow predisposing to type 1 diabetes. Addison's disease, adrenal gland insufficiency, is found more commonly in patients with type 1 diabetes; about 1 in 200 to 250 patients with type 1 diabetes will also develop adrenal insufficiency. This can be a very serious problem in a person with diabetes, because it can be life threatening and is often missed. So it's worth asking about getting tested.

Some experts believe that vitiligo is a skin marker for propensity to autoimmunity, especially thyroid problems, adrenal insufficiency, and type 1 diabetes.

In some cases, if a disease has a strong genetic component, genetic counseling may be needed. You also need to ask questions about the chances of passing along an autoimmune disease to your child. Physicians should be board certified in Medical or Clinical Genetics by the American Board of Medical Genetics. A genetic counselor (who could be a social worker or other health professional) is usually trained in a graduate program. (See Appendix A.)

Keep Track of Details

Just as physicians keep an up-to-date file on each patient, so should you keep a medical file for yourself. This can be a notebook or a file folder, and it should contain a record of doctor visits, copies or records of lab reports and other diagnostic tests, and a list of medications you're taking (the dose, when and how each drug is taken, and so on).

You should have a section for a diary of symptoms. Because knowledge of autoimmune clusters is just beginning to reach physicians who are not specialists in rheumatology or endocrinology, you need to keep track of symptoms, even those that don't appear to be related to your specific diagnosis. An unusual symptom may be the very first clue that you have a second (or third) autoimmune disease.

If your clinic or medical center provides access to your electronic health records (EHR), do take advantage of it. With these systems you'll be able to see all of your lab results and even imaging reports. Ask about it at your next medical visit. You may also be able to obtain copies of MRI or x-ray images.

At each doctor visit, bring a list of symptoms you're experiencing; review that list with your doctor and give him or her a copy to keep in your file. As you've learned from reading this book, when you have an autoimmune disease you can often experience a number of symptoms that may seem unrelated. So let your doctor know about any new symptom. And don't worry that your doctor will think you're a chronic complainer, or that you'll just end up with another prescription. Be honest. You only hurt yourself if you don't speak up.

Autoimmune diseases are not simple. And many times, especially during the first physician visits, you may get a lot of information to process in a short amount of time. Bring your medical diary or a pad and paper, or use your smart phone or a digital tape recorder to record the visit.

Make sure you understand unfamiliar terms, the tests you may need, and treatment options. And before you leave, go over what was discussed so you're clear about the details.

You need someone who not only knows about your disease, but who's alert to the other complications and other diseases. When you have a symptom, they have to think it may not just be your disease acting up. You have to be very alert, you have to know your body, and you have to speak up when there's something bothering you. We may not always be good at articulating exactly what's wrong, but there are also too many things that doctors will say are "all in your head."

Laura, 46

After I was first diagnosed with Crohn's, I had to have surgery. They removed a foot of my small intestine, my appendix, and some of my colon. But the gastroenterologist I was seeing in the hospital didn't really explain what any of the follow-up was going to entail and basically discharged me without any medication or anything. And about a month after I got out of the hospital, I started having trouble again. I tried to call him, but he never returned any of my phone calls. About two years later I started developing some symptoms, and they finally put me on medication. But that was a gap of two years, which allowed my disease to get worse again. Now I know to ask questions and find out as much as I can.

Janine

A Team Effort

The American College of Rheumatology (ACR) and other experts advocate "shared decision making," and so do we.

The time is long past when patients blindly accepted doctors' pronouncements. And that's a good thing. You need to form an active partnership with your doctor. Ask questions from the outset. Make sure you get a thorough clinical examination and ask if your test results are being stored in an electronic health records database that you can access (even individual practices are adopting these systems).

Be sure to describe symptoms in detail (again, make a list) and emphasize how your symptoms impact your daily functioning. Don't allow any physician to dismiss your symptoms as "stress."

If you've ever hesitated to speak up in your doctor's office, you're not alone. Many people are afraid to ask their doctor too many questions, worrying they'll be seen as "difficult" patients.

In fact, a survey conducted among almost 4,000 adults with rheumatoid arthritis in 13 countries by the Harris Poll reveals that 41 percent of patients feel uncomfortable discussing their concerns and fears with a healthcare provider.[9] Almost one-quarter worry that asking a lot of questions and being perceived as "difficult" will affect the quality of their care, according to the RA NarRAtive survey. Only 35 percent feel like they have any control over their treatment.

"Unfortunately, patients may default to a submissive role with their doctor when they are in pain or losing some of their function," comments

Allan Gibofsky, MD, professor of clinical medicine and public health at the Weill Cornell Medical College.

There are ways to improve communication with your physician. "For one thing, make eye contact; too many patients discuss their concerns while a doctor is looking down and writing in their file or looking at a screen while they enter information on a computer, which can be a distraction for both parties," says Dr. Gibofsky, an attending rheumatologist at the Hospital for Special Surgery in New York.

Be mindful that many physicians have time constraints, so ask about making an appointment when there will be some extra time for discussion, he advises.

Keep asking what *else* could be going on (and with autoimmunity a lot can be going on), and explore your potential diagnosis together. Carefully fill out the assessment forms and questionnaires that help determine disease activity.

"Don't consider the office visit over until your concerns are addressed," adds Dr. Gibofsky, who served as cochair of an advisory panel of physicians and patient advocates who devised the RA NarRAtive survey with a major pharmaceutical company.

During your exam, or if you're asked to go for extra tests or imaging, do ask your doctor what he or she is looking for.

As you've seen, tests vary for different autoimmune diseases, and often there's no single test that can diagnose your condition. You may be faced with the prospect of undergoing a battery of tests, and you need to ask what each is for and whether there are any alternatives. Will a diagnostic procedure be done on an outpatient or inpatient basis? Will there be any pain or discomfort? Will you need anesthesia? If you suffer from claustrophobia and need an MRI (which means spending 30 minutes inside a magnetic tube), ask about medications to make you more comfortable during the procedure. Ask how much a procedure costs, and whether it will be covered by your health insurance. Who will get the test results, and what will they tell us about your condition? Although diagnostic criteria can define a disease, your particular array of symptoms may be uncertain.

Get a second, third, or fourth opinion if need be. Because autoimmunity is still just being recognized as an underlying cause of many diseases, and because symptoms can be vague, many doctors don't initially think to test for autoimmune diseases.

Ask questions about treatment options. What are the advantages and disadvantages? How long will the treatment last? Make sure all your questions are answered so that you thoroughly understand the risks *and* benefits.

"I tell my patients that the only 'silly' question is the one that you don't ask. If it's important enough for you to make note of it, then it's important enough to discuss," stresses Dr. Gibofsky.

> *I was seriously depressed from the prednisone, though I didn't know it at the time. Prednisone increases anger, anxiety, and depression—none of which any doctor ever told me. And the methotrexate was even worse. When I had a period I thought I was hemorrhaging, and twice I almost went to the hospital just thinking, "This is it. This is the end." Again, no one spoke to me about any of this. I'd look it up in a medical guide and find out what the hell was going on for myself. And I would wake up each morning in this rage, and have to tell myself, "OK, wait a minute. This is not me. I'm not angry. I don't have any reason to be angry other than life, and what was going on with my disease, but there's nothing to be angry at. Just chill out. Calm down. It's the medication, it's not me." Which I needed to do . . . I was risking personal relationships all over the place. I have wonderful friends and a wonderful husband, but there's only so far you can go before they say, "Would you please stop?" And I wish someone had spoken to me about the possible effects of the medication on my thinking, my emotions.*
>
> Kathleen Turner

Find Out All You Can About Your Medications

As Kathleen Turner found out the hard way, medications can have unexpected side effects. And in all likelihood you're going to be taking several medications, all of which have side effects. So you need to know how they can affect you, and how they may interact with other drugs you may be taking (including over-the-counter drugs, supplements, and herbs).

Write down the name of each drug, what it's used for (an immunosuppressant or a pain reliever, for example), the dose you need to take and how often, if it needs to be taken with (or without) food, and any potential side effects.

To be as informed as possible, read the pharmacy information sheet that came with your prescription (or check the web page for the specific medication). It's also wise to check the FDA web site (www.fda.gov) for any updated warnings and look at a current edition of the consumers' version of the Physician's Desk Reference or check your library's copy of the PDR or the online version (see Appendix A) to obtain complete information on medications that have been prescribed for you.

If you're seeing more than one doctor, make sure they *all* know what medications you're taking, including over-the-counter drugs and herbal preparations. Sit down once a year with your physician to review those medications to make sure you still need the same drug and the same dose.

Save drug information package inserts in your medical folder at home for reference. Even commonly used medications may, in very rare cases, cause severe, possibly fatal reactions. There's usually a section that says "Contact your doctor immediately if . . . ." This contains key information about potential side effects and interactions. Your risk of serious side effects may be small, but you need to know the warning signs. If you don't get an insert, ask for it, or get a computer printout of drug instructions and precautions from your pharmacy. If you have any reaction to a drug, call your doctor immediately.

Don't be surprised if your questions about how medications affect women prompt a response of "We don't know—there haven't been any studies on that."

In writing this book and talking to preeminent experts around the country, many of them concede that knowledge is very limited about the effects of female and male sex hormones, and even the effects on pregnancy or menopause of medications that have been used for long periods of time. Clinical trials of medications sponsored by the National Institutes of Health have only been required to include women since 1989 (women had been excluded because of concerns about potential birth defects and the notion that female hormones could confuse trial results). Reporting of those clinical trials to include sex differences in responses and side effects of medications has only been mandated by the Food and Drug Administration since 1999.

Investigate Drug Costs

Medication costs are escalating at an alarming rate, especially for the newest brand-name drugs but also for generics.

Biologic disease-modifying antirheumatic drugs (DMARDs) have become part of standard care for rheumatoid arthritis, and even the first biologics such as etanercept (Enbrel, approved in 1998) now cost upwards of $42,000 a year.[10] Multiple sclerosis patients face annual bills for Avonex (approved in 1996) of more than $62,000 a year, about on par with newer drugs like Tecfidera (approved in 2013).[11] These drugs are typically taken for long periods (if not for life). And for many patients, a big chunk of those costs are out-of-pocket, whether you have private insurance or Medicare.

Researchers at the University of California, San Francisco (UCSF) and the University of Hawaii conducted the first national investigation of stand-alone Medicare Part D coverage for DMARDs in RA compared with Medicare Advantage plans.[12] They looked at whether prior authorization was required, what was covered under specialty "tiers," and co-payment amounts versus fixed-dollar co-pays in January 2013. The analysis looked at costs and coverage for nine conventional DMARDs (such as leflunomide and methotrexate) and nine biologic DMARDs (including adalimumab, certolizumab, etanercept, rituximab, and tocilizumab).

At the time of the study, several biologics were available only by intravenous infusion, usually given under physician supervision. Medicare Part D covers self-administered biologics dispensed by pharmacies.

During the initial period of an RA patient's drug coverage under Part D, patients were expected to pay almost a third of the cost of biologics out-of-pocket.[12]

That's not a trivial amount. The study found that RA patients starting just a single biologic faced more than $2,700 in annual co-pays. The average monthly tab for DMARDs under standard Part D coverage was $835 per month. Medicare Advantage plans ran a little more, about $862 per month, but they covered more DMARDs. In contrast, the fixed co-pay for nonbiologic DMARDs was about $5 to $10 a month.[8]

The least expensive biologic listed in the report was the older TNFα inhibitor *infliximab (Remicade)*, at around $270 per month; *anakinra (Kineret)* costs patients almost $3,000 a month. Not only that, but patients were almost always expected to have prior authorization—which can mean paying for extra office visits.

Then there's the Medicare coverage gap known as the "donut hole," which patients can tumble into by February or March of a given year. In the donut hole, cost-sharing escalated to 45 percent until "catastrophic coverage" eligibility kicked in (usually by July).[8] After that, patients paid 5 percent of drug costs. But that's six or seven months of higher costs—every year.

All this can affect whether patients take medications as prescribed. An earlier study of 1,100 adults with RA found that one in six decreased their medication dose because of cost.

Patients not covered by Medicare face a different problem.

Even if you have health insurance, there's no guarantee that you'll easily be able to get the medications your doctor prescribed. Insurance plans have devised "formularies" under which newer, more expensive medications are either not covered or covered at higher co-pays, depending on whether the plan is a low-cost basic plan or a "platinum" top-tier. Additionally, many insurers require what's called "step therapy," in which you must first try less-expensive therapies (like methotrexate) before you can be prescribed drugs such as biologicals. As a consequence, many autoimmune patients are finding themselves unable to obtain the best medications for their condition, says AARDA's Virginia Ladd.

Many pharmaceutical companies have programs or discount cards to help patients obtain medications at low or no cost. Check whether your state has a State Pharmaceutical Assistance Program, which helps eligible patients obtain subsidies and drug discounts. (Sources are listed in Appendix A.) However, be aware that discount cards may not help if a medication is excluded or restricted by a formulary.

New studies are also underway to see whether reduced doses or other treatment regimens can be disease-effective as well as cost-effective.

According to the FDA, generic drugs are supposed to be chemically equivalent to brand-name medications. "Biosimilar" drugs are also becoming available, ostensibly with equivalent effects at lower costs.

However, AARDA cautions that biosimilars are not "generics" and may never be *identical* to the original approved branded product and may cause a negative immune reaction in people with autoimmune diseases. "Known as immunogenicity, this response can cause further disease and damage to the cells, tissues and organs of AD patients," the AARDA statement explained.[13]

There's a lot you need to learn on your own. I had to learn how to adjust my insulin intake to match my natural appetite, which is something most doctors don't encourage diabetics to do. They want to get everyone on the same schedule, which makes it easier for them to explain. I had to find endocrinologists and doctors who understood, who would spend the time with me to work this out. No one told me to increase the amount of blood testing when I started on estrogen for my hot flashes. I knew about gestational diabetes and I thought there could be a reaction that could increase the need for insulin. But when my gynecologist prescribed estrogen, she never mentioned it and she knew I was a diabetic. I just started testing more on my own. I almost did that automatically. There's a lot that you have to find out for yourself.

Mary Kay

I was extremely lucky to find a gynecologist who worked closely with the MS center. She wanted me to take estrogen because she thought it would help my disease, even though there hadn't been many clinical studies at the time. So the choice of a gynecologist can be critical.

Ana

Find a Gynecologist Familiar with Autoimmune Disease

As Mary Kay and Ana discovered, having a gynecologist who's knowledgeable and up to date on your particular autoimmune disease is extremely important, since you'll need expert guidance and follow-up should you choose to have a child or take estrogen (or its alternatives).

For example, says Mount Sinai diabetologist Dr. Carol Levy regarding decisions about taking oral contraceptives or hormone replacement, "Up until a few years ago there was this misconception among doctors that women couldn't go on birth control pills because it would cause fluctuations in blood sugar levels. That misconception has been passed along to patients, and it often makes them fearful. Oral contraceptives can make glucose fluctuations more predictable, but we need to be able to work with the gynecologist."

Information may not be offered, or your questions about postmenopausal hormones may (again) be answered with "We don't know" or "That's a question you need to take up with your gynecologist." "Rheumatologists may not discuss it, and the gynecologist may not know anything about autoimmune disease," remarks Lila E. Nachtigall, MD, of the NYU School of Medicine, who has been researching estrogen for decades. "The question of hormones, be it birth control pills or hormone therapy, is part of the whole patient picture. So a woman needs to get answers somewhere. For our part, we find it extremely helpful when a woman keeps track of her symptoms, because it can help us individualize care."

Keep a symptom diary during the menstrual cycle, pregnancy, or menopause, and bring it with you to doctor visits and ask questions. Don't ignore regular pelvic exams and Pap smears, and periodically have pelvic floor muscle function assessed, especially in diseases that affect muscle and nerve function. Many women who become disabled as a result of their disease have difficulty finding a gynecologist who's not only knowledgeable but also has adequate equipment (like specially designed examining tables that can adjust to women who must use wheelchairs). Incontinence and sexual problems can be side effects of multiple sclerosis, myasthenia gravis, and other diseases and require special and empathetic attention. The specialist treating your disease can often help with a referral to a gynecologist. Sources of information include the American College of Obstetricians and Gynecologists (ACOG). Your specialist can often make a referral to an OB/GYN.

I decided to combine drug therapy with the natural treatments. I had been seeing a naturopathic doctor before I was diagnosed with autoimmune hepatitis, and she had recommended milk thistle for my liver. Milk thistle is an herb that contains Silybum marianum, which has been shown to help regenerate liver cells. It doesn't cure the hepatitis. She also told me to avoid fatty foods and alcohol, and had also recommended acupuncture before I was diagnosed. That made me feel better, psychologically at least. Thanks to that naturopath, I was also taking calcium from the beginning. When I moved to New York I started seeing a liver specialist, who told me there was no harm in my taking milk thistle, but it was probably a waste of my money. I've continued to take it, and I think it's helped.

Hannah

Complementary and Alternative Medicine (CAM) Therapies

Up to 90 percent of arthritis and autoimmune patients are using some form of CAM. But this widespread practice is often based not on medical evidence but on word of mouth—and hope.

Some studies of CAM for autoimmune diseases, notably RA, have been published in respected, peer-reviewed journals. However, many widely publicized remedies are promoted by Internet advertising, relying heavily on patient "anecdotes" with little or no basis in fact.

In writing this book, we made a decision not to delve too deeply into the myriad of complementary therapies being used by women with autoimmune diseases. That's a subject for another book.

A number of CAM therapies that have been investigated and found to be effective for some patients include acupuncture and omega-3 fish oil.

Fortunately, there's the NIH *National Center for Complementary and Integrative Health (NCCIM)*, where you can find descriptions of complementary therapies, herbal remedies, and supplements (see Appendix A). But there are many cautions.

While many women find complementary therapies extremely helpful, it's important to remember that "natural" doesn't always mean safe, and that supplements are largely unregulated. There's no guarantee that you'll get what you pay for. And studies have found that some herbal supplements contain little or none of the active ingredient listed on the label and may even be contaminated.

We urge you to investigate everything carefully, consult the physician managing your care, and don't be afraid to discuss herbs and other things you've tried. (After all, glucosamine was once on the fringes, and now it's a widely accepted therapy for osteoarthritis.) Some drugs may make your condition worse or cause interactions with medications you're taking (such as evening primrose oil and anticoagulants); many herbs should not be taken before surgery; and some herbs (like kava) may even be toxic.

This is one area where you need to do your homework. Realize that many remedies have a powerful placebo effect—in other words, if you *believe* something is going to help you, chances are *it will.*

It sounds weird, but if you have to have one of these diseases, this is a great time.

They have made leaps and bounds in research. There is some real hope for MS and other diseases, and you need to hang on to that hope. They've made more progress in the last few years than they have in the last 25 years. Because of AIDS, they've learned a great deal about the immune system and the central nervous system that will benefit people with autoimmune disease. We also have the Internet, which is a godsend. You get a lot of support and information. There are bulletin boards and chat rooms. And there's tons of information. Even if you have a handicap, so much more is accessible than before, and I thank God I was born now rather than 25, 30 years ago. I would tell women, don't shut yourself in, get out and be part of the world you live in. The more you isolate yourself, the scarier the world becomes. That can be quite a rut, and it's easy to slip into that when you have a chronic disease. The Internet is also a great place to make contact with people, and women should get in touch with support groups, because they can give you so much. Whatever you do, don't isolate yourself.

MARIANA

With a Little Help from Some Friends

As Mary Kay puts it, you almost have to make a profession out of your own healthcare. But you can't go it alone, and any chronic disease can have its rough spots. Support groups can be lifesavers. It may be hard to walk into that group meeting for the first time, but once you get over that hurdle, a group can be a source of information, friendship, and emotional support. Find a support group that avoids a "pity party" atmosphere, advises Ladd.

Millions of people find valuable resources on the Internet. You can do a surprising amount of research right from your own home. You can find information that can help clarify symptoms, uncover sources for finding a good diagnostician, and share your experiences with others. Many libraries provide access to the Internet through their computers and will even help guide your search. Contact your hospital's community education or outreach program to find out about support groups.

A comprehensive listing of resources and self-help groups appears in Appendix A, and a list of recommended reading is included in Appendix B.

As Virginia Ladd tells AARDA patient forums: "Be your best advocate."

I'm obviously a success story, but what I really want women to know is not to give up, not to think that this is going to be the only controlling factor of their lives from now on.

Because that's not necessary at all. . . . They find their way to fight it, whether it's through exercise or medication. I think exercise is totally essential. I can't imagine doing without it. I would put that right on par with medication, frankly. But you need to take action. There's so much fear of being crippled, or permanently damaged, or not being able to pursue the work you love and being dependent on loved ones. You need to keep moving and be as strong as you can be; you can't feel helpless. They told me I would never recover, but here I am.

Kathleen Turner

Notes

1. American Autoimmune Related Diseases Association (AARDA). Autoimmune diagnosis surveys 2013. Presented March 18, 2014, Washington, D.C., National Coalition of Autoimmune Patient Groups (NCAPG) news briefing.
2. Singh JA, Saag KG, Bridges SL, et al. 2015 American College of Rheumatology guideline for the treatment of rheumatoid arthritis. *Arthritis Rheumatol.* 2015;67(12). doi:10.1002/art.39480. Published online at http://onlinelibrary.wiley.com/doi/10.1002/art.39480/epdf.
3. Smolen JS, Landewé R, Breedveld FC, et al. EULAR recommendations for the management of rheumatoid arthritis with synthetic and biological disease-modifying antirheumatic drugs: 2013 update. *Ann Rheum Dis.* 2014;73:492–509.
4. http://kff.org/health-costs/issue-brief/patient-cost-sharing-in-marketplace-plans-2016/. Accessed November 20, 2015.
5. Health Insurance Marketplace. How to choose Marketplace insurance: type of plan and provider network. 2015. https://www.healthcare.gov/choose-a-plan/plan-types/.
6. www.healthcare.gov. Accessed November 20, 2015.
7. National Coalition of Autoimmune Patient Groups survey on ACA. Presented March 18, 2014, Washington, D.C., National Coalition of Autoimmune Patient Groups (NCAPG) news briefing.
8. Hempstead K, Sung I, Gray J, Richardson S. Tracking trends in provider reimbursements and patient obligations. *Health Aff.* 2015;34(7):1220–1224. doi:10.1377/hlthaff.2015.0105.

9. RA NarRAtive patient survey. 2015. Pfizer Inc, New York, NY. www.Pfizer.com/RANarRAtive.
10. Feurstein A. Amgen indulges in another rheumatoid arthritis drug price increase. *TheStreet.com.* May 5, 2015. http://www.thestreet.com/story/13139368/1/amgen-indulges-in-another-rheumatoid-arthritis-drug-price-increase.html.
11. Hartung DM, Bourdette DN, Ahmed SM, Whitham RH. The cost of multiple sclerosis drugs in the US and the pharmaceutical industry. *Neurology.* 2015;84(21):2185–2192. doi:10.1212/WNL.0000000000001608.
12. Yazdany J, Dudley RA, Randi Chen R, et al. Coverage for high cost specialty drugs for rheumatoid arthritis in Medicare Part D. Drug coverage for rheumatoid arthritis. *Arthritis Rheum.* 2015;67(6):1474–1480. doi:10.1002/art.39079.
13. American Autoimmune Related Diseases Association white paper and press release: leading autoimmune patient advocacy group survey finds overwhelming majority of patients lack understanding of biosimilar drugs. http://www.aarda.org/wp-content/uploads/2015/02/BiosimilarsWhitePaperPressRelease.pdf.

Afterword

When I first learned I had an autoimmune disease I had just completed my MD and was moving along on my PhD training in the laboratory. Just like the stories contained in this book, the diagnosis took a long time in coming, probably a good 6 to 12 months. Ironically I was studying autoimmunity in mice at the time, and as the old adage goes, if you study it long enough you will finally get it.

It was a senior and very seasoned laboratory technician who noticed I was turning yellow. Indeed, I ate lots of carrots every day (my excuse) and was pale from long hours in the lab instead of the summer sun. The consensus lab diagnosis, a dangerous concept in and of itself, was that I must have been coming down with hepatitis from some patient encounter over the past year. After much prodding I dutifully went to the student health service (a highly risky venture). It took many trips to rule out the common causes of yellowed skin, but eventually I was diagnosed as having severe hypothyroidism. My yellow skin represented very longstanding disease.

I was relieved to know what was wrong, but my PhD advisor was stressed. He personally called the physician in charge of health service to let her know that she needed to reevaluate her diagnosis (this was prior to HIPPA rules!) or that I must have misunderstood her words and I had hyperthyroidism. My thesis advisor was certain I had *hyper*thyroidism (overactive thyroid). My nickname in the lab was "fireball," and it was hard for everyone to believe that the corrective therapy might actually supercharge the already energetic Faustman. My story had a happy ending. If there is one autoimmune disease that is almost entirely corrected by a little pill, it is hypothyroidism. (And yes, I did get my PhD done on time.)

But for millions of women, diagnosis and treatment do not come as easily. One of my long-term acquaintances, who herself worked in the field of autoimmunity for 25 years, had three major surgical interventions, all mistakes. Her dentist later correctly diagnosed her as having multiple sclerosis. You can be fully educated and be in the care of smart doctors, and those smart doctors can miss these diseases time and time again.

If you have autoimmune disease or know someone close to you who has one of these dreadful diseases, consider becoming a lay advocate. You can have a significant impact on influencing funding for research. You have unique motivation that distinguishes you from the scientists who do the research work; you do not care *who* discovers the cure, you only want the cure and with as great a speed as possible.

I think as scientists we must do significantly better at coming up with cures for these diseases. In my lifetime, I want to hear someone say: "I had type I diabetes 10 years ago." Over the next decade, I think it is highly feasible that we may be able to actually cure some of these diseases.

Because there are so many different aspects to autoimmunity, we will be attacking these diseases on a number of fronts. As this book outlines, there will be new ways to diagnose these diseases before they occur. This may be by a simple blood sample. There may be ways to stop certain forms of autoimmunity prior to severe end organ damage, and there is hope, yes hope, that even once these diseases occur, there may be ways beyond treatment of symptoms to actually reverse the disease.

As our work highlights, the now global push to move multi-dosing BCG "vaccine" (which may block the action of defective T cells, see page 213) into established type 1 diabetes, multiple sclerosis, and Sjögren's syndrome highlights the ability to take generic drugs and recycle them for new indications. BCG vaccine therapy also has another advantage—perhaps safety and affordability could be features of this drug too.

In this book you've learned about inflammatory cytokines and the damage they can cause. We have already developed medicines to disable some of these cytokines, but the task is now to uncover and interfere with the pathways that lead to their release. The anti-cytokine therapies in their many forms are on the pharmacy shelves, but just remember they do not stop the disease, they only treat the symptoms.

We must also target the cells that cause destruction in autoimmunity. It was long thought that once the disease was fully established identifying markers of only "bad" cells would not exist. On the research and clinical trial side, these "bad" cells can now be uniquely identified and monitored. And in our clinical trials with the 100-year-old generic drug called BCG, we can even see the death of these cells.

Finally we need a greater understanding of the antigens that provoke autoimmunity to begin. This research is moving forward, albeit more slowly. It was long thought there would only be one antigen per disease, but perhaps the more typical picture is that there are many antigens that trigger disease.

The challenge will be to make the agents that target these pathways nontoxic (or at least less toxic). Corticosteroids are an example of a wonderful medicine that has devastating effects. The cost of a cure should not be another disease or disability.

Indeed, there are medications in the pipeline and in research laboratories that appear for the first time to not only be specific for the "bad" cells but also to selectively eliminate the "bad" cells. The remarkable data in autoimmune diabetes show that disease can be permanently eliminated by a short course of these drugs, and the end organ, in this case the insulin-secreting islet cells, regrows in adult animals. This sort of research opens up new opportunities for all afflicted with autoimmunity but also opens up the paths for identifying the adult stem cells with unrecognized potential for treating many diseases and perhaps even slowing the aging process that we all experience.

Why talk about all of this work? Much of this work is actually in various stages of clinical trials, both in academia for the recycled generic drug approaches and in the pharma world for the new drugs. We need to find the right drugs, the specific drugs, and if these drugs already exist for other diseases, immediately "recycle" generic drugs to needy autoimmune patients. I believe public opinion and public pressure is necessary and extremely helpful at keeping the research, both clinical trials and pharmaceutical lab research, around the world on track. Which leads me to my final thought: do not be discouraged, and be an advocate and volunteer.

Denise L. Faustman, MD, PhD
Associate Professor of Medicine
Harvard Medical School

Appendix A

Where to Go for Help—Information and Support Groups

Autoimmune Diseases

American Autoimmune Related Diseases Association, Inc.
National Office
22100 Gratiot Ave.
Eastpointe, MI 48021
(586) 776-3900
(586) 776-3903 (fax)
(800) 598-4668
www.aarda.org

National Coalition of Autoimmune Patient Groups (NCAPG)

The NCAPG was founded and is facilitated by AARDA.
NCAPG members' individual websites:
American Behcet's Disease Association
www.behcets.com

American Vitiligo Research Foundation
www.avrf.org/

APS Foundation of America
www.apsfa.org/

Arthritis Foundation
www.arthritis.org/

Celiac Disease Foundation
https://celiac.org/

Celiac Support Association
www.csaceliacs.org/

Coalition for Pulmonary Fibrosis
www.coalitionforpf.org/

Crohn's and Colitis Foundation of America
www.ccfa.org/

Dysautonomia International
www.dysautonomiainternational.org/

Endometriosis Association
www.endometriosisassn.org/

Gluten Intolerance Group
www.gluten.org/

Graves' Disease & Thyroid Foundation
www.gdatf.org/

Immune Deficiency Foundation
http://primaryimmune.org/

International Foundation for Autoimmune Arthritis
www.ifautoimmunearthritis.org/

International Pemphigus & Pemphigoid Foundation
www.pemphigus.org/

Lupus Foundation of America
www.lupus.org/

Lupus and Allied Diseases Association
www.nolupus.org/

Myasthenia Gravis Foundation of America
www.myasthenia.org/

Myasthenia Gravis Foundation of Illinois
www.myastheniagravis.org/

National Adrenal Diseases Foundation
www.nadf.us/

National Alopecia Areata Foundation
www.naaf.org/

National Foundation for Celiac Awareness
www.celiaccentral.org/

National Kidney Foundation
www.kidney.org/

National Multiple Sclerosis Society
www.nationalmssociety.org/

National Psoriasis Foundation
www.psoriasis.org/

National Sleep Foundation
http://sleepfoundation.org/

PANDAS Network.org
Pediatric Autoimmune Neuropsychiatric Disorders
http://pandasnetwork.org/

Platelet Disorder Support Association
www.pdsa.org/

Relapsing Polychondritis Awareness and Support Foundation, Inc.
www.polychondritis.org/

Scleroderma Foundation
www.scleroderma.org/

Sjögren's Syndrome Foundation
www.sjogrens.org/

The Myositis Association
www.myositis.org/

Transverse Myelitis Association
http://myelitis.org/

U.S. Pain Foundation, Inc.
www.uspainfoundation.org/

Vasculitis Foundation
www.vasculitisfoundation.org/

Vitiligo Support International
www.vitiligosupport.org/

Autoimmune Disease Centers

Johns Hopkins Autoimmune Disease Research Center
Ross Building, Room 659
School of Medicine, Pathology Department
720 Rutland Avenue
Baltimore, MD 21205
http://autoimmune.pathology.jhmi.edu

Barbara Volcker Center for Women & Rheumatic Diseases
The Hospital for Special Surgery
535 East 70th Street
New York, NY 10021
(212) 606-1461 or (212) 774-2291
Fax: (212) 774-2374
www.hss.edu/barbara-volcker.asp
E-mail: volckerctr@hss.edu

The Arthritis Center
Boston University Medical Center
72 East Concord Street, Evans 501
Boston, MA 02118
(617) 638-4312, Clinic (617) 638-7460
Fax: (617) 638-5226
www.bmc.org/arthritis.htm

NYU Center for Arthritis & Autoimmunity
NYU Langone Medical Center
333 East 38th Street, 4th Floor
New York, New York 10016
(646) 501-7400
http://nyulangone.org/locations/center-for-arthritis-autoimmunity

In Canada

Rebecca MacDonald Centre for Arthritis and Autoimmune Disease
Mount Sinai Hospital
Joseph and Wolf Lebovic Health Complex
60 Murray Street, 2nd Floor (Main)
Toronto, Ontario, Canada M5T 3L9
Fax for appointments: (416) 586-8766
www.mountsinai.on.ca/care/rmcad/

Alopecia Areata

National Alopecia Areata Foundation
714 "C" Street
San Rafael, CA
(415) 456-4644
www.naaf.org

Antiphospholipid Syndrome

APS Foundation of America, Inc.
www.apsfa.org/

Arthritis

American College of Rheumatology
60 Executive Park South, Suite 150
Atlanta, GA 30329
(800) 346-4753
www.rheumatology.org

Arthritis Foundation
1330 West Peachtree Street
Atlanta, GA 30309
(800) 283-700
www.arthritis.org

National Institute of Arthritis and Musculoskeletal and Skin Diseases
www.niams.nih.gov

Complementary and Alternative Medicine

National Center for Complementary and Integrative Health
https://nccih.nih.gov/

Celiac Disease

American Celiac Society
Dietary Support Coalition
www.americanceliacsociety.org/index.html

Celiac Disease Foundation
20350 Ventura Boulevard, Suite 240
Woodland Hills, CA 91364
(818) 716-1513
Fax: (818) 267-5577
www.celiac.org

Celiac Support Association
413 Ash Street
Seward, NE 68434
P.O. Box 31700
Omaha, NE 68131-0700
(402) 643-4101 or 877-CSA-4CSA (toll-free)
Fax: (402) 643-4108
E-mail: celiacs@csaceliacs.org
www.csaceliacs.org/

Gluten Intolerance Group
31214 124th Avenue SE
Auburn, WA 98092
(253) 833-6655
Fax: (253) 833-6675
E-mail: Customerservice@gluten.org
www.gluten.org

Celiac Society
www.celiacsociety.com/

Chronic Fatigue Syndrome

Solve ME/CFS Initiative (formerly the CFIDS Association of America)
Solve ME/CFS Initiative
P.O. Box 36007
Los Angeles, CA 90036-0007
(704) 364-0016
E-mail: SolveCFS@SolveCFS.org
http://solvecfs.org/

Crohn's Disease and Ulcerative Colitis

Crohn's & Colitis Foundation of America, Inc.
733 Third Avenue, Suite 510
New York, NY 10017
(800) 932-2423 or (212) 685-3440
www.ccfa.org

National Institute of Diabetes and Digestive and Kidney Diseases
www.niddk.nih.gov/health/digest/niddic.htm
United Ostomy Associations of America
P.O. Box 512
Northfield, MN 55057-0512
www.ostomy.org/Home.html

Diabetes

American Diabetes Association
1701 North Beauregard Street,
Alexandria, VA 22311
1-800-DIABETES (800-342-2383)
www.diabetes.org

Juvenile Diabetes Research Foundation International
120 Wall Street
New York, NY 10005-4001
(800) 533-CURE or (212) 785-9500
Fax: (212) 785-9595
www.jdrf.org

National Institute of Diabetes and Digestive and Kidney Diseases
National Institutes of Health
www.niddk.nih.gov

Endometriosis

The Endometriosis Association
International Headquarters
8585 North 76th Place
Milwaukee, WI 53223
(800) 992-3636 or (414) 355-2200
Fax: (414) 355-6065
www.endometriosisassn.org

Fibromyalgia

Fibromyalgia Alliance of America
P.O. Box 21988
Columbus, OH 43221-0988
www.php.com/fibromyalgia-alliance-america-fhaa

National Fibromyalgia Research Association, Inc.
P.O. Box 500
Salem, OR 97308
(503) 588-1411
www.nfra.net

Lupus (Systemic Lupus Erythematosus)

Lupus Foundation of America
1300 Piccard Drive, Suite 200
Rockville, MD 20850
(800) 74-LUPUS or (800) 558-0121
www.lupus.org

S.L.E. Lupus Foundation
330 Seventh Avenue, Suite 1701
New York, NY 10001
(212) 685-4118
Fax: (212) 545-1843
E-mail: Lupus@LupusNY.org
www.lupusny.org

Lupus and Allied Diseases Association, Inc.
P.O. Box 170
Verona, NY 13478
(866) 258-7874 (toll-free) or (315) 829-4272
Fax: (315) 829-4272
E-mail LupusInnovators@aol.com
http://nolupus.org

LupusLine®
Telephone counseling offered in coordination with S.L.E. Foundation, Inc. and The Hospital for Special Surgery, New York City.
(866) 375-1427 (toll-free)
https://www.hss.edu/LupusLine.asp

National Kidney Foundation, Inc.
30 East 33rd Street, New York, NY 10016
(800) 622-9010
www.kidney.org/

Immunology

American Academy of Allergy, Asthma & Immunology
E-mail: info@aaaai.org
www.aaaai.org

Multiple Sclerosis

National Multiple Sclerosis Society
(800) 344-4686
www.nmss.org

American Academy of Neurology
www.aan.com

National Institute of Neurological Disorders and Stroke (NINDS)
www.ninds.nih.gov

Myasthenia Gravis

Myasthenia Gravis Foundation of America
5841 Cedar Lake Road, Suite 204
Minneapolis, MN 55416
(800) 541-5454 or (952) 545-9438
Fax: (952) 545-6073
www.myasthenia.org

Myositis (Polymyositis, Dermatomyositis)

The Myositis Association
755 Cantrell Avenue, Suite C
Harrisonburg, VA 22801
(540) 433-7686
Fax: (540) 432-0206
www.myositis.org

Pemphigus

International Pemphigus & Pemphigoid Foundation
Atrium Plaza, Suite 203
828 San Pablo Avenue
Albany, CA 94706
(510) 527-4970
www.pemphigus.org

Thrombocytopenia (ITP)

Platelet Disorder Support Association
8751 Brecksville Road, Suite 150
Cleveland, OH 44141
1-87-PLATELET or (440) 746-9003 (toll-free)
Fax: (844) 270-1277
www.pdsa.org
E-mail: pdsa@pdsa.org

National Heart, Lung, and Blood Institute
Information Center
P.O. Box 30105
Bethesda, MD 20824
(301) 251-1222
www.nhlbi.nih.gov

Psoriasis/Psoriatic Arthritis

National Psoriasis Foundation
6600 SW 92nd Avenue, Suite 300
Portland, OR 97223
(800) 723-9166 or (503) 244-7004
Fax: (503) 245-0626
www.psoriasis.org

Genetic and Rare Disease (GARD) Information Center
National Institutes of Health
http://rarediseases.info.nih.gov

Scleroderma

Scleroderma Foundation
300 Rosewood Drive, Suite 105
Danvers, MA 01923
(800) 722-HOPE (4673)
E-mail: sinfo@scleroderma.org
www.scleroderma.org

Scleroderma Family & DNA Repository
5431 Fannin Street, Suite 5.245
Houston, TX 77030
(713) 500-7196 Fax: (713) 500-0718
E-mail: sclerodermaregistry@uth.tmc.edu
https://med.uth.edu/scleroderma-registry/

International Scleroderma Network
www.sclero.org/isn/a-to-z.html

Sjögren's Syndrome

Sjögren's Syndrome Foundation, Inc.
6707 Democracy Blvd, Suite 325
Bethesda, MD 20817
(800) 475-6473 (toll free) or (301) 530-4420
Info line: (800) 475-6473
Fax: (301) 530-4415
www.sjogrens.org

Thyroid Disease

American Foundation of Thyroid Patients
P.O. Box 572472
Houston, TX 77257
E-mail: thyroidfoundation@yahoo.com
http://thyroidfoundation.cfsites.org/

American Thyroid Association
6066 Leesburg Pike, Suite 550
Falls Church, VA 22041
E-mail: thyroid@thyroid.org
www.thyroid.org

Vasculitis

Vasculitis Foundation
P.O. Box 28660
Kansas City, MO 64188
(816) 436-8211 or (800) 277-9474
Fax: (816) 656-3838
www.vasculitisfoundation.org/

Affordable Care Act Information

Healthcare.gov

Federal law requires that insurers planning to significantly increase plan premiums (by more than 10 percent) submit their rates to the federal government (or states) for review.

To find rate review information for your insurance plan, follow this link:
https://ratereview.healthcare.gov/

Kaiser Family Foundation (KFF)

KFF is a nonprofit organization following healthcare trends. Its website offers a wealth of information, including an insurance marketplace rate calculator:

Health Insurance Marketplace Calculator www.kff.org/interactive/subsidy-calculator

Information and Help with Medications

NeedyMeds

A national clearinghouse for information on State Pharmaceutical Assistance Programs, drug discount cards (including its own card), medication pricing.

www.needymeds.org/state_programs.taf

HealthFinder.gov—Prescription Assistance

This site is run by the U.S. Department of Health and Human Services and even provides a link to apply for Medicare.

http://healthfinder.gov/rxdrug

Partnership for Prescription Assistance
Provides a listing of free drug savings cards.
https://www.pparx.org/prescription_assistance_programs/savings_cards

Assistance Fund
This nonprofit group also provides patient advocates for live chats.
4700 Millenia Boulevard, Suite 310
Orlando, FL 32639
(855) 845-3363 Fax: (866) 254-9411
www.theassistancefund.org

PDR Health, Physicians' Desk Reference online
www.pdrhealth.com/

Medline Plus
Information from the NIH on drugs, herbs, and supplements.
www.nlm.nih.gov/medlineplus/druginformation.html

Appendix B
Selected Reading

Arthritis

Living with Rheumatoid Arthritis, Tammi L. Shlotzhauer, MD, and James L. McGuire, MD. 2003, Johns Hopkins University Press, Baltimore, MD.

Good Living with Rheumatoid Arthritis, Arthritis Foundation, Dorothy Foltz-Gray. 2006, Arthritis Foundation, Atlanta, GA.

The First Year: Rheumatoid Arthritis: An Essential Guide for the Newly Diagnosed, M. E. A. McNeil. 2005, DaCapo Press, Boston, MA.

Your Life with Rheumatoid Arthritis: Tools for Managing Treatment, Side Effects and Pain, Lene Andersen. 2013, Two North Books.

A Resilient Life: Learning to Thrive, Not Just Survive with Rheumatoid Arthritis, Kat Elton, OTR. 2010, Kat Elton (self-published).

What to Do When the Doctor Says It's Rheumatoid Arthritis, Harry D. Fischer, MD, and Winnie Yu. 2005, Fair Winds Press, BC, Canada.

The Hospital for Special Surgery Rheumatoid Arthritis Handbook, Stephen A. Paget, MD, Michael D. Lockshin, MD, and Suzanne Loebl. 2002, John Wiley & Sons, New York.

The Arthritis Sourcebook, 3rd ed., Earl J. Brewer, MD, and Kathy Cochran Angel. 2000, Contemporary Books, New York.

The Arthritis Bible: A Comprehensive Guide to Alternative Therapies and Conventional Treatments for Arthritic Diseases, Leonid Gordon and Craig Weatherby. 1999, Inner Traditions, Rochester, VT.

The Arthritis Foundation's Guide to Alternative Therapies, Judith Horstman. 1998, Arthritis Foundation, Atlanta, GA.

The Duke University Book of Arthritis, David S. Pisetsky, MD, PhD, and Susan Flamholtz Trien. 1992, Fawcett Columbine, New York.

Autoimmunity

Intolerant Bodies: A Short History of Autoimmunity, Warwick Anderson and Ian R. Mackay. 2014, Johns Hopkins University Press, Baltimore, MD.

The Autoimmune Epidemic: Bodies Gone Haywire in a World Out of Balance—and the Cutting-Edge Science That Promises Hope, Donna Jackson Nakazawa. 2008, Touchstone Books, New York.

Women and Autoimmune Disease: The Mysterious Ways Your Body Betrays Itself, Robert G. Lahita, MD, and Ina L. Yalof. 2005, William Morrow Paperbacks, New York.

An Epidemic of Absence: A New Way of Understanding Allergies and Autoimmune Diseases, Moises Velasquez-Manoff. 2012, Scribner, New York.

The Encyclopedia of Autoimmune Disease, Dana K. Cassell and Noel R. Rose, MD, PhD. 2003, Facts on File, New York.

Autoimmune Diseases and Their Environmental Triggers, Elaine A. Moore. 2002, McFarland & Company, Jefferson, NC.

Complementary/Dietary Approaches

The Autoimmune Solution: Prevent and Reverse the Full Spectrum of Inflammatory Symptoms and Diseases, Amy Myers, MD. 2015, Harper Collins, New York.

The Immune System Recovery Plan: A Doctor's 4-Step Program to Treat Autoimmune Disease, Susan Blum, MD, MPH, with Michelle Bender. 2013, Scribner, New York.

Living Well with Autoimmune Disease: What Your Doctor Doesn't Tell You . . . That You Need to Know, Mary J. Shomon. 2002, William Morrow, New York.

Autoimmune: The Cause and the Cure, Annesse Brockley and Kristin Urdiales. 2011, Nature Had It First.

What Your Doctor May Not Tell You About Autoimmune Disorders: The Revolutionary Drug-free Treatments for Thyroid Disease, Lupus, MS, IBD, Chronic Fatigue, Rheumatoid Arthritis, and Other Diseases, Stephen B. Edelson, MD, and Deborah Mitchell. 2003, Grand Central Publishing, New York.

The Wahls Protocol: How I Beat Progressive MS Using Paleo Principles and Functional Medicine, Terry Wahls and Eve Adamson. 2014, Avery Paperbacks, New York.

Help, My Body Is Killing Me: Solving the Connections of Autoimmune Disease to Thyroid Problems, Fibromyalgia, Infertility, Anxiety, Depression, ADD/ADHD and More, Kevin Conners. 2010, Authorhouse, Bloomington, IN.

Up the Creek with a Paddle: Beat MS and Many Autoimmune Disorders with Low Dose Naltrexone (LDN), Mary Boyle Bradley. 2009, Outskirts Press, Denver, CO.

The Paleo Approach: Reverse Autoimmune Disease and Heal Your Body, Sarah Ballantyne, PhD. 2014, Victory Belt Publishing, Las Vegas, NV.

Thriving with Your Autoimmune Disorder: A Woman's Mind-Body Guide, Simone Ravicz, PhD. 2000, New Harbinger, Oakland, CA.

Celiac Disease/Gluten

Celiac Disease: A Hidden Epidemic, rev. and updated ed., Peter H. R. Green, MD, and Rory Jones. 2010, William Morrow, New York.

The First Year: Celiac Disease and Living Gluten-Free: An Essential Guide for the Newly Diagnosed, Jules E. Dowler Shepard. 2008, Lifelong Books, Perseus, Boston, MA.

Healthier Without Wheat: A New Understanding of Wheat Allergies, Celiac Disease, and Non-Celiac Gluten Intolerance, Stephen Wangen. 2009, Innate Health Publishing, Fishpond, NZ.

Crohn's Disease and Ulcerative Colitis

Crohn's Disease and Ulcerative Colitis: Everything You Need to Know, Fred Saibil and Frederic G. Saibil. 1997, Firefly, New York.

Controlling Crohn's Disease the Natural Way, Virginia M. Harper and Tom Monte. 2002, Kensington Publishing Corp., New York.

The New Eating Right for a Bad Gut: The Complete Nutritional Guide to Ileitis, Colitis, Crohn's Disease, and Inflammatory Bowel Disease, James Scala, PhD. 2001, Plume/Penguin Putnam, New York.

The First Year: Crohn's Disease and Ulcerative Colitis Handbook: An Essential Guide for the Newly Diagnosed, Jill Sklar and Michael Sklar. 2002, Marlowe & Co., New York.

Diabetes

The American Diabetes Association Complete Guide to Diabetes, 5th ed. American Diabetes Association. 2011, Bantam Books, New York.

The Joslin Guide to Diabetes, Richard S. Beaser, MD, with Amy P. Campbell, RD, CDE. 2005, Fireside Books, New York.

Dr. Bernstein's Diabetes Solution: The Complete Guide to Achieving Normal Blood Sugars, updated ed., Richard K. Bernstein, MD. 2011, Doctor's Option, New York.

Endometriosis

Endometriosis: Endometriosis Guide to Understanding Endometriosis and Treating Endometriosis, Amanda Hollingsworth. 2015, Kindle Edition (e-book).

Stop Endometriosis and Pelvic Pain: What Every Woman and Her Doctor Need to Know, Andrew S. Cook, MD, FACOG. 2012, Femsana Press LLC, India.

Endometriosis for Dummies, Joseph Krotec, MD, and Sharon Perkins, RN. 2006, John Wiley & Sons, New York.

Living Well with Endometriosis: What Your Doctor Doesn't Tell You . . . That You Need to Know, Kerry-Ann Morris. 2006, Harper Collins, New York.

Endometriosis: The Complete Reference for Taking Charge of Your Health, Mary Lou Ballweg and the Endometriosis Association. 2003, McGraw-Hill Professional, New York.

Coping with Endometriosis: Sound, Compassionate Advice for Alleviating the Challenges of This Chronic Disorder, Robert Philips, PhD, and Glenda Motta, RN. 2000, Penguin Books, New York.

Fibromyalgia

The Complete Idiot's Guide to Fibromyalgia, 2nd ed., Lynne Matallana, PhD, and Laurence A. Bradley, PhD. 2009, Penguin Books, New York.

Fibromyalgia: An Essential Guide for Patients and Their Families, Daniel J. Wallace, MD, and Janice Brock Wallace. 2003, Oxford University Press, New York.

Autoimmune Hepatitis

Dr. Melissa Palmer's Guide to Hepatitis and Liver Disease: What You Need to Know, rev. ed., Melissa Palmer, MD. 2004, Avery, New York.

Lupus

Lupus: Everything You Need to Know, Sasha Bernatsky, MD, and Jean-Luc Senécal, MD, editors. 2005, Firefly Books, LTD, New York.

Coping with Lupus: A Practical Guide to Alleviating the Challenges of Systemic Lupus Erythematosus, 4th ed., Robert H. Phillips, PhD. 2012, Penguin Group, New York.

Taking Charge of Lupus: How to Manage the Disease and Make the Most of Your Life, Maureen Pratt and David Hallequa, MD. 2002, New American Library, Trade, New York.

Lupus and Me: Living Well with an Autoimmune Illness: Healthy Nutrition, Jenn Schoch. 2013, CreateSpace Independent Publishing Platform (On-Demand book).

The Lupus Book, 5th ed., Daniel J. Wallace, MD. 2013, Oxford University Press, New York.

Medications

Consumer Drug Reference, Consumer Reports and the American Society of Health-System Pharmacists, 2009 ed. 2009, Consumer Reports/Consumers Union, Yonkers, New York.

Multiple Sclerosis

Multiple Sclerosis for Dummies, Rosalind Kalb, PhD, Nancy Holland, EdD, RN, and Barbara Giesser, MD. 2011, John Wiley & Sons, New York.

Multiple Sclerosis: A Guide for the Newly Diagnosed, 4th ed., T. Jock Murray, MD, and Nancy Holland, RN, EdD. 2012, Demos Medical Publishing, New York.

Multiple Sclerosis: The Questions You Have, the Answers You Need, 5th ed., Rosalind C. Kalb, MD. 2011, Demos Medical Publishing, New York.

What Nurses Know . . . Multiple Sclerosis: The Answers You Need from the People You Trust. Carol Saunders, BA, BSN, MSCN. 2011, Demos Medical Publishing, New York.

When the Diagnosis Is Multiple Sclerosis: Help, Hope, and Insights from an Affected Physician, Kym Orsetti Furney, MD. 2008, Greenwood Publishing Group, Westport, CT.

The Everything Health Guide to Multiple Sclerosis: An Authoritative Guide to Help You Understand Symptoms, Decide on Treatment, and Enhance Your Well-Being, Margot Russell and Allen C Bowling, MD, PhD. 2008, Adams Media, Avon, MA.

Scleroderma

The Scleroderma Book: A Guide for Patients and Families, 2nd ed., Maureen D. Mayes, MD. 2005, Oxford University Press, New York.

Scleroderma, Coping Strategies, B. Bianca Podesta. 2001, Two Harbors Press, Minneapolis, MN.

Sjögren's Syndrome

The Sjögren's Syndrome Survival Guide, Terri P. Rumph, PhD, and Katherine Moreland Hammitt. 2003, New Harbinger, Oakland, CA.

A Body Out of Balance: Understanding and Treating Sjögren's Syndrome, Nancy Carteron, MA, and Ruth Fremes, MD. 2003, Penguin Publishing Group, New York.

Sjögren's Syndrome: Cause and Recovery in Ten Simple Steps, Hannah Yoseph, MD. 2013, Hannah Yoseph (self-published).

Positive Options for Sjögren's Syndrome: Self-Help and Treatment, Sue Dyson. 2005, Hunter House, Alameda, CA.

The Sjögren's Book, 4th ed., Daniel J. Wallace, MD. 2011, Oxford University Press, New York.

Thyroid Disease

Graves' Disease: A Practical Guide, Elaine A. Moore, Lisa Moore, and Kelly R. Hale. 2001, McFarland & Co, New York.

Advances in Graves' Disease and Other Hyperthyroid Disorders, Elaine A. Moore and Lisa Marie Moore. 2013, Mcfarland Health Topics, Jefferson, NC.

Living Well with Hypothyroidism: What Your Doctor Doesn't Tell You . . . That You Need to Know, rev. ed., Mary J. Shomon. 2005, Harper Resource, New York.

Why Do I Still Have Thyroid Symptoms? When My Lab Tests Are Normal, Datis Kharrazian, DHSc, DC, MS. 2010, Elephant Printing, LLC, East Sussex, UK.

Thyroid Balance: Traditional and Alternative Methods for Treating Thyroid Disorders, Glenn S. Rothfield, MD, MAC, and Deborah Romaine. 2002, Adams Media, Avon, MA.

Self-Help/Personal Journeys

When Doctors Don't Listen: How to Avoid Misdiagnoses and Unnecessary Testing, Leana Wen, MD. 2013, St. Martin's Press, New York.

As My Body Attacks Itself: My Journey with Autoimmune Disease, Chronic Pain and Fatigue, Kelly Morgan Dempewolf, PhD. 2014, K2CS Books, Tecumseh, KS.

Why I Used to Hate Tomorrow: My Story About Rheumatoid Arthritis, Depression, Friends, Family and Love, Anthony Driggers. 2012, Kindle Edition.

If You Have to Wear an Ugly Dress, Learn to Accessorize: Guidance, Inspiration, and Hope for Women with Lupus, Scleroderma, and Other Autoimmune Illnesses, Linda McNamara and Karen Kemper. 2011, Wheatmark Publishing, Tucson, AZ.

SHOWgrins: Women Who Walk on Water, Betty Collier. 2013, Xlibris, Kindle Edition.

Women, Work, and Autoimmune Disease: Keep Working, Girlfriend! Rosalind Joffe and Joan Friedlander; L. G. Mansfield, ed. 2008, Demos Medical Publishing, New York.

Tales from the Dry Side: The Personal Stories Behind the Autoimmune Illness Sjögren's Syndrome, Christine Molloy. 2013, Outskirts Press, Denver, CO.

Jennifer's Way: My Journey with Celiac Disease, Jennifer Esposito with Ed Adamson. 2014, DeCapo Press, Boston, MA.

Index

About the Authors

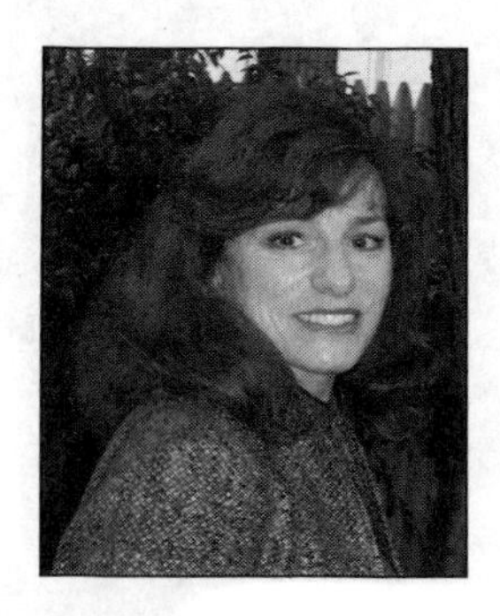

Rita Baron-Faust, MPH, CHES, is an award-winning medical journalist and author of five books on women's health, who has been a regular contributor to the *Rheumatology Network.com*. She is an adjunct professor in the department of Biology and Health Promotion at St. Francis College in Brooklyn, NY, and serves as a national educator for the American Autoimmune Related Diseases Association. During her career, Ms. Baron-Faust has been the recipient of more than two dozen awards for medical journalism.

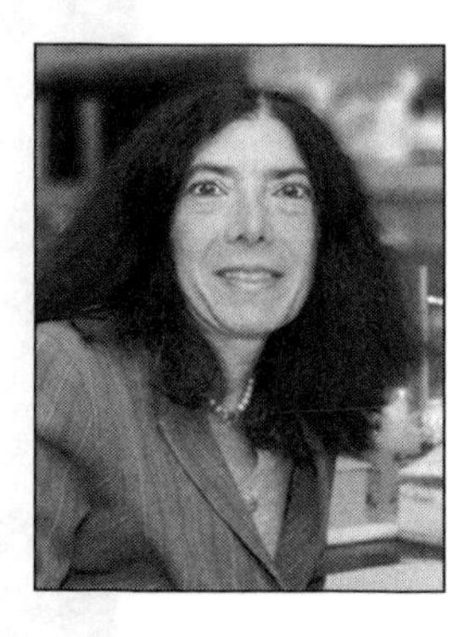

Jill P. Buyon, MD, is director of the Division of Rheumatology at the NYU School of Medicine/NYU Langone Medical Center, and the Lady Va and Sir Deryck Maughan Professor of Medicine. She is the founder and Director of the NYU Lupus Center at the NYU/Hospital for Joint Diseases. She has devoted her career to the study of Lupus with a focus on issues related to reproductive health. Her work has been supported by continuous funding from the National Institutes of Health. Dr. Buyon is Editor-In-Chief of the newly launched journal *Lupus Science & Medicine* and is an internationally-recognized researcher in the field of neonatal lupus.